HEALTH CARE EMERGENCY MANAGEMENT

PRINCIPLES AND PRACTICE

Michael J. Reilly, DrPH, MPH, NREMT-P

Director, Graduate Program in Emergency Preparedness
Assistant Director, Center for Disaster Medicine
Assistant Professor, Public Health Practice
New York Medical College
School of Health Science and Practice
Valhalla, New York

David S. Markenson, MD, FAAP, FACEP, EMT-P

Medical Director and Vice President
Disaster Medicine and Regional Emergency Services
Westchester Medical Center
Director, Center for Disaster Medicine
Associate Professor, Public Health Practice
Professor of Pediatrics
New York Medical College
Valhalla, New York

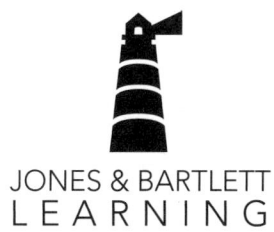

JONES & BARTLETT
L E A R N I N G

World Headquarters
Jones & Bartlett Learning
5 Wall Street
Burlington, MA 01803
978-443-5000
info@jblearning.com
www.jblearning.com

Jones & Bartlett Learning books and products are available through most bookstores and online booksellers. To contact Jones & Bartlett Learning directly, call 800-832-0034, fax 978-443-8000, or visit our website, www.jblearning.com.

Substantial discounts on bulk quantities of Jones & Bartlett Learning publications are available to corporations, professional associations, and other qualified organizations. For details and specific discount information, contact the special sales department at Jones & Bartlett Learning via the above contact information or send an email to specialsales@jblearning.com.

Production Credits
Publisher: Michael Brown
Editorial Assistant: Catie Heverling
Editorial Assistant: Teresa Reilly
Production Manager: Tracey Chapman
Associate Production Editor: Kate Stein
Senior Marketing Manager: Sophie Fleck
Manufacturing and Inventory Control Supervisor: Amy Bacus
Composition: Achorn International
Art: diacriTech
Associate Photo Researcher: Sarah Cebulski
Cover Design: Kristin E. Parker
Cover Image: Top left: Courtesy of Andrea Booher/FEMA; Top Right: Courtesy of Win Henderson/FEMA; Bottom left: Courtesy of Jocelyn Augustino/FEMA; Bottom right: Courtesy of Cynthia Hunter/FEMA
Printing and Binding: Edwards Brothers Malloy
Cover Printing: Edwards Brothers Malloy

Library of Congress Cataloging-in-Publication Data
Health care emergency management : principles and practice / [edited by] Michael J. Reilly and David S. Markenson.
    p. ; cm.
 Includes bibliographical references and index.
 ISBN-13: 978-0-7637-5513-3 (pbk.)
 ISBN-10: 0-7637-5513-3 (pbk.)
 1. Emergency medical services. 2. Emergency management—Planning. 3. Hospitals—Emergency services. I. Reilly, Michael J. II. Markenson, David S.
  [DNLM: 1. Disaster Planning—organization & administration. 2. Emergencies. 3. Emergency Service, Hospital—organization & administration. WX 185 H4336 2011]
 RA645.5.H38 2011
 362.18068—dc22
                                                                 2010001554
6048

Printed in the United States of America
18 17 16 15 14   10 9 8 7 6 5 4 3 2

Dedication

MICHAEL REILLY

I dedicate this text to my family and friends who have supported me throughout this project. I especially thank my parents, who have provided their unwavering advice and support throughout my life and career. I also dedicate this text to my professional mentors Dr. Linda Degutis and Dr. Robyn Gershon, who continue to give me invaluable guidance throughout my professional development. Finally, I dedicate this book to my coauthor David, who has provided me with the opportunity to pursue academic emergency and disaster medicine professionally, and who continues to encourage and support my development as a scientist and scholar in this evolving area of medicine and public health.

DAVID MARKENSON

This text is dedicated to my parents, who have always guided, supported, and encouraged me, and who, as physicians, have shown me through their work that providing care to others in a compassionate and knowledgeable way can be a rewarding endeavor. This text is also dedicated to my brothers, sister, and sisters-in-law, who are a constant source of advice, support, and energy; without their help and involvement in my life none of my efforts could have been accomplished. Most importantly this text is dedicated to my wife Heidi and my wonderful children, Emily, Rachel, and George, who not only support me but who were willing to give of their time with me to allow me to write this text.

MICHAEL REILLY AND DAVID MARKENSON

Lastly, this text is dedicated to all healthcare providers, emergency managers, and those in their care. Healthcare providers and emergency managers work each day in an environment that is unpredictable, often dangerous, and constantly challenging. They have become champions in changing the system to become better prepared. They dedicate their lives to aid the sick and the injured and prepare for any disaster, terrorism event, or public health emergency, driven only by their care for others and their devotion to this profession we call healthcare emergency management. We salute all of you in your professionalism and dedication. Also, we dedicate this to our patients who, in allowing us the privilege to provide them care, teach us each day about humanity.

Contents

About the Authors

MICHAEL J. REILLY, DRPH, MPH, NREMT-P

Dr. Michael Reilly is currently the Assistant Director of the Center for Disaster Medicine at New York Medical College in Valhalla, New York. Additionally, he is an Assistant Professor of Public Health Practice and the Director of the Graduate Program in Emergency Preparedness at the School of Health Science and Practice.

Dr. Reilly has over a decade of multidisciplinary experience in emergency preparedness, public safety, intergovernmental relations, public health, and emergency management. He has been published in the world's leading disaster medicine and public health preparedness journals, and received international awards and recognition for his work on trauma systems and health systems in the context of disaster and public health preparedness. Dr. Reilly is an internationally recognized expert in the areas of emergency medical services, and health system preparedness and response, with direct experience in responding to mass casualty events and public health emergencies. Dr. Reilly is frequently called upon to provide expert consultation, subject matter expertise, and to evaluate healthcare systems preparedness, emergency planning, and drills and exercises.

Dr. Reilly has designed numerous educational curricula and training programs for a variety of preparedness functional roles for public health, emergency management, and public safety audiences at the professional and graduate levels. He is a senior lecturer for multiple federal agencies including the Department of Justice, Department of Homeland Security, and the Occupational Safety and Health Administration. Additionally, he is an active member of several state and national committees on homeland security and emergency management programs.

He received his undergraduate education at Northeastern University in paramedic technology and health science. He earned his Masters of Public Health from Yale University, and a doctorate in public health from New York Medical College.

Dr. Reilly remains active as a paramedic in the Metro New York City region and maintains numerous specialty and technical certifications and instructor credentials in the areas of emergency medical services, worker safety, environmental health, hazardous materials emergency response, emergency management, counterterrorism, and weapons of mass destruction preparedness and response.

DAVID SAMUEL MARKENSON, MD, FAAP, FACEP, EMT-P

Dr. David Markenson is a board-certified pediatrician with Fellowship training in both pediatric emergency medicine and pediatric critical care. He is the Vice President and Medical Director of Disaster Medicine and Regional Emergency Services at the Westchester Medical Center and Maria Fareri Children's Hospital. In addition, he is the Director of the Center for Disaster Medicine and the Interim Chair of Epidemiology and Community Health at the School of Health Sciences and Practice at New York Medical College. Dr. Markenson is also a Professor of Pediatrics and an Associate Professor of Public Health at the School of Health Sciences and Practice at New York Medical College in Valhalla, New York.

He is an active member of, and has served in leadership positions within, multiple professional societies, including the American Academy of Pediatrics (AAP), the American College of Emergency Physicians, the Society of Critical Care Medicine, the American College of Physician Executives, and the National Association of EMS Physicians. Dr. Markenson has been actively involved with the American Red Cross for over 20 years and currently serves as the National Chair of the Advisory Council which oversees disaster health, preparedness, and health and safety. In this role he directs the scientific and technical aspects of all programs and products in these areas including their development, implementation, and research. Prior to coming to Westchester Medical Center and New York Medical College he was the Deputy Director of the National Center for Disaster Preparedness at the Mailman School of Public Health, Columbia University, and was also the Director of the Program for Pediatric Preparedness of the National Center, a program dedicated to improving the care children receive in times of disasters or acts of terrorism.

His career has been dedicated to improving the approach to pediatric care, disaster medicine, EMS, and emergency medicine. He is the principal investigator on several federal grants related to pediatric disaster medicine, including Model Pediatric Component for State Disaster Plans and National Consensus Conference on the Needs of Children in Disasters. He has also addressed the needs of other special and vulnerable populations and directed a federal grant to develop the first and only national guidelines for emergency preparedness for persons with disabilities. In addition to this, he has conducted research on healthcare preparedness and healthcare provider and student education. In this area he was the principal investigator for a federal grant which developed the first competencies for all healthcare students in emergency preparedness and then piloted this set of competencies in a medical, dental, public health, and nursing school. Dr. Markenson has been recently appointed to the FEMA National Advisory Council as the In-Patient Medical Provider representative. The FEMA NAC is comprised of emergency management and law enforcement leaders from state, local, and tribal government and the private sector to advise the FEMA Administrator on all aspects of disaster preparedness and management to ensure close coordination with all partners across the country.

He is a frequent presenter and lecturer at medical conferences across the country, serves in editorial roles for multiple professional scientific journals, and has authored numerous articles and books on pediatric care, disaster medicine, and prehospital medicine. His work in disaster medicine started during his college career when he worked in disaster services in upstate New York providing direct services and education to other disaster services workers on behalf of the local Red Cross and county office of emergency management. Dr. Markenson is a graduate of Albert Einstein College of Medicine in the Bronx, New York.

Contributors

Lindsey P. Anthony, MPA, CEM, CHEC-III
Operational Medicine Education Coordinator
Center for Operational Medicine
Medical College of Georgia
Augusta, Georgia

Peter Arno, PhD
Professor
Department of Health Policy and Management
New York Medical College
School of Health Sciences and Practice
Valhalla, New York

Ariadne Avellino, MD, MPH
Research Associate
Center for Disaster Medicine
New York Medical College
Valhalla, New York

Lauren Babcock-Dunning, MPH
Research Associate
Center for Transportation Safety, Security and Risk
Rutgers, The State University of New Jersey
New Brunswick, New Jersey

Barbara A. Butcher, MPH
Chief of Staff
Office of the Chief Medical Examiner
City of New York
New York, New York

Nicholas V. Cagliuso, Sr., MPH
Corporate Director
Emergency Management
Continuum Health Partners, Inc.
New York, New York

Arthur Cooper, MD, MS
Professor of Surgery
Columbia University College of Physicians & Surgeons
Director of Trauma and Pediatric Surgical Services
Harlem Hospital
New York, New York

Elizabeth A. Davis, JD, EdM
Principal
EAD & Associates, LLC
Brooklyn, New York

Linda C. Degutis, DrPH, MSN
Associate Professor of Surgery (Emergency Medicine) and Public
    Health
Director, Center for Public Health Preparedness
Yale University School of Medicine
New Haven, Connecticut

Frank DePaolo, RPA–C
Director
Special Operations Division
Office of the Chief Medical Examiner
City of New York
New York, New York

Garrett T. Doering, MS, EMT-P, CEM, MEP
Director of Emergency Management
Westchester Medical Center
Valhalla, New York

Tony Garcia, RN, CCEMT-P
Training Specialist
Texas Engineering Extension Service
Texas A&M University System
College Station, Texas

Rebecca Hansen, MSW
Senior Project Manager
EAD & Associates, LLC
Brooklyn, New York

Nathaniel Hupert, MD, MPH
Associate Professor of Public Health and Medicine
Weill Cornell Medical College
New York, New York

Sean M. Kelly, MA, CCEMT-P
Lecturer
New York Medical College
School of Health Sciences and Practice
Valhalla, New York

Nicole E. Leahy, RN, MPH
Manager
Burn Outreach and Professional Education
New York-Presbyterian Hospital / Weill Cornell Medical Center
New York, New York

E. Brooke Learner, PhD
Associate Professor
Department of Emergency Medicine
Department of Population Health
Medical College of Wisconsin
Milwaukee, Wisconsin

David S. Markenson, MD, FAAP, FACEP, EMT-P
Medical Director and Vice President
Disaster Medicine and Regional Emergency Services
Westchester Medical Center
Director, Center for Disaster Medicine
Associate Professor, Public Health Practice
Professor of Pediatrics
New York Medical College
Valhalla, New York

Jennifer Mincin, PhD (ABD)
Senior Project Manager/Director
EAD & Associates, LLC
Brooklyn, New York

John A. Muckstadt, PhD
Acheson/Laibe Professor
Business Management and Leadership Studies
School of Operations Research and Industrial Engineering
Cornell University
Ithaca, New York

Kobi Peleg, PhD, MPH
Director, Israel National Center for Trauma and Emergency Medicine
Gertner Institute for Epidemiology and Health Policy Research
Sheba Medical Center
Co-chair, The Multi-disciplinary Program for Emergency and
    Disaster Management
School of Public Health
Tel-Aviv University
Tel-Aviv, Israel

Michael J. Reilly, DrPH, MPH, NREMT-P
Director, Graduate Program in Emergency Preparedness
Assistant Director, Center for Disaster Medicine
Assistant Professor of Public Health Practice
New York Medical College
School of Health Sciences and Practice
Valhalla, New York

John Rinard, BBA, MSCPI
Milano, Texas

Ramon Rosal, PhD
Chemical Response Director
Public Health Laboratory
New York City Department of Health and Mental Hygiene
New York, New York

Michael Rozenfeld, MA
Researcher
National Center for Trauma & Emergency Medicine Research
Gertner Institute for Epidemiology and Health Policy Research
Sheba Medical Center
Tel Hashomer, Israel

Marcelo Sandoval, MD
Faculty, Department of Emergency Medicine
Co-Chair, Emergency Management Committee
Beth Israel Medical Center / Petrie Division
New York, New York

Robert Michael Schuler, BGS, NREMT-P
Training Coordinator
Texas Engineering Extension Service
The Texas A&M University System
College Station, Texas

Richard B. Schwartz, MD
Chair and Professor
Department of Emergency Medicine
Medical College of Georgia
Augusta, Georgia

Veronica Senchak Snyder, MHS, MBA
Emergency Management Coordinator
Emergency Management Services
Geisinger Health System
Geisinger Medical Center
Danville, Pennsylvania

Doris R. Varlese, JD
Visiting Lecturer
New York Medical College
School of Health Sciences and Practice
Valhalla, New York

Deborah Viola, PhD, MBA
Associate Professor of Public Health Practice
Department of Health Policy and Management
New York Medical College
School of Health Sciences and Practice
Valhalla, New York

Isaac B. Weisfuse, MD, MPH
Deputy Commissioner
Division of Disease Control
New York City Department of Health and Mental Hygiene
New York, New York

Wei Xiong, PhD, MS
Instructor in Public Health
Weill Cornell Medical College
New York, New York

Acknowledgments

The material contained in this text reflects the contributions of many authors, editors, emergency managers, healthcare providers, reviewers, and others who provided assistance and valuable suggestions. While here we acknowledge them, our sincere appreciation for all of their efforts is truly hard to express in this limited space. In addition, we could not possibly acknowledge all those who participated in this important endeavor, and so we would like to also extend our sincere appreciation to every person who helped with this project, whether listed by name or not.

Many talented people at Jones & Bartlett Learning have been involved in developing and producing this new text. As authors and editors, we turned our manuscript to the exceptional editorial staff and publishers at Jones & Bartlett Learning to create this finished product. We are fortunate to have been able to work with this team of people, who have contributed so much and had such a tremendous impact on the quality of the textbook you now have in your hands. Specifically Michael Brown, Publisher, assisted by Catie Heverling and Kate Stein, has been our support at Jones & Bartlett Learning. As Publisher, Mike is committed to publishing quality books; his energy, intelligence, patience, and helpful efforts have enabled us to create an exceptional product. With the additional day-to-day support and guidance of both Catie Heverling and Kate Stein we were able to keep our project on track and ultimately produce this important text.

A significant amount of coordinating and operational support in moving this project forward would not have been possible without the tireless work of our administrative assistant Patience Ameyaw. We thank her for her hard work and support of this project along with Geordana Roa, Nina Luppino, and our numerous disaster medicine interns over the past several years.

Components of this text have been based on the exceptional work of the Center for Disaster Medicine at the New York Medical College, School of Health Sciences and Practice for which we serve as the Director and Assistant Director. Without the support of our Center, the prior research and models developed, and the strong and supportive academic environment of New York Medical College, this work would not have been possible. We would like to specifically thank Dean Robert Amler of the New York Medical College, School of Health Sciences and Practice, who in his own right is an internationally recognized expert in public health and healthcare preparedness, for providing his personal expertise and his leadership in creating an academic environment where work such as this text is not only encouraged but supported, and for his continued dedication to providing education to improve emergency preparedness.

We would like to also acknowledge the Westchester Medical Center and its Maria Fareri Children's Hospital, which serves as the regional center for healthcare emergency preparedness. The source and real-world testing of many of the theories and models in this text come from the preparedness efforts of this institution, which is recognized as not only a regional but as a national leader in emergency preparedness. We would like to thank the leadership of this institution for allowing us to use the wonderful preparedness work they have done as models for others to follow. While not being able to list all, we would like to acknowledge the members of the senior leadership who day in and day out support the preparedness activities: Mr. Michael Israel, Mr. Gary Brudnicki, Dr. Renee Garrick, Dr. Michael Gewitz, Ms. Marsha Casey, and Mr. Anthony Costello. Lastly, we would especially like to thank the institution's Director of Emergency Management and chapter contributor Mr. Garrett Doering for sharing his professional insight and experience with us as we completed this project.

Finally, we are extremely grateful to the numerous healthcare providers, emergency managers, educational consultants, and members of the preparedness academic community who carefully critiqued the manuscript to ensure that the information in this text would be both relevant and appropriate. Many more dedicated professionals than we could name here gave unstintingly of their own time and expertise. Their enthusiastic participation has been a motivating force behind this project, and they received no compensation beyond the knowledge that they were helping to create a greatly needed resource. We hope the final product lives up to their efforts, hopes, and expectations.

Our warmest and kindest regards,
Michael and David

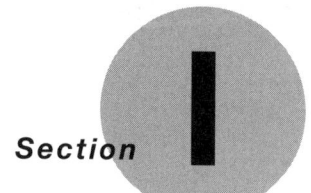

Section **I**

Principles of Emergency Management for Healthcare Facilities

Chapter 1

Introduction to Hospital and Healthcare Emergency Management

Michael J. Reilly, DrPH, MPH, NREMT-P and

David S. Markenson, MD, FAAP, FACEP, EMT-P

Photo by Jocelyn Augustino/FEMA News Photo

Learning Objectives

- Describe the need for and responsibilities of healthcare emergency management.
- Describe the role of the hospital emergency manager.
- Identify the activities performed by healthcare emergency management.

Emergence and Growth of Healthcare Emergency Management

The concept of healthcare emergency management is not entirely new, but may seem strange and foreign to those who have worked in healthcare or emergency management and, until recently, have not known anyone working in this profession. If one looks back more than 30 years, it would be almost impossible to find a hospital role called hospital emergency management or even a position for a healthcare emergency manager in a hospital or medical center. Yet healthcare emergency management responsibilities have always been addressed by hospitals, such as fire safety, backup power, and the ability to handle victims from a mass casualty event.

A fundamental tenet of emergency management is that institutions must prepare for events that may rarely occur while taking protective actions to mitigate any likelihood that they will occur at all. Due to the low frequency of events testing the health system's ability to respond to a disaster, an act of terrorism, or a public health emergency, the ability to evaluate the strengths and weaknesses of hospital emergency preparedness is limited. In addition, the public has strong expectations of the roles hospitals should play during times of disaster. Healthcare institutions are expected to provide both emergency care and continuance of the day-to-day healthcare responsibilities regardless of the volume and demand. Recently, they have also become sites of community refuge, bastions of safety in a threatening and dangerous environment. The public believes that hospitals will have light, heat, air conditioning, water, food, and communications capabilities, regardless of the fact that the institution may itself be affected by the calamity. During the terrorist attacks in the fall of 2001 and the Northeast Blackout of 2003, the public flocked to hospitals, even when they did not require medical care. Furthermore, with increased intelligence of the vulnerabilities of the healthcare infrastructure and the desire of terrorists to exploit this, institutions have been forced to focus limited resources on safety and security rather than on comprehensive emergency management efforts.

A major change in the way hospitals plan for hazards and vulnerabilities includes less planning for specific single issues or threats but rather the adoption of an all–hazards comprehensive emergency management planning process. Additionally, hospitals need to look beyond their emergency department doors and engage community stakeholders to assist in this process, reaching out to local and regional emergency planners to assist in larger communitywide emergency preparedness planning. The interest of nonhospital entities in health system emergency preparedness can be seen through several examples, including emergency management and public health initiatives on mass vaccination, pandemic planning, increasing hospitals' ability to perform decontamination of casualties contaminated with hazardous materials, etc. Recent reflection of the role of the hospital in emergency management and population health can been seen in revised laws, regulations, and even accreditation standards. An example of this is The Joint Commission on the Accreditation of Healthcare Organizations' (JCAHO) change from placing emergency preparedness standards in the Environment of Care section to placing the standards in a separate and distinct section with specific goals and requirements, as well as the release of the Occupational Safety and Health Administration (OSHA) document *Best Practices for Hospital-Based First Receivers*.[1-3]

Over the past eight years we have embarked on an interesting marriage of these two separate disciplines—health care and emergency management—whose common ground has historically been brought together in the street or on the disaster scene by emergency medical services workers, or sometimes brought into the emergency departments of hospitals and trauma centers across the country. Both disciplines have separate roles and responsibilities, but where the seemingly disparate goals of these fields come together is the reduction of morbidity and mortality following disasters, acts of terrorism, and public health emergencies.

Emergency management agencies have traditionally been responsible for bringing first responders, government agencies, and community stakeholders together to assist with comprehensive emergency planning or disaster response and recovery. A common cornerstone of emergency management has been to protect life, then property, then the environment. As a result, when conducting emergency planning activities, the health and medical needs of the population are among the most significant and are considered with basic public health and human needs including sheltering, mass care, sanitation, environment health, food and water, and other essential services. In addition, as public health professionals, we also believe that population health activities include the mitigation of increased morbidity and mortality during and following a disaster, act of terrorism, or public health emergency.

In healthcare delivery, we attempt to meet the health and medical needs of the community by providing a place for individuals to seek preventative medicine, care for chronic medical conditions, emergency medical treatment, and rehabilitation from injury or illness. While a healthcare institution serves the community, this responsibility occurs at the level of the individual. Each individual expects a thorough assessment and treatment if needed, regardless of the needs of others. This approach is different than that practiced by emergency managers, whose goal is to assist the largest number of people with the limited resources that are available. As such, emergency management principles are focused on the needs of the population rather than the individual. When either planning for a disaster or operating in a disaster response mode, the hospital should be prepared at some point to change its focus from the individual to the community it serves and to begin weighing the needs of any individual patient versus the most good for the most patients with scarce resources. Moving from the notion of doing the most for each individual to doing the best for the many is a critical shift in thinking for healthcare institutions considering a program of comprehensive emergency management. While the initial planning for emergencies by hospitals is focused on maintaining operations and handling the care needs of actual or potential increased numbers of patients and/or different presentations of illness or injury than is traditionally seen, there is also the need to recognize that at some point during a disaster, act of terrorism, or public health emergency there may be an imbalance of need versus available resources. At this point the approach to delivering healthcare will need to switch from a focus on the individual to a focus on the population. This paradigm shift is one of the core unique aspects of hospital emergency management that allows the hospital to prepare to maximize resources in disasters and then to know when to switch to a pure disaster mode of utilizing its limited and often scant resources to help the most people with the greatest chance of survival.

The healthcare delivery system is vast and comprised of multiple entry points at primary care providers, clinics, urgent care centers, hospitals, rehabilitation facilities, and long-term care facilities. The point of entry for many individuals into the acute healthcare system is through the emergency department (ED). Since the late 1970s, the emergency medical services (EMS) system has allowed victims of acute illness and injury to receive initial stabilization of life-threatening medical conditions on the way to the emergency department. Among the many strengths of the ED is the ability to integrate two major components of the healthcare system: prehospital and definitive care. The emergency department maintains constant communications with the EMS system and serves as the direct point of entry for prehospital providers into the hospital or trauma center. Emergency physicians represent a critical link in this process by anticipating the resources that ill and injured patients will need upon arrival at the ED, and initiating appropriate life-saving medical care until specialty resources become available.[4-11] In this context, the healthcare system is an emergency response entity.

Healthcare Emergency Management Activities

Hospital emergency management activities vary and can be categorized in many ways, however some common areas of focus within healthcare emergency management include the following areas:

- communication
- surge capacity
- volunteer management
- security issues
- hazmat/CBRNE preparedness
- collaboration and integration with public health
- education and training

- equipment and supplies
- worker safety
- drills and exercises
- emergency department disaster operations
- trauma centers

COMMUNICATION

Communication issues in disaster preparedness and response are cited throughout the literature as a major source of frustration and inadequacy for coordinating and executing disaster operation plans.[4–5,8,11–16] By identifying the vulnerabilities in the existing system of healthcare communication systems, we can take steps to address these issues and further increase our health system preparedness. Addressing the vulnerabilities in communication systems and planning how to overcome them is an essential responsibility of a hospital emergency manager. Many of the criticisms of the current state of health systems' communication systems center around the inability to communicate easily with external agencies and share critical information. Disaster after-action reports and exercise improvement plans almost universally cite poor communication as one of the problems associated with incident management and the event being reviewed.

Infrastructure support is an important consideration when examining whether adequate safeguards are in place to support the systems we will rely upon during a disaster. On September 11, 2001, while one New York City hospital was preparing to treat a large number of (anticipated) casualties from the disaster, they experienced a loss of their computer and information systems.[17] This unplanned event arose because the communication system line that supported their system's infrastructure ran beneath the World Trade Center.[17] Additionally, other reports have cited problems with battery failure and the lack of a prolonged power supply as limiting communication systems' abilities during an event.[14] This example illustrates a major point in emergency communication systems: hospitals need the ability to connect all significant parties during a disaster or other emergency and the system should be based on a redundant infrastructure.[5] Clearly, from a planning perspective, this would be a desirable option. However, the reality remains that investing in communication systems is a significant financial burden on already underfunded hospitals and healthcare systems.

Risk communication is often overlooked during the planning phase of an event, and this can lead to frustration and confusion during disaster operations. Risk communication is sometimes the only way for the public to gain an understanding of the scope and severity of an incident. Additionally, risk communication information provided by hospitals may be used to help families of disaster victims find information about their loved ones' condition. Reviews of risk communication have shown that a predesignated public information officer (PIO), who will liaise with the media and the public and who has specific training and experience in giving briefings and fielding questions, should perform all risk communication tasks during disaster operations.[13] Specific elements of risk communication that may be conveyed to the public may include information on evacuations, scope and breadth of the event, where and how to obtain assistance if needed, whom to call for specific information, location of postexposure prophylaxis or vaccination clinics, and what to expect over the next several hours and/or days of the event. This is discussed in more detail in Chapter 12.

SURGE CAPACITY

The General Accounting Office (GAO), which changed its name to the Government Accountability Office (GAO) in 2004, finalized reports during 2003 on the public health and hospital preparedness for bioterrorism and emerging infectious diseases.[9,16] These reports found that most hospitals in the United States do not have the means to care for a surge of patients during a public health emergency.[9,16] They stated that, based on the national emergency department diversion rates in urban and suburban areas, shortages in the healthcare workforce, and the general lack of available supplemental medical equipment and supplies in hospitals, the medical community is not prepared to handle a patient surge caused by an infectious disease outbreak or bioterrorism related event.[9,16] Emergency departments are being utilized more often as urgent care centers because the growing population utilizes the ED as their point of primary care. This increasing phenomenon is contributing to ED overcrowding and diversionary status (hospital EDs asking that ambulances refrain from bringing patients to their facility for a period of time) in virtually every healthcare and trauma system in the country. The current state of affairs in the nation's EDs makes it very difficult to prepare for surge capacity when many hospitals cannot effectively handle their daily patient volume.[18]

Referral patterns of patients presented to medical facilities will vary in terms of how they arrive at the facility (EMS or self-transport) as well as which facilities they access (hospital ED or physician's office), depending on the type of disaster or public health emergency. In cases of natural disasters, explosions, and acute catastrophic events where there is a clear and defined "scene," many patients will be triaged, treated, and perhaps transported to hospitals or trauma centers by EMS personnel. In cases of bioterrorism or infectious disease outbreaks, patients would normally exhibit minor signs and/or symptoms of an illness (e.g., fever, rash, flu-like symptoms, etc.). These patients may be presented to their primary care physician or an urgent care center to receive initial diagnosis and treatment. The patients that can be expected to arrive at the ED in these cases would be those who could not access a private physician, those too acutely ill to seek care in an office setting, those referred to the ED by their physicians, and those patients who called EMS for assistance. This latter group would yield the least number of ED arrivals.[19–20]

Incidents of chemical and biological terrorism as well as pandemic or epidemic incidents of infectious diseases may arguably produce the most significant burden on the healthcare system.[9,13,16,18,21] A main reason for this is the unpredictable referral patterns of patients who fall victim to a chemical or biological hazard. Although some disaster after-action reports do suggest that even victims of conventional disasters will self-refer to medical facilities, the issues of delayed onset of symptoms, cross-contamination, and person-to-person disease transmission that are associated with a chemical, biologic, or radiologic incident call for more detailed contingency plans. An example of hospital referral patterns after a chemical agent event can be seen in the post-event summary of the sarin attack in the Tokyo subways in March of 1995.[22] In this incident 12 people were killed, but more than 5000 people sought medical attention, and only 688 of them were medically transported to area hospitals.[22]

At some point during the evolution of a disaster or other public health emergency, patients will converge on acute care hospitals. Studies have consistently shown that despite rigorous planning initiatives, hospitals and emergency departments are not prepared to handle the mass influx of patients that a bioterrorism event or infectious disease outbreak would produce.[9,16,19–20] During the sarin attack on the Tokyo subway in 1995, the nearest hospital had 500 patients in the first hour after the incident and more than 20% of its staff was secondarily contaminated.[22] It is important that planners additionally recognize that in certain catastrophic disasters involving bombings, building collapse, etc., mass injuries and a patient surge may not occur as anticipated because of the high rate of mortality.[17,23] The hospital emergency manager and all those involved in hospital emergency management must ensure that their hospital has adequate plans for the surge of patients that will arrive during a disaster, terrorism event, or public health emergency.

VOLUNTEER MANAGEMENT

The use of volunteers in disasters and public health emergencies presents a unique set of considerations for the hospital emergency manager. Volunteers can be utilized in several ways to assist in disaster relief services. However, the problems of volunteer management, credentialing, safety, and security often preclude their utility in the acute disaster environment unless significant pre-planning for their use has occurred and their arrival is through a pre-defined system. Cone et al. describe "convergent volunteerism" (the influx of citizens and/or health providers to a major incident) as a "critical problem" in disaster management.[24] Intuitively, you may think that the outpouring of community support to assist in rendering aid during a disaster or other public health emergency is a welcome show of support for disaster victims. However, the reality is that convergent volunteerism brings with it security, resource, and worker safety problems that require personnel and critical resources to manage.

In their discussion of convergent volunteerism in the September 11 terrorist attacks in NYC, Cone and colleagues discuss the myriad of additional challenges and problems that the unsolicited and often intrusive behavior of "Good Samaritans" imposed on the NYC responders. Issues included the unsupervised practice of medicine and paramedicine; credential verification of certified and/or licensed personnel; the performance of search and rescue operations by lay responders; the need to feed, shelter, and provide sanitary facilities for volunteers; potential injury and illness to volunteers who were unsupervised and lacked proper personal protective equipment; and personal vehicle congestion on scene access and egress.[24]

Many of these concerns may seem trivial to some who view a community response to a disaster as being the quintessential demonstration of altruism and support for fellow citizens. However, as mentioned by Cone and colleagues, untrained and unauthorized volunteers can ultimately put themselves and others in danger, and deplete emergency response resources by attempting to provide assistance at disaster scenes. This was most poignantly illustrated during the 1995 bombing of the Alfred P. Murrah Federal Building in Oklahoma City, when an untrained and unprotected volunteer nurse was crushed by falling debris while trying to assist with urban search and rescue operations.[24]

SECURITY ISSUES

Hospitals frequently overlook the need to maintain adequate security of the healthcare facility and overall medical operations as part of both daily operations and emergency planning. The concept of "locking down" or restricting access to a healthcare facility is often contradictory to the typical hospital design and approach of open access to both patients and their families and other visitors. But during a disaster this type of control is essential for many reasons, which include but are not limited to: control of the flow of patients to the areas where care will be provided; access to the facility only by authorized staff; accounting for staff and patients in time of evacuation; prevention of potentially contaminated patients entering the hospital from contaminating staff, other patients, and facilities; and prevention of acts of terrorism.

Security resources generally vary among hospitals. Some hospitals and trauma centers have sworn police officers present in their facilities 24 hours a day, and others may hire a private security firm to maintain safety or simply serve a concierge or customer service role. Security concerns during disasters and public health emergencies can become significant when considering the potential vulnerabilities associated with the chaotic response environment.[15,17,24–25] Specifically cited issues with security during the response to a disaster or public health emergency include access control to medical facilities; credentialing of employees, responders, and volunteers; crime scene and evidence preservation; infrastructure and resource protection; and crowd control.[15,17,24–25]

HAZMAT/CBRNE PREPAREDNESS

There is no question that in the current state of health system and public health preparedness the medical community is ill-prepared to deal with an incident that involves the management and treatment of multiple potentially contaminated victims, including those from chemical, biological, radiological, nuclear, and explosive (CBRNE) events. Multiple recent reports of hospital preparedness cite decontamination capabilities as a serious weakness of disaster readiness plans.[4–5,8–9,11,15–16,26–27] One study cites as few as 6% of Level I trauma centers as having the necessary equipment on hand to safely decontaminate a single patient.[26] Planning for these events has traditionally centered around the fallacy that patients will be decontaminated at the scene by first responders and then be triaged, treated, and transported to the ED. The decontamination process serves a dual purpose.

First, it removes the potential agent that is causing harm to the patient, and second, it prevents the spread of secondary contamination to other patients and hospital staff. We have come to realize from recent incidents involving victim contamination that many ambulatory victims will leave the scene and bypass EMS decontamination and triage, seeking medical care on their own.[11,15,19–20] The reality of dealing with an intentional release of chemical, biological, or radiological agent is that by the time acute care facilities can be made aware that an event has taken place, they may have already been contaminated themselves.[22] The specifics of hospital decontamination and worker safety are discussed in Chapter 14.

Throughout the nation, trauma systems, acute care hospitals, and first responders are unprepared for handling an event involving the release of a nuclear, biological, or chemical (NBC) agent.[8,15,26] Largely, this is due to ineffective planning and relying on resources that may not be available during a disaster or public health emergency.[15] The most often cited weaknesses are an overall lack of training, lack of personal protective equipment (PPE), lack of resources and equipment to rapidly and reliably perform preliminary agent detection, and lack of appropriate medical facilities, equipment and supplies to effectively isolate infectious patients and manage them through the course of their illnesses.[8,15,21–22,26]

COLLABORATION AND INTEGRATION WITH PUBLIC HEALTH

In order for disaster preparedness and response to be successful, it must involve interagency resources and consider the 3C's of emergency response planning: Collaboration, Cooperation, and Coordination. Response plans cannot be designed and implemented in a vacuum. Disaster response and recovery operations will certainly consist of a multiagency response at the local, state, and federal levels. In order to ensure that the response plan is valid, and will operationally integrate with other key responding agencies, the planner must collaborate with fellow agencies and develop plans that involve aspects of interagency response. Interagency planning groups, such as the Local Emergency Planning Committee (LEPC), operate under the assumption that if a hazardous event occurs, all key public safety and health agencies will respond in a unified approach with common goals to protect the welfare and safety of the community. These principles of collaboration, cooperation, and coordination among the agencies that will likely respond to a disaster or other public health emergency will minimize unnecessary redundancy in response plans and create partnerships with agencies that can provide expertise and resources during the public health emergency response.

In a large-scale disaster or act of terrorism, such as the World Trade Center attacks in 1993 and 2001, the Oklahoma City bombing in 1995, and the 1994 and 1995 sarin attacks in Tokyo, continuous medical monitoring and follow-up of the survivors, responders, and participants in these events is needed to detect the associated long-term health effects. With the exception of large academic medical institutions that may perform epidemiologic analysis on specific cohorts of individuals, the public health community must recruit and maintain a database of affected individuals so they can study the long-term impact of these events on the health of the population. It is important to note that although the imminent threat of danger may no longer be present, the need for medical care, disease surveillance, and follow-up studies is essential to the completion of the public health role in a disaster or other public health emergency.

Additionally, public health agencies at the federal, state, and local levels have the responsibility under the National Response Framework (NRF) to coordinate and serve as the lead agency for disasters involving mass care. This may include assisting both hospitals and communities to establish alternate care sites (ACS) where patients can be directed to receive medical treatment during a public health emergency, which will allow a hospital to use its resources to treat higher acuity patients and remain open to handle routine emergencies during a pandemic or other public health emergency.

EDUCATION AND TRAINING

Reports have suggested that healthcare workers lack the knowledge to detect and manage a patient who has been exposed to a chemical or biological agent.[6,27–28] The Health Resources and Services Administration (HRSA) survey helped to illustrate the lack of training and education among trauma center and hospital staff by reporting that only eight states required employees to be trained in disaster-related topics, two states required training in biological agent topics, and two states required training for chemical-related topics.[8] Additionally, training for EMS personnel was equally poor because only six states required prehospital providers to have education on disaster-related topics, only one state required biological agent training, and three states required education on chemical agents.[8]

EQUIPMENT AND SUPPLIES

In the GAO's report of hospital preparedness in August 2003, they reported several findings on hospital equipment and supply resources. The survey showed that for every 100 beds, 50% of hospitals had fewer than 6 ventilators, fewer than 3 PPE suits, fewer than 4 isolation beds, and could only handle fewer than 6 patients per hour through a 5-minute decontamination shower, given their current state of preparedness.[9] Additionally, the GAO reports that most first responders lack a reliable means to detect chemical and/or biological agents in the field, and do not typically have the proper PPE to protect themselves from agent exposure.[9] The HRSA evaluation of state trauma systems showed that the availability of PPE for healthcare workers was significantly lacking among states because only one state (Ohio) had enough PPE resources immediately available for its EMS personnel, and only one state (New Jersey) had enough PPE resources immediately available for its hospital personnel if a chemical or biological agent release occurred.[8]

In addition to PPE issues, hospitals and trauma centers often lack the inventory of equipment and supplies necessary to effectively treat an influx of potentially affected patients.[8–9,14–16,26] Many hospitals, in a strategy to reduce overall costs, replenish their central supply on a "just-in-time" basis, clearly ineffective in preparing to treat a mass influx of patients.[18] Pharmaceutical access is another concern among healthcare facilities. As demonstrated in the fall 2001 anthrax scare, hundreds of postal and healthcare workers required postexposure prophylaxis after potential exposure to the agent. Maintaining an adequate pharmaceutical stock of essential antibiotics, antidotes, and specialty medications in case of a disaster is often viewed as cost prohibitive due to the shelf life and daily usefulness of certain drugs.[18] Although this has improved slightly over the past 6 years, hospitals around the country still struggle to build the internal capacity necessary to perform emergency decontamination of patients from hazardous substance incidents and properly protect their staff, patients, and visitors from secondary contamination.

WORKER SAFETY

A report released by HRSA on the national state of the trauma system and EMS preparedness for disasters and mass causality events showed that only one state in the country thought that its hospital workers would be adequately protected in the event of a biological (but not chemical) agent attack.[8] Additionally, only one state reported that its EMS system would have access to PPE in the event of a bioterrorism event.[8] Similar research has underscored a general lack of protection for the public health workforce against any type of chemical, biological, or radiological contamination in the event of a disaster.[8] A major role for the public health community during an event is to ensure the health and safety of all disaster workers.[13,15]

DRILLS AND EXERCISES

Criticisms regarding drills and exercises are notable throughout the preparedness literature.[6,9,11,15,21,26] Comments include statements that exercises are not realistic, drills tend to be conducted with advanced warning on shifts with favorable staffing levels, and with equipment and resource levels at their best, etc. Therefore, the drills bias any useful results from the exercise.[15] The purpose of conducting drills and exercises (besides remaining in compliance with accrediting bodies) is to assess whether or not a facility is adequately prepared to handle an incident with relatively low probability, but with extremely significant impact on the health system, and to identify areas that need improvement on an operational and planning level.[15] Exercises that simply go through the motions or are conducted with limited realism, under optimal conditions, or are simply haphazardly conducted to meet regulatory or legal requirements are futile and worthless assessment tools that will only perpetuate a hospital's state of unpreparedness.[15]

EMERGENCY DEPARTMENT DISASTER OPERATIONS

The importance of the ED's role in disaster and emergency preparedness is discussed in several sources.[4–12] The American College of Surgeons mentions that the ED is a major strength of a trauma center.[12] They refer to the ED staff as "highly competent" and often "experts" in the medical management of chemical, biological, and radiological casualties.[12] Among the many strengths of the ED is the ability to integrate two major components of the trauma system: prehospital and definitive care. The emergency department maintains constant communications with the EMS system and serves as the direct point of entry for prehospital providers into the hospital or trauma center. Emergency physicians represent a critical link in the chain of survival by anticipating the resources that ill and injured patients will need upon arrival at the ED, and initiating appropriate lifesaving medical care until specialty resources become available.[4–11]

TRAUMA CENTERS

The roles of trauma centers during a disaster or public health emergency are consistent with their daily activities in the treatment of injured patients. Triage and treatment of injured victims after a disaster is frequently discussed as a central role of the trauma center in the aftermath of a disaster.[6,8–11,13,15–16,18,23,25–29] It is well documented that trauma centers are adept at the care of the injured victim, and are viewed as the best choice for the triage and treatment of disaster-related injured victims.[4–10,12,14,17,23,25–31] Trauma care is identified most frequently as the major strength of the trauma center and the trauma system. Another expectation is that trauma centers and acute care hospitals will be able to treat mass numbers of affected patients as well, including the rapid triage and treatment of all casualties (including those from CBRNE events), decontamination and/or isolation, and quarantine of contaminated or potentially infectious patients. Trauma centers are also expected to have access to essential equipment, supplies, and pharmaceutical agents.[4–6,8,14–15,17,23,27–29,32]

The Role of the Hospital/Healthcare Emergency Manager

What then, is a hospital or healthcare emergency manager? A hospital or healthcare emergency manager is an individual employed by a healthcare organization whose job is to coordinate the emergency management functions of the hospital. This may include many responsibilities depending on the hospital or healthcare system, the location of the facility, the size and type of facility or organization, and specific local issues or threats and activities. While there may be variation in the role, almost universally the hospital/healthcare emergency manager will perform hazard vulnerability analysis, planning activities, coordination of the hospital's disaster and other emergency management planning groups or committees, design and conduct training programs, perform drills and exercises, interact with other agencies and organizations involved in healthcare emergency management (e.g., local public health department, local office of emergency management, EMS, local law enforcement, and state agencies), and maintain compliance with regulatory agencies and accreditation organizations such as the JCAHO. Many hospital or healthcare emergency managers are individuals who have these duties in addition to their normal occupational roles in the healthcare organization. Typical positions within healthcare organizations that also perform emergency preparedness activities include nursing managers, educators, administrators, security managers, environmental health and safety administrators, facilities or physical plant directors, or emergency medical services coordinators.

Few hospitals have taken the initiative to hire a full-time emergency preparedness coordinator for several reasons. First, there is no direct revenue return on investment in hospital preparedness. Emergency management is rather a fixed but necessary operating cost. In the United States, hospitals and healthcare organizations need to generate a profit. Even in not-for-profit hospitals, CEOs need to be able to show that profit increased in order to justify growth and add services for their patients. Activities that cannot improve the profitability of the organization often remain unfunded. Second, there is a shortage of qualified individuals to fill these positions. As mentioned before, most hospitals have added the duties and responsibilities of preparedness onto an existing full-time employee and this individual had to teach themselves how to perform these added duties. Most individuals who serve in full-time hospital emergency manager positions have a public safety background or a clinical background and have had to learn the discipline of emergency management.

Until recently there have been few higher educational opportunities for people who wish to learn the discipline of healthcare emergency management. In 2010, the Federal Emergency Management Agency's (FEMA) Higher Education Program listed only 10 undergraduate and graduate programs combined that focus on both healthcare and emergency management. Many of these are new programs that have only been in existence for a few years. There have been degree programs in general emergency management, but only a few that apply this discipline to the public health or hospital environment.

If you don't seek out a formal degree, how do you become knowledgeable in hospital emergency planning? Initially, it begins with your current role. If you are a healthcare worker who needs to learn the finer points of emergency planning, drills and exercises, and incident management, then you could benefit from FEMA's independent study program or professional development series. On the other hand, if you are an emergency management professional with little knowledge of the healthcare environment, you may benefit from continuing education in health and medical issues such as the strategic national stockpile, emerging infectious diseases and pandemics, the health and medical impact of terrorism and weapons of mass destruction, and the health impact on populations displaced as the result of disasters.

This text is designed specifically for individuals who wish to learn the applied discipline of healthcare emergency management, and for all other personnel in a hospital or from other disciplines who will work with either a hospital or any other aspect of a healthcare system in planning for and responding to disasters, terrorism, and public health emergencies. Whether you are a college or graduate student learning the fundamentals of public health or healthcare emergency management, or a current healthcare professional looking to increase your current knowledge in order to apply emergency management principles to your trade, this book is designed to meet your needs. There is a lot to learn, and this text is just the beginning. This emerging field is exciting, challenging, and rewarding. We wish you luck on your journey!

References

1. U.S. Department of Labor, Occupational Safety and Health Administration. *Best Practices for Hospital-Based First Receivers of Victims from Mass Casualty Incidents Involving the Release of Hazardous Substances.* Washington, DC: OSHA; 2005. OSHA publication 3249–08N.

2. Joint Commission Resources. Emergency management standards. *Environ Care News.* 2007;10(12):2–8.

3. Joint Commission Resources. Preparing for catastrophes and escalating emergencies. *Environ Care News.* 2008;11(1):1–3, 11.

4. American College of Surgeons. *Resources for Optimal Care of the Injured Patient: 1999.* Chicago: American College of Surgeons; 1999.

5. American Trauma Society and U.S. Department of Transportation, National Highway Traffic Safety Administration. *Trauma System Agenda for the Future.* National Highway Traffic Safety Administration; October 2002. Report #3P0138.

6. American College of Surgeons. [ST-42] Statement on disaster and mass casualty management [by the American College of Surgeons]. American College of Surgeons Web site. http://www.facs.org/fellows_info/statements/st-42.html. Published 2003. Accessed December 28, 2009.

7.   Bledsoe BE, Porter RS, Cherry RA. *Essentials of Paramedic Care.* Upper Saddle River, New Jersey: Brady/Prentice Hall Health; 2003.

8.   U.S. Department of Health and Human Services, Health Resources and Services Administration. *A 2002 National Assessment of State Trauma System Development, Emergency Medical Services Resources, and Disaster Readiness for Mass Casualty Events.* Washington, DC: Health Resources and Services Administration; 2002.

9.   U.S. General Accounting Office. *Hospital Preparedness: Most Urban Hospitals Have Emergency Plans but Lack Certain Capacities for Bioterrorism Response.* Washington, DC: U.S. General Accounting Office; August, 2003. Report GAO-03-924.

10.   Frykberg ER. Disaster and mass casualty management: a comment on the ACS position statement. *Bulletin of the American College of Surgeons.* 2003;88(8):12–13.

11.   White SR. Hospital and emergency department preparedness for biological, chemical, and nuclear terrorism. *Clin Occup Environ Med.* 2002;2(2):405–425.

12.   Trunkey DD. Trauma centers and trauma systems. *JAMA.* 2003;289:1566–1567.

13.   Landesman LY. *Public Health Management of Disasters: The Practice Guide.* Washington, DC: American Public Health Association; 2001.

14.   May AK, McGwin G Jr, Lancaster LJ, et al. The April 8, 1998 tornado: assessment of the trauma system response and the resulting injuries. *J Trauma.* 2000; 48(4):666–672.

15.   Rubin, JN. Recurring pitfalls in hospital preparedness and response. *J Homeland Security.* January, 2004. http://www.homelanddefense.org/journal/Articles/rubin.html. Accessed August 18, 2009.

16.   U.S. General Accounting Office. *SARS Outbreak: Improvements to Public Health Capacity Are Needed for Responding to Bioterrorism and Emerging Infectious Diseases.* Washington, DC: U.S. General Accounting Office; May 7, 2003. Publication GAO-03-769T.

17.   Feeney J, Parekh N, Blumenthal J, Wallack MK. September 11, 2001: a test of preparedness and spirit. *Bulletin of the American College of Surgeons.* 2002;87(5).

18.   Barbera JA, Macintyre AG, DeAtley CA. Ambulances to nowhere: America's critical shortfall in medical preparedness for catastrophic terrorism. In: Howitt AM, Pangi RL, eds. *Countering Terrorism: Dimensions of Preparedness.* Cambridge, MA: MIT Press; 2003:283–297.

19.   Reilly MJ, Markenson D. Hospital emergency department referral patterns in a disaster. *Prehosp Disast Med.* 2009;24(2):s29–s30.

20.   Reilly MJ. Referral patterns of patients in disasters—who is coming through your emergency department doors? *Prehosp Disast Med.* 2007;22(2):s114–s115.

21.   Kellerman A. A hole in the homeland defense. *Modern Healthcare.* 2003;33(16):23.

22.   U.S. Department of Defense, Army, SBCCOM, Federal Domestic Preparedness Program. *NBC Domestic Preparedness Senior Officials' Workshop (SOW)* [CD-ROM]. SBCCOM; 1999.

23.   Cushman JG, Pachter HL, Beaton HL. Two New York City hospitals' surgical response to the September 11, 2001, terrorist attack in New York City. *J Trauma.* 2003;54:147–155.

24.   Cone DC, Weir SD, Bogucki S. Convergent volunteerism. *Ann Emerg Med.* 2003;41(4):457–462.

25.   Feliciano DV, Anderson GV Jr, Rozycki GS, et al. Management of casualties from the bombing at the Centennial Olympics. *Am J Surg.* 1998;176(6):538–543.

26.   Ghilarducci DP, Pirallo RG, Hegmann KT. Hazardous materials readiness of United States Level 1 trauma centers. *J Occup Environ Med.* 2000;42(7):683–692.

27. American College of Surgeons. Disasters from biological and chemical terrorism—what should the individual surgeon do?: a report from the Committee on Trauma. American College of Surgeons Web site. http://www.facs.org/civiliandisasters/trauma.html. Accessed December 30, 2009.

28. American College of Surgeons. Statement on unconventional acts of civilian terrorism: a report from the Board of Governors. American College of Surgeons Web site. http://www.facs.org/civiliandisasters/statement.html. Accessed December 30, 2009.

29. Jacobs LM, Burns KJ, Gross RI. Terrorism: a public health threat with a trauma system response. J Trauma. 2003;55(6):1014–1021.

30. MacKenzie EJ, Hoyt DB, Sacra JC, et al. National inventory of hospital trauma centers. JAMA. 2003;289:1515–1522.

31. Mann NC, Mullins RJ, MacKenzie EJ, Jurkovich GJ, Mock CN. Systematic review of published evidence regarding trauma system effectiveness. J Trauma. 1999; 47(3);S25–S33.

32. Peterson TD, Vaca F. Commentary: Trauma systems: a key factor in homeland preparedness. Ann Emerg Med. 2003;41(6):799–801.

Chapter 2

Healthcare Incident Management Systems

Arthur Cooper, MD, MS

Learning Objectives

- Discuss the fundamental principles of healthcare incident management systems.
- Describe the incident command system structure and its application to the healthcare environment.
- Discuss the importance of interagency cooperation and collaboration when managing disasters and public health emergencies that impact the healthcare system.

Overview

Making method out of madness

The aim of this chapter is to arm the busy healthcare staff, clinician, or emergency manger with a basic understanding of incident management systems as applied to the healthcare and hospital environment, including the Hospital Incident Command System (HICS), not as a substitute, but as a rationale for incident management training and the need to understand the application to a hospital or healthcare system. This chapter will cover the fundamental principles of healthcare incident management systems, including one system modified specifically for the hospital, the Hospital Incident Command System. Such systems are vital to the management of disasters, acts of terrorism, and public health emergencies involving healthcare organizations because, without the effective coordination of resources achieved through use of a healthcare incident management system, chaos, rather than order, will prevail. After a concise introduction to set the stage, the chapter will consider the historical background, foundational principles, incident leadership, command structures, HICS organization, training systems, HICS implementation, logistic concerns, practical concerns, and interagency relationships essential to successful healthcare incident management, before delivering its conclusions.

Case Study

A Cloud in the Midnight Sky

You are the administrator on duty (AOD) when you are called by the physician in charge of the emergency department, who reports that numerous arriving patients are exhibiting spasms of severe coughing triggered by "something in the air." While you consider your next steps, your spouse calls to tell you there has been a large explosion at a nearby tank farm adjacent to a large industrial facility. Television reports document widespread panic at the scene and in the immediate vicinity of your hospital, which is located about two miles (three kilometers) east of the site. It is past midnight; only caretaker staff are on duty (except in your critical and acute care units) and hospital staff await your orders.

The following questions race through your mind. How would you begin to answer them?

- Does a bona fide disaster exist?
- Should I declare a disaster now?
- Should I seek additional information before declaring a disaster?
- Should I implement the hospital's emergency operations plan?
- Should I activate the hospital's command center?
- How will I ensure the safety of staff and patients?
- Should I mobilize additional hospital staff?
- Should I lock down the facility?
- Should all emergency patients be decontaminated?
- Should public health agencies be notified?

- Who should I ask for necessary additional resources?
- Are there potential threats to the hospital itself?
- How will I coordinate and supervise all the staff?

The decisions are yours to make. The answers may be found in this chapter.

Introduction

"Who's in charge? They're all in charge!"[1]

Understanding the Incident Command System (ICS) applied during disasters may prove a daunting task, even for healthcare executives experienced in interpreting complex tables of organization that baffle other managers, clinicians accustomed to solving and treating complex medical problems, and staff prepared to work in the complex healthcare environment. However, as recently stated so eloquently by Lieutenant Thomas Martin of the Virginia State Police in the illuminating video, *The Many Hats Of Highway Incident Command* (http://cts .virginia.edu/incident_mgnt_training.htm), the principles of incident command are fundamentally no different from the everyday manners children learn as youngsters, as elegantly and clearly described in the poignant work by author Robert Fulghum, *All I Really Need To Know I Learned In Kindergarten.*[1,2] Within this simple framework, the responsible healthcare emergency manager can readily answer the question, "Who's in charge?" The answer, of course, is that *they're all in charge, of what they're in charge of*—because all those involved in the disaster response are responsible for their immediate tasks, their communication with others, and *first and foremost, their own and others' safety*.

Historical Background

"The best way to predict the future is to create it."[3]

Modern incident command grew from the experience of firefighters in combating the California wildfires of the mid 1970s. Inadequate communication and ineffective collaboration between the numerous agencies battling these natural disasters led to the deaths of many firefighters whose lives need not have been lost. The subsequent after-action reports identified numerous critical weaknesses in the organization and delivery of many responders' agencies and efforts, including lack of accountability, barriers to communication, poor planning processes, overloaded incident commanders, and absent response integration. The dawning realization that deficient and defective command and control were mostly responsible for these tragic fatalities led California fire chiefs to develop an "interoperable" system for emergency response, whereby all the involved agencies could communicate with one another and collaborate in the field, based upon a common organizational structure that all such agencies could understand and apply.

This new system, called FIRESCOPE (Firefighting Resources of California Organized for Potential Emergencies), was based upon principles gleaned from military experience and management theory, especially the management by objectives concepts introduced in 1954 by Peter F. Drucker in his classic work, The Practice of Management.[4] Its core purpose was to provide a standardized, on-scene, all-hazard incident management dogma that allowed its users to quickly implement an integrated organizational structure that was not impeded by jurisdiction boundaries, and was flexible and scalable enough to match the needs and resources for single, expanding, multiple, and complex incidents, despite their special circumstances and unique demands. It rapidly evolved into the Incident Command System (ICS) that has gradually been adopted by most fire and emergency services nationwide, the purposes of which are to ensure the (1) safety of responders and others, (2) achievement of tactical objectives, and (3) efficient use of resources. As a result, ICS was subsequently designated for use throughout the United States by the federal Superfund Amendments and Reauthorization Act (SARA) of 1986 (PL 99-499), Occupational Health and Safety Administration (OSHA) rule 1910.120, and, most recently, Homeland Security Presidential Directive 5 (HSPD 5),[5] in addition to numerous other state and local regulations. Its early success also led the California Emergency Medical Services Authority to adapt and periodically revise it for use in all disasters involving hospitals, such that it now serves as the basis of the Hospital Incident Command System (HICS) used by most hospitals in the Americas and, increasingly, worldwide. Specific instruction in HICS is available through both the California Emergency Medical Services Authority HICS Web site (http://www.emsa.ca.gov/HICS/default.asp), and the Emergency Management Institute's Web site (http://training .fema.gov), within the independent study ICS courses IS-100.HC and IS-200.HC revised in 2007 for healthcare providers.[6]

Foundational Principles

"Management by objectives"[4]

The three key strategies of the disaster response, in order, are to (1) protect and preserve life, (2) stabilize the disaster scene, and (3) protect and preserve property. Healthcare providers intuitively understand the first purpose, and intellectually understand that the third purpose is essential to the first because healthcare providers cannot perform their lifesaving tasks without the appropriate facilities, equipment, and resources. The second purpose, however, may be less obvious. This is because an organized disaster response can occur only within the context of a stable work environment—an environment that is difficult to achieve in the first minutes after disaster strikes, when chaos is the rule, even in greatly complex work environments, such as hospitals, that are highly self-regulated.

Thus, an incident management system is needed to bring order to the chaos, the *sine qua non* of which is an incident command structure characterized by the three key tactics that must underlie all of incident command—*unity of command*, *span of control*, and *clarity of text*. Unity of command refers to the principle that sharing of information among all personnel involved in a disaster response is vital, but such individuals receive formal orders from, and make formal reports to, a single supervisor in order to preserve the viability of the chain of command. Span of control refers to the principle that in a high stress environment, no line supervisor can effectively coordinate the efforts of more than three to seven, and ideally no more than five, subordinate personnel. Clarity of text refers to the principle that all communications, written and spoken, must be transmitted in the simplest, most generic language possible, avoiding the use of words or jargon likely beyond the understanding of many emergency responders, so as to ensure that all personnel involved in the disaster response understand both the general strategy of the Emergency Operations Plan (EOP) and the special tactics being applied to combat the disaster.

Incident Leadership

"Coordination, Communication, Cooperation"[1]

Healthcare incident management systems achieve their goals by ensuring what have been termed the "3 Cs" of incident command: *coordination, communication*, and *cooperation*, of which the most important is cooperation, because it makes coordination and communication feasible. However, effective incident management requires not only universal education in disaster management appropriate to the functional job description of the individual healthcare employee—awareness, technical, and professional—but also frequent drilling in the implementation of the hospital disaster plan, especially its incident command structure. Most texts and training rightly emphasize that the individuals designated to fulfill specific functional job descriptions must be appropriately trained to do so; therefore, hospital executives who perform similar tasks during routine hospital business must step aside and yield these responsibilities to those who have been trained to do so. However, this notion ignores long-established realities of human behavior—the boss is still the boss, even if untrained in disaster management—so every effort should be made by senior executives to ensure that all hospital executives receive training in disaster management and incident command that will enable supervisors to function in their assigned roles even when disaster strikes.

Physicians commonly presume that because the first key purpose of incident management is to protect and preserve life, they should be in charge of emergency operations. However, physicians often overlook the fact that while they must clearly be in charge of all aspects of medical care, they generally comprise no more than approximately 10% of the total number of hospital personnel. Typically, the healthcare needs of the hospitalized patient require an average of 10 other personnel to support the treatments prescribed and the operations performed by a single physician or surgeon. Moreover, the physician's expertise—and most valuable contribution to the hospital disaster response—lies in the medical care of the hospitalized patient, rather than its operational, logistical, or planning support.

Command Structure

"[ICS is] the system to achieve the coordination necessary to carry out an effective and efficient response."[7]

Two basic command structures, and variations thereof, are utilized worldwide: (1) the Hospital Incident Command System (HICS), developed by the California Emergency Medical Services Authority and promulgated both by its originator (http://www.ems.ca.gov/HICS/default.asp) and by the Domestic Preparedness Consortium of the Federal Emergency Management Agency (http://training.fema.gov), has been adopted for use by most hospitals in the Americas (Figure 2-1), while (2) nation-specific templates are used by hospitals in Europe and Australasia, which are promulgated chiefly through the extensive disaster medicine training programs of the Emergo Train System (ETS), developed by the Linköping University Trauma Center in Sweden (http://www.emergotrain.com)[8,9] (Figure 2-2). These various systems differ chiefly in the relative independence of their medical operations units, and the specificity of their tables of organization, the former tending to be more hierarchical and the latter tending to be more collegial. In the United States, the Hospital Incident Command System (HICS) has been adopted by the Department of Homeland Security as the system most congruent with the Incident Command System (ICS) designated by the National Incident Management System (NIMS) under the authority of Homeland Security Presidential Directive

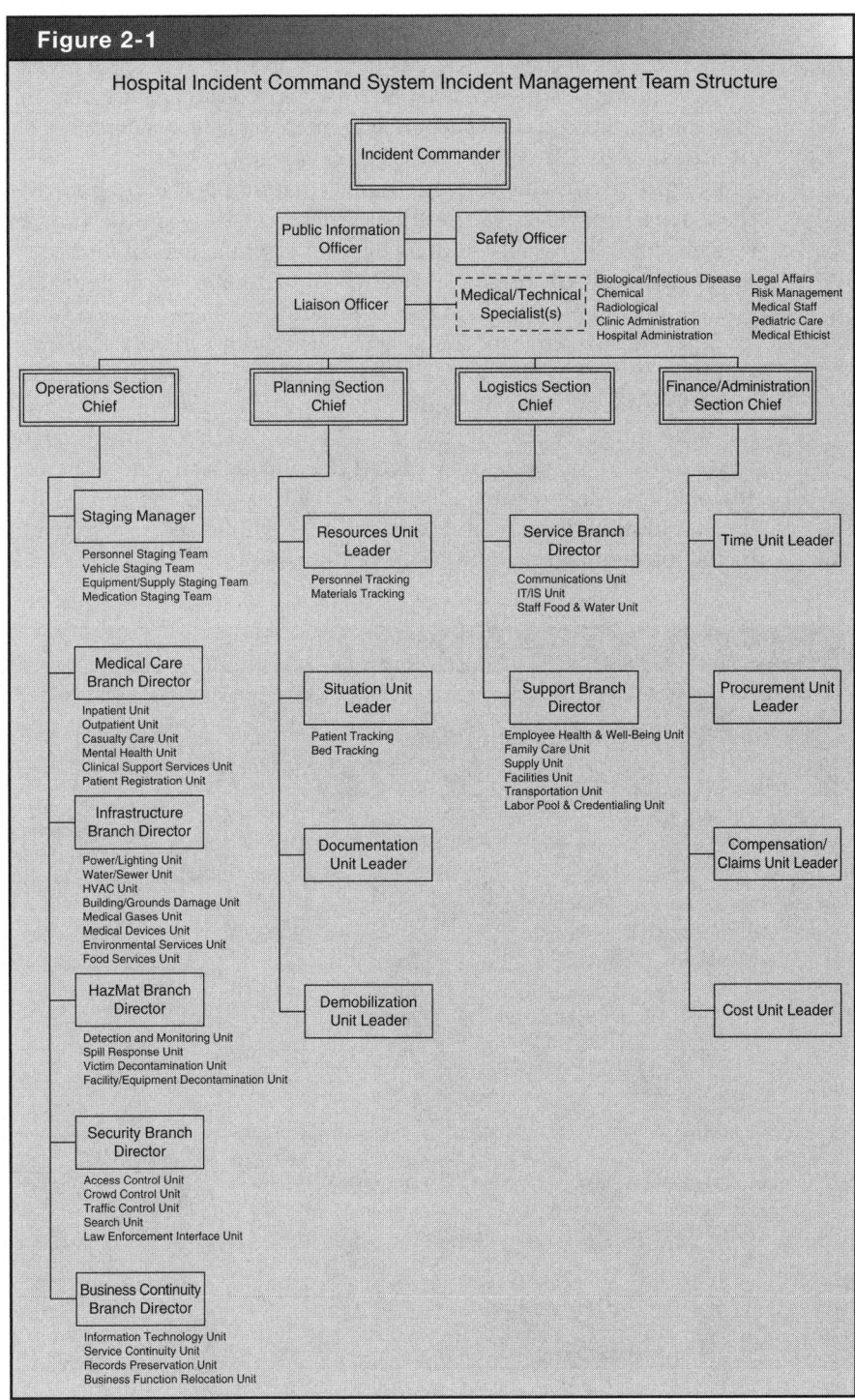

Figure 2-1

Hospital Incident Command System Incident Management Team Structure

California Emergency Medical Services Authority

5 (HSPD 5).[5] However, it is less important which system is utilized than the fact that the chosen system has the support of both hospital executives and hospital staff—cooperation depends upon acceptance of a single approach to hospital incident management by all hospital personnel, because they are the ones who must implement it.

Regardless of which system is utilized, it is important to note that there are far more similarities than differences between the various systems. All systems must address the four key functions of the emergency management response: finance and administration, logistics, operations, and planning and intelligence. Moreover, with the passage of time, all disaster response systems have been evolving toward a common model for incident command that emphasizes the fundamentally different tasks of medical and logistic operations. For example, the most recent iteration of HICS includes appropriate medical/technical specialists within the command staff who assist and advise the incident commander within the hospital command center, thereby ensuring that medical concerns directly inform decisions made by the incident command team in real time.

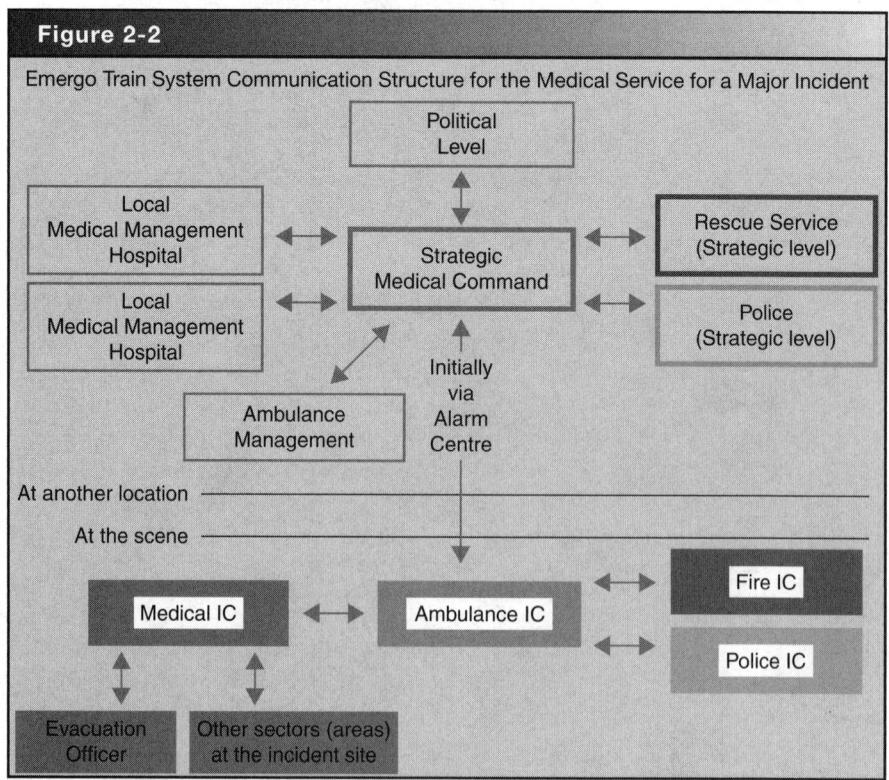

Figure 2-2

Emergo Train System Communication Structure for the Medical Service for a Major Incident

Rüter A, Nilsson H, & Vikström T. *Medical Command and Control at Incidents and Disasters*. Lund: Studentlittatur, 2006.

Hospital Incident Command System (HICS)

"[HICS is] a methodology for using ICS in a hospital/healthcare environment."[8]

The functional job action categories that must be addressed under HICS include incident **command** and staffing, **finance** and administration, **logistics**, **operations**, and **planning** and intelligence. (Remember these categories by the mnemonic "**CFLOP**," for without ICS, one will **"C"** [see] the disaster response **"FLOP**.") The additional command staff functions that must be addressed under HICS include **liaison**, **medical/technical**, **public information**, and **safety**. (Remember these categories by the mnemonic "[Mount O]**LMPS**," indicating their physical proximity to the incident commander.) Each of these categories is described in the following sections in greater detail. Utilization of HICS in a disaster is not intuitive, and requires far more than anecdotal familiarity with its structure and terminology for its successful implementation. Detailed presentations and all requisite forms to guide the implementation of HICS may be downloaded from its Web site free of charge (http://www.emsa.ca.gov/HICS/default.asp).

COMMAND

A single *incident commander* (IC) is responsible for all aspects of the disaster response, whether operational or medical. The initial responsibilities of the IC are to declare an internal disaster (originating within the facility) or an external disaster (originating outside the facility), to activate the *hospital emergency operation center* (HEOC), to implement the hospital *Emergency Operations Plan* (EOP), and, based upon the nature and extent of the disaster, to organize the disaster response through designation of the various section chiefs (general staff) and staff officers (command staff). All ICS section chiefs report directly to the IC and must be in constant communication with the IC, either in person or by telecommunications, for hospital incident command to be effective and efficient. In addition to coordinating and supervising the disaster response through the four ICS section chiefs, the IC is responsible for the provision of the following four key command functions: *liaison*, *medical/technical*, *public information*, and *safety*. The decision to designate section chiefs and staff officers to fulfill the various functional roles required for incident command rests solely with the IC. Not every response will require all positions to be filled, based on the size and scope of the event. In addition, in the early stages there may insufficient personnel to fill all roles, so several may be held by a single person. In fact, in the beginning one could say the IC is fulfilling all roles until they are assigned. This is a key principle in that the IC must assume personal responsibility for any function not so assigned.

Liaison

The liaison officer interfaces with all appropriate government and non-governmental agencies and health system organizations. At a minimum, these should include local public health, office of emergency management, police, fire, and emergency medical services, as well as state, county, and local departments of public health, and regional healthcare associations.

Medical/Technical

The medical/technical specialists are chiefly responsible for providing the IC with medical and technical advice. The medical/technical specialists may vary based on the type of disaster (infectious disease specialist for biological agents, hazardous materials specialist or medical toxicology physician for chemical agents, radiation safety physician for nuclear agents, and trauma or burn surgeon for explosive or incendiary agents).

Public Information

The public information officer interfaces with all appropriate communications media to provide regular reports on the progress of the disaster response. The public information officer also offers advice and assistance in developing and instituting communications to staff and families of patients potentially or actually hospitalized after a disaster to ensure that information is accurate and uniformly presented, and to provide regular reports of the outcome of each individual patient's care to the approapite parties.

Safety

The safety officer is chiefly responsible for the integrity of the disaster response through situational awareness of potential hazards, surveillance of staff and victims safety, and making recommendations to the IC with regard to safety. This is accomplished via review of the **S**ituation (of hospital facilities), **P**rotection (of hospital personnel), **I**dentification (of possible risks), and **N**otification (of appropriate authorities), or **SPIN**.

FINANCE

The finance and administration section monitors and tracks costs incurred in mounting the disaster response. It also identifies potential legal issues and liabilities, and maintains the records of the HCC, such that extraordinary expenses, legal risks, and after-action reports can be accurately determined, delineated, and developed for reimbursement, reconsideration, and review.

LOGISTICS

The *logistics* section is the "quartermaster" of the disaster response. It obtains and manages all staff, facilities, and equipment needed to support the disaster response, such as food, supplies, equipment, facilities, and sanitation, as well as transport vehicles, fuel, physical space, and equipment repair.

OPERATIONS

The *operations* section is the central component of the disaster response and all other components are designed to support it. It executes the disaster plan and is responsible for all necessary medical, nursing, and ancillary functions at patient-care sites, as well as decontamination and waste control, ground and air rescue, evacuation of casualties, and crisis management.

PLANNING

The *planning and intelligence* section formulates instant changes in the response plan based upon feedback obtained from administrative, logistical, and operation personnel. The role of this section is to always be thinking several events ahead of the current time and providing the IC with the information and approach to these future eventualities and possibilities. It is responsible for the collection, organization, evaluation, and dissemination of information on the present status of, and future needs for, staff, facilities, and resources in the disaster response.

Training and Education in ICS

Talking the talk vs. walking the walk

Although disaster professionals and emergency managers have adopted a nomenclature that is unique to disaster medical and mass casualty management, it follows a pattern that can be compared to terms recognized by anyone in healthcare familiar with the principles of public health and/or injury control. Still, one must be knowledgeable of the specialized terminology used in emergency management for the principles of emergency preparedness to be fully mastered: (1) preparation is analogous to *primary* injury prevention, which seeks to avoid injuries before they occur, chiefly through targeted educational programs; (2) mitigation (or protection) is analogous to *secondary* injury prevention, which seeks to attenuate injuries as they occur, mainly through system or product engineering strategies; (3) response is analogous to *tertiary* injury prevention, which seeks to ameliorate the effects of injury through timely application of sustentative, followed by definitive, prehospital and in-hospital emergency medical care; (4) recovery is analogous to what might be called *quaternary* injury prevention, which seeks to (re)activate local public health and healthcare systems to effectively manage intercurrent or recurrent injuries and illnesses using surviving or restored community-based resources. Note that many experts use the term "mitigation" to refer to the interdisaster phase of emergency response planning, but, in the opinion of the author, this is an incorrect usage of the word because planning efforts undertaken during this period are designed to attenuate the effects of disasters after they occur. Regardless of the terminology adopted, it is vital that all hospital personnel seek to understand and practice their disaster roles, because the cost of failure to learn is the inability to adequately prepare, respond and recover from a disaster.

It is self-evident that hospitals can no longer afford *not* to invest in disaster management training, including ICS, but portable, inexpensive training programs in hospital disaster management have yet to be developed, let alone disseminated. Among the best of those currently available are (1) the *Hospital Disaster Life Support I and II* (HDLS I and HDLS II) courses offered by the SiTEL program of the ER One Institute of the Washington Hospital Center (http://www.web.sitelms.org); (2) the *Hospital Emergency Response Training* and the *Healthcare Leadership and Decision-Making* courses, both still offered free of charge as of January 2010, at the Noble Training Facility of the Center for Domestic Preparedness of the Federal Emergency Management Agency in Anniston, Alabama (https://cdp.dhs.gov); and (3) the programs offered by the Emergo Train System (ETS) of the Linköping University Trauma Center in Sweden, including its *European Master in Disaster Medicine* (EMDM) program (http://www.emergotrain.com).[9–11] As stated, both the California Emergency Medical Services Authority (http://www.emsa.ca.gov/HICS/default.asp) and the Emergency Management Institute of the Federal Emergency Management Agency (http://training.fema.gov) offer independent study options online that can educate hospital executives in the fundamental principles of HICS, but *there is no substitute for frequent disaster simulations* that force hospital employees to learn and practice the roles they must play in actual disasters (see the following role descriptions). Regardless of the training program used, the functional job action categories that must be addressed are shown in Exhibit 2-1.[9]

Exhibit 2-1

Emergo Train System: Responsibilities of Incident Command in the Hospital

Logistic Commander

- personnel and their requirements
- hospital beds
- premises
- operation, electricity, water, heating, etc.
- safety
- collaboration with external authorities
- information to the media and the logistic commander's personnel
- documenting the work of the staff
- economic issues that need to be handled

Medical Commander

- contact with the strategic command (alternatively, contact with the incident site if the current staff form a part of the strategic command)
- intensive care
- emergency department
- operating theatre
- surgical wards in the widest sense (neurosurgery, thorax surgery, vascular surgery, etc.)
- contact with other groups within the unit
- psychological and psychosocial management (PPM)
- informing relatives

Rüter A, Nilsson H, & Vikström T. *Medical Command and Control at Incidents and Disasters*. Lund: Studentlittatur, 2006.

Implementing Hospital Incident Management

"Failing to plan is planning to fail."[12]

The hospital or healthcare system's Incident Command System (ICS) is but one component of the incident management system (IMS), which embraces all phases of readiness for both internal (originating within the hospital) and external (originating outside the hospital) disasters.[8] While beyond the scope of this chapter, all healthcare systems and organizations, and each constituent unit, must develop, implement, test, and refine both facility-wide and unit-specific Emergency Operations Plans (EOPs) that are comprehensive enough to embrace all foreseeable hazards—identified via a formal hazard vulnerability analysis (HVA), a probabilistic evaluation of the internal and external dangers to which it is most likely to be exposed—yet simple enough to be rapidly implemented by all levels of staff. The facility-wide EOP must specify (1) who has the responsibility and authority to implement it, usually the hospital chief operating officer (COO) or designee—it is generally best not to include the chief executive officer (CEO) as part of the ICS because this individual has ultimate responsibility for the entire hospital, not only the incident, and must therefore be answerable on an ongoing ("24/7/365") basis to the governing entity—and (2) the steps to be taken to establish the *hospital emergency operation center* (HEOC), recognizing that successful implementation of the IMS depends upon the education and training of all hospital personnel in its use, based on the expected competencies of all hospital workers and leaders, as shown in Exhibits 2-2 and 2-3.[13] The "DISASTER Paradigm" developed and disseminated by the National Disaster Life Support (NDLS) courses of the National Disaster Life Support Foundation—the *Core Disaster Life Support* (CDLS) and *Basic Disaster Life Support* (BDLS) levels of which have recently been made available online (http://www.bdls.com)—provides a useful approach to implementation of the IMS, the first step of which, following detection and declaration of an internal or external disaster, is the activation of the HICS and the establishment of the HEOC, as shown in Exhibit 2-4.[14]

Exhibit 2-2

Emergency Preparedness and Response Competencies for Hospital Workers[13]

The ability of a hospital to respond to an emergency depends upon having staff who know what to do and have the needed skills. As a hospital employee, you should be able to complete the following tasks:

- Locate and use the section of the hospital emergency response plan that applies to your position.
- Describe your emergency response role and be able to demonstrate it during drills or actual emergencies.
- Demonstrate use of any equipment (such as personal protective equipment or special communication equipment) required by your emergency response role.
- Describe your responsibilities for communicating with or referring requests for information from other employees, patients and families, media, general public, or your own family, and demonstrate these responsibilities during drills or actual emergencies.
- Demonstrate the ability to seek assistance through the chain of command during emergency situations or drills.
- Demonstrate the ability to solve problems that arise while carrying out your role during emergency situations or drills.

Courtesy of the National Center for Disaster Preparedness, Center for Public Health Preparedness

Exhibit 2-3

Emergency Preparedness and Response Competencies for Hospital Leaders[13]

The following core emergency competencies are those you need as a hospital leader (hospital-wide manager, department head, or senior manager in a large department), though you may demonstrate them in a variety of ways depending upon your exact role and the specific emergency or drill. These competencies provide a template for your continued development and can be used flexibly with other emergency preparedness activities within your institution:

- Describe the mission of the hospital during response to emergencies of all kinds, including the disaster response chain of command and emergency management system (e.g., Hospital Incident Command System, Incident Command System) used in your hospital.
- Demonstrate the ability to review, write, and revise as needed those portions of the hospital emergency response plan applicable to your management responsibilities and participate in the hospital's hazard vulnerability analysis on a regular basis.
- Manage and implement the hospital's emergency response plan during drills or actual emergencies within your assigned functional role and chain of command.
- Describe the collaborative relationship of your hospital to other facilities or agencies in the local emergency response system and follow the planned system during drills and emergencies.
- Describe the key elements of your hospital's emergency preparedness and response roles and policies to other agencies and community partners.
- Initiate and maintain communication with other emergency response agencies as appropriate to your management responsibilities.
- Describe your responsibilities for communicating with other employees, patients and families, media, the general public, or your own family, and demonstrate them during drills or actual emergencies.
- Demonstrate use of any equipment (such as personal protective equipment or special communication equipment) required by your emergency response role.
- Demonstrate flexible thinking and use of resources in responding to problems that arise while carrying out your functional role during emergency situations or drills.
- Evaluate the effectiveness of the response within your area of management responsibility in drills or actual emergencies, and identify improvements needed.

Courtesy of the National Center for Disaster Preparedness, Center for Public Health Preparedness

---

Exhibit 2-4

National Disaster Life Support Program

"DISASTER Paradigm"[14]

Detect/**D**eclare
Incident Command
Safety/**S**ecurity
Assess Hazards
Support Resources
Triage/**T**reatment
Evacuation
Recovery

Courtesy of the American Medical Association

The HEOC is established in a secure location that is located at a distance from any potential event, but has ready access to communication with and monitoring of the decontamination unit, emergency department, operating suites, intensive care units, acute care areas, facilities plant, information systems, and family waiting areas at a minimum. The location should be isolated from potential hazards, such as contaminated heating/ventilation/air conditioning (HVAC) and drainage/sewage systems, but close enough to the environments of care that reports can be physically received and orders can be physically transmitted if electronic communication or transport systems fail—a surprisingly frequent occurrence, even in disasters limited to hospitals, giving rise to the oft repeated and highly valuable advice to ensure redundancy of all communications systems and equipment among the HCC and all hospital departments, whether based on landline telephones, cellular telephones, an intranet, or the Internet. Because incident command structures such as HICS are designed to be both flexible and scalable, only those elements of the incident command structure and staff deemed essential to the disaster response need be activated—and likewise deactivated after the disaster has been brought under control—upon determination of the incident commander (IC) or designee. The HEOC, at the direction of the IC, next activates the hospital's Emergency Operations Plan (EOP), an "all-hazards" plan with branch points designed to address not only specific threats identified by the hospital's HVA, but also generic threats, such as chemical, biological, radiological, nuclear, or explosive (CBRNE) events that may result from industrial mishaps or intentional mischief. Although a detailed iteration of the critical elements of hospital EOPs is beyond the scope of this chapter, the EOP should be kept as simple as possible, as shown in Exhibit 2-5, and should rely on individual Job Action Sheets to be distributed among hospital personnel assigned to affected units as soon as possible after the disaster is declared by the IC.[15]

Exhibit 2-5

Example of Simple Hospital Disaster Plan Printed on Reverse of Hospital Identification Card[15]

Styner Memorial Medical Center
In *Case of Disaster*

- C—Cease nonacute patient care activity
  - Delay elective operations, procedures, infusions
- A—Activate unit-specific disaster plan
  - Assign caretaker staff, reassign others
- R—Report to assigned workstation
  - Review assignment, Job Action Sheet
- E—Ensure your own and others' safety
  - Don PPE appropriate to assignment

Courtesy of the American College of Surgeons

Logistical Concerns

"Amateurs study tactics. Experts study logistics."[16]

Emergencies become disasters when the existing needs outstrip available resources. Three levels of medical disasters creating multiple casualties in a fixed time period are generally recognized:

1. "Multiple casualty incidents" (MCIs) typically involve five or more patients. Available medical assets are strained but not overwhelmed.

2. "Mass casualty events" (MCEs) typically involve 20 or more patients. Available medical assets are overwhelmed, but can be reinforced through mobilization of additional medical assets, known as surge capability. (MCEs are termed "limited" if available medical assets can be expeditiously reinforced through provision of additional staff, equipment, and resources; no specific terminology currently exists to define more egregious circumstances.)

3. Catastrophic medical disasters (also called "complex humanitarian emergencies" or CHEs), typically involve 500 or more patients per million population, thereby affecting public as well as personal health. Available medical assets are overwhelmed or destroyed, with no prospect of early reinforcement of staff, facilities, equipment, or resources.

Computer simulations have demonstrated that emergency department throughput that exceeds approximately five to seven critical casualties per hour will cause most critical care processes to become unmanageable (critical imaging studies are most often the rate-limiting step), unless specific measures are taken through rapid mobilization of surge resources (medical response teams, provision only of minimal acceptable care, and strict reliance on unidirectional patient flow).[17] If such measures are not adopted, the critical mortality rate (the best measure of quality of medical care in disasters) can be expected to rise beyond acceptable limits, but if they are adopted, it will decrease as triage precision increases.[18]

The Joint Commission on the Accreditation of Healthcare Organizations (JCAHO) now requires that every healthcare organization seeking its accreditation engage its community (including all locally involved public safety, health, education, and works services such as police, fire, emergency medical services, health departments, hospital associations, school districts, colleges and universities, water, and sanitation, as well as executives of businesses and industries from which logistical support may be called forth) in each of the four specific phases of its internal and external disaster planning—preparation, mitigation, response, recovery—and that it participate in a minimum of one communitywide disaster drill annually. Such drills must evaluate the communication, coordination, and command elements of the hospital's EOP developed by the healthcare organization in partnership with its community, and range from discussion-based exercise, such as seminars and workshops, to operations-based exercises, such as functional and full-scale (or field) exercises, as shown in Exhibit 2-6.[19] Assessment of each facility's ICS is best evaluated through the use of specially developed and validated performance indicators by trained observers, as well as structured review of after-action reports, both during and following hospital disaster exercises.[20–22] The Homeland Security Exercise and Evaluation Program (HSEEP) of the Federal Emergency Management Agency (FEMA) seeks to establish a national standard for all disaster management and emergency preparedness exercises through provision of a standardized methodology and terminology for exercise design, development, conduct, evaluation, and improvement planning. Extensive resources are available on its Web site (https://hseep.dhs.gov/pages/1001_HSEEP7.aspx).[22]

Exhibit 2-6

Exercise Types Defined by the Homeland Security Exercise and Evaluation Program[22]

Discussions-based exercises familiarize participants with current plans, policies, agreements, and procedures, or may be used to develop new plans, policies, agreements, and procedures. Types of discussion-based exercises include the following examples:

    seminar: A seminar is an informal discussion designed to orient participants to new or updated plans, policies, or procedures (e.g., a seminar to review a new evacuation standard operating procedure).

- **workshop**: A workshop resembles a seminar, but is employed to build specific products, such as a draft plan or policy (e.g., a training and exercise plan workshop is used to develop a multi-year training and exercise plan).
- **tabletop exercise (TTX)**: A tabletop exercise involves key personnel discussing simulated scenarios in an informal setting. TTXs can be used to assess plans, policies, and procedures.
- **games**: A game is a simulation of operations that often involves two or more teams, usually in a competitive environment, using rules, data, and procedures designed to depict an actual or assumed real-life situation.

Operations-based exercises validate plans, policies, agreements, and procedures; clarify roles and responsibilities; and identify resource gaps in an operation environment. Types of operations-based exercises include the following examples:

- **drill**: A drill is a coordinated, supervised activity usually employed to test a single, specific operation or function within a single entity (e.g., a fire department conducts a decontamination drill).
- **functional exercise (FE)**: A functional exercise examines and/or validates the coordination, command, and control between various multiagency coordination centers (e.g., emergency operation center, joint field office, etc.). A functional exercise does not involve any "boots on the ground" (i.e., first responders or emergency officials responding to an incident in real time).
- **full-scale exercises (FSX)**: A full-scale exercise, previously known as a field exercise, is a multiagency, multijurisdiction, multidiscipline exercise involving functional (e.g., joint field office, emergency operation centers, etc.) and "boots on the ground" response (e.g., firefighters decontaminating mock victims).

United States Department of Homeland Security

Practical Concerns

"Don't fight against chaos. Use chaos."[23]

Perhaps the most important tools with which healthcare emergency managers can equip hospital employees are *situational awareness* and *systematic reporting*, as shown in Figure 2-3 and Exhibit 2-7. The oft repeated phrase, "If you see something, say something," is at the heart of situational awareness. All hospital employees must be regularly

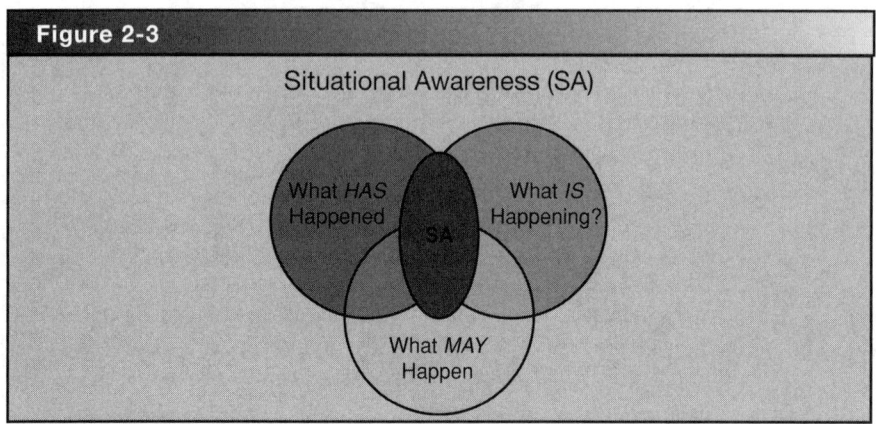

Figure 2-3

Situational Awareness (SA)

encouraged to report to their immediate supervisors any activity that seems out of place (or time), based on their assessment of *what has happened, what is happening,* and *what may happen* if the item or event that seems unusual, atypical, or out of place or time is not immediately investigated and appropriate action taken. Information is best transmitted using a standardized format known as "SBAR," which was originally developed for use by nuclear submariners. Information to be transmitted includes decisions made regarding the potential nature of any possible hazard by the individual named in the EOP as responsible for declaring a disaster, usually the COO or designee, often the administrator on duty (AOD). A useful approach for determining whether or not an identified hazard may warrant activation of the EOP has been

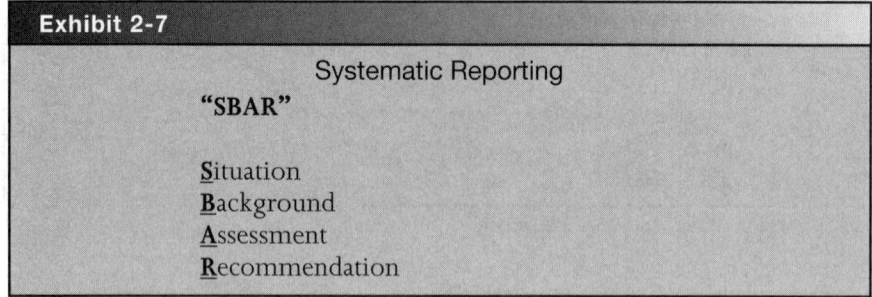

Exhibit 2-7

Systematic Reporting

"SBAR"

Situation
Background
Assessment
Recommendation

described for field use, as shown in Figure 2-4, but is readily adaptable to the hospital environment.[24]

The Harvard Law of Animal Behavior, originally applied to laboratory animals used in medical experiments, pertains equally to *Homo sapiens* during disasters that threaten personal or public health: "Despite the most rigorous of experimental conditions, the animal does as it

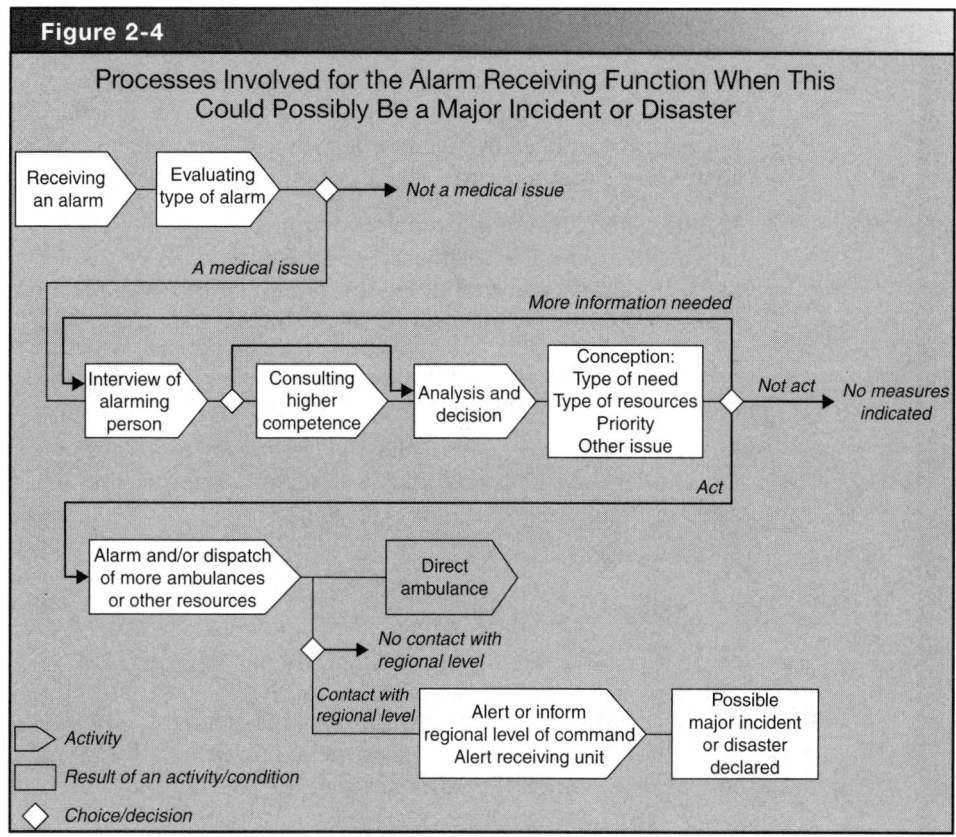

Figure 2-4

Processes Involved for the Alarm Receiving Function When This Could Possibly Be a Major Incident or Disaster

Rüter A, Lundmark T, Ödmansson E, & Vikström T. The Development of a National Doctrine for Management of Major Incidents and Disasters. Scandinavian Journal of Trauma Resuscitation and Emergency Medicine. 2006;14:177–181.

damn well pleases." Under the stress of a major disaster that may involve their families, hospital employees cannot be expected to function optimally if the safety or welfare of their families is uncertain. Because all hospital emergency response plans depend upon mobilization of adequate staff, hospitals can best ensure continuity of operations during disasters by assisting their employees in meeting their responsibilities to their families by (1) helping to identify alternative resources for care of dependent children and adults, and (2) ensuring that all employees develop and discuss family disaster plans. The following elements should be included in every family disaster plan:

1. Maintain a well-stocked first aid kit.

2. Keep waterproof flashlights and radios with extra batteries.

3. Stockpile a four-day supply of prepared food, bottled water, and necessary medications for each family member, including pets, and

at least one gallon of potable water per individual per day for drinking. (At least five extra gallons per person per day will be needed if washing and bathing are contemplated because fuel and other means to sterilize water may be in short supply. Note that poisoning of children by ingestion of hydrocarbons and bleach is an all-too-common occurrence following major disasters.)

4. Identify alternative means of telecommunication with one another, often through distant relatives, because local telephone lines, both land and mobile, will typically be overwhelmed, while long distance lines will usually be intact.

5. Establish a secure place and time to meet after a disaster if it proves impossible to reach one another by telephone.

6. Keep current photographs of all family members, especially infants and young children, to assist in family reunification in case family members become separated.

Interagency Relationships

"The problem with public health is that it's in government."[25]

For most external disasters, and some internal disasters, the hospital does not function independently, but is rather one element of what is described by the *National Response Framework* of the United States (http://www.fema.gov/emergency/nrf)—similar plans having been established by most local, regional, state, and other governments worldwide—as *Emergency Support Function #8* (ESF #8): the Public Health and Medical Service component of the disaster response (http://www.fema.gov/emergency/nrf/nrf-esf-08.pdf). While most disasters will not rise to the level of national significance and require the assets of a federal government, most states and provinces have adopted similar terminology and structures for statewide and provincial emergency management of disasters at a regional or local level. Under such circumstances, the activities of all healthcare organizations will be coordinated by the regional or local *Emergency Operations Center* (EOC), which, for disasters requiring a public health or medical service response, will activate a "desk" for ESF #8. Assigned to such a "desk" will be an emergency manager with responsibility for coordination of healthcare functions and resources, including healthcare organizations such as hospitals, nursing homes, and urgent care centers, as well as medical transport services, including emergency medical services (EMS) as well as nonemergency, wheelchair-accessible, "ambulette" services. Each entity may send a liaison representative to assist the responsible emergency manager with asset coordination.

In complex humanitarian emergencies (CHEs), coordination of public health and medical service assets may become so complicated that a separate, but integral, *hospital emergency operations center* (HEOC) may be established by the IC. Under such circumstances, the HEOC will virtually always be a unified incident command (UIC) entity comprised of the officers in charge of all major activated public safety and public health services who make collective decisions about incident management that are duly transmitted via an appointed spokesperson.[26] Such activities are well beyond the scope of this chapter, but you can follow the same principles of emergency management for multiple or expanding, and multiagency or complex, incidents promulgated by the *Intermediate ICS for Expanding Incidents* (ICS-300) and *Advanced ICS for Complex Incidents* (ICS-400) courses of the National Wildfire Coordinating Group (NWCG) recognized by FEMA, but offered at a state level by state emergency management offices (SEMOs). It is self-evident that all such HEOCs, whether free-standing or co-located with the regional EOC, depend upon robust communications with all healthcare assets to function and succeed. It is, therefore, essential that reliable and redundant communications systems be available, because events of such magnitude as to require the activation of HEOCs are likely to be of such a scope that public utilities, including communication networks, may already have failed.

Summary

"So that next time, we respond like it's not the first time."[10]

The purposes of the response to medical disasters, in order, are to (1) protect and preserve life, (2) stabilize the disaster scene, and (3) protect and preserve property. The Incident Command System (ICS) provides a tested means to achieve the second desired purpose, which in turn facilitates achievement of the first and third. All hospital workers must be educated and trained, meaning drilled, in their expected roles within ICS. Such efforts will ensure, to quote the HDLS program of SiTEL, the ER One Institute, and the Washington Hospital Center, "So that next time, we respond like it's not the first time."[10]

References

1. Martin JT. *The Many Hats of Highway Incident Command* [video]. University of Virginia: Center for Transportation Studies. http://cts.virginia.edu/incident_mgmt_training.htm. Accessed January 1, 2010.
2. Fulghum R. *All I Really Need to Know I Learned in Kindergarten*, Fifteenth Anniversary Edition. New York: Ballantine Books; 2003.

3.   Attributed to Peter F. Drucker.

4.   Drucker PF. *The Practice of Management*. New York: Harper & Row; 1954.

5.   Bush GW. Homeland Security Presidential Directive 5: Management of Domestic Incidents. Homeland Security Web site. http://www.dhs.gov/xabout/laws/gc_1214592333605.shtm. Published February 28, 2003. Accessed January 2, 2010.

6.   Emergency Management Institute. Introduction to the Incident Command System for Healthcare/Hospitals (IS-100.HC) and Applying Incident Command System (ICS) to Healthcare Organizations (IS-200.HC). Emergency Management Institute. http://training.fema.gov. Published May 24, 2007. Accessed January 2, 2010.

7.   National Response Team. Incident Command System/Unified Command (ICS/UC) Technical Assistance Document. The U.S. National Response Team Web site. http://www.nrt.org/production/NRT/NRTWeb.nsf/AllAttachmentsByTitle/SA-52ICSUCTA/$File/ICSUCTA.pdf?OpenElement. Updated 2000. Accessed January 2, 2010.

8.   California Emergency Medical Services Authority. *Hospital Incident Command System Guidebook*. Sacramento, California: California Emergency Medical Services Authority; 2006. http://www.emsa.ca.gov/HICS/default.asp. Accessed January 3, 2010.

9.   Rüter A, Nilsson H, Vikström T. *Medical Command and Control at Incidents and Disasters*. Lund: Studentlittatur; 2006.

10.   Simulation and Training Environment Lab (SiTEL), ER One Institute, Washington Hospital Center. *Hospital Disaster Life Support I and II* (HDLS I and HDLS II) student course manuals. 2nd ed. Washington: Washington Hospital Center; 2008. Courses accessed at http://www.web.sitelms.org.

11.   Center for Domestic Preparedness, Federal Emergency Management Agency, United States Department of Homeland Security. *Hospital Emergency Response Training and Healthcare Leadership and Decision-Making* student course manuals. Washington: United States Department of Homeland Security; 2009. Courses accessed at https://cdp.dhs.gov.

12.   Attributed to Benjamin Franklin.

13.   Center for Public Health Preparedness, Columbia University Mailman School of Public Health, Center for Health Policy, Columbia University School of Nursing, in collaboration with Greater New York Hospital Association. Emergency Preparedness and Response Competencies for Hospital Workers. New York: Columbia University; 2004. http://www.ncdp.mailman.columbia.edu/files/hospcomps.pdf. Accessed January 3, 2010.

14.   National Disaster Life Support Executive Committee, National Disaster Life Support Foundation and American Medical Association. *Advanced, Basic, Core, and Decontamination Life Support* provider manuals. Chicago: American Medical Association; 2007. Courses accessed at http://www.bdls.com.

15.   American College of Surgeons Committee on Trauma. Disaster management and emergency preparedness (optional lecture) and Appendix H. In: American College of Surgeons Committee on Trauma. *Advanced Trauma Life Support for Doctors Student and Faculty Manuals with DVD*, 8th ed. Chicago: American College of Surgeons; 2008. Courses accessed at http://www.facs.org/trauma/atls/index.html.

16.   Attributed to Dwight D. Eisenhower.

17.   Hirshberg A, Scott BG, Granchi T, Wall MJ Jr, Mattox KL, Stein M. How does ca-

sualty load affect trauma care in urban bombing incidents? A quantitative analysis. *J Trauma.* 2005;58(4);686–695.

18. Frykberg ER, Tepas JJ III. Terrorist bombings: lessons learned from Belfast to Beirut. *Ann Surg.* 1988;208(5):569–576.

19. Thomas TL, Hsu EB, Kim HK, Colli S, Arana G, Green GB. The incident command system in disasters: evaluation methods for a hospital-based exercise. *Prehosp Disast Med.* 2005;20(1):14–23.

20. Arnold JL, Paturas J, Rodoplu U. Measures of effectiveness of hospital incident command system performance [letter]. *Prehosp Disast Med.* 2005;20(3): 202–205.

21. Rüter A, Nilsson H, Vilkström T. Performance indicators as quality control for testing and evaluating hospital management groups: a pilot study. *Prehosp Disast Med.* 2006;21(6):423–426.

22. Federal Emergency Management Agency. *An Introduction to Exercises* (IS-120.A) and *Exercise Evaluation and Improvement Planning* (IS-130). Washington: United States Department of Homeland Security; 2008. Courses accessed at https://hseep .dhs.gov/pages/1001_HSEEP7.aspx.

23. Attributed to Yoel Donchin.

24. Rüter A, Lundmark T, Ödmansson E, Wikström T. The development of a national doctrine for management of major incidents and disasters. *Scand J Trauma Resusc Emerg Med.* 2006;14:189–194.

25. Attributed to Ronald J. Waldman.

26. Burkle FM Jr, Hsu EB, Loehr M, et al. Definition and functions of health unified command and emergency operations centers for large-scale bioevent disasters within the existing ICS. *Disaster Med Public Health Prep.* 2007;1(2): 135–141.

Chapter 3

Improving Trauma System Preparedness for Disasters and Public Health Emergencies

Michael J. Reilly, DrPH, MPH, NREMT-P

Photo by Win Henderson / FEMA Photo

Learning Objectives

- Investigate the role of the trauma system and trauma centers in the preparedness and response to disasters and other public health emergencies.
- Discuss strategies to integrate better trauma systems and trauma centers in the emergency management and public health emergency response system.

Introduction

During the fall of 2001, the United States experienced the most devastating acts of terrorism in its history. These incidents caused the important issue of public health and hospital emergency preparedness to be examined more thoroughly. As a result, the public safety and public health communities have made domestic preparedness and medical counterterrorism a national priority for health care and public policy. One of the most difficult issues for the health system to address is how to deliver health care to the victims of disasters while struggling to cope with issues such as lack of funding for health system infrastructure, a national nursing shortage, decreasing reimbursement rates, healthcare reform, and the challenge of delivering health care to more than 44 million uninsured Americans.[1] In order to improve our capacity to respond to disasters, it is necessary to evaluate and clearly define the roles of each component of the healthcare emergency response infrastructure.

Since the creation of the first trauma center in Baltimore, Maryland in 1969, trauma centers have been recognized as the optimal point of entry for critically injured patients into the healthcare system.[2] In the past 40 years, the development of trauma systems and the evolution of the specialties of trauma surgery and emergency medicine have put the trauma center in a position to deliver some of the most comprehensive and skilled treatment of patients with injuries in the healthcare system. Trauma centers set themselves apart from other hospitals by maintaining a comprehensive network of resources geared toward optimal care of the injured patient through the entire spectrum of an injury event.

The American College of Surgeons (ACS) released a position statement stating that due to the trauma center's integral role in the emergency medical services (EMS) system, and because the trauma center specializes in the treatment of traumatic injuries, the trauma center should be the leader of the hospital preparedness initiative, and benchmark the quality delivery of disaster medical care.[3] This statement has generated debate on what the role of the trauma center and trauma system should be during a disaster or public health emergency. For example, what should be the role of the trauma center in a bioterrorism attack, pandemic, public health emergency, or infectious disease outbreak?

In addition to the perceived strengths of the trauma system, reports have shown significant gaps in the national state of hospital and trauma system preparedness.[4–17] Many healthcare disparities exist in the healthcare system of the United States, most commonly among those residing in rural and underserved areas, or in low socioeconomic brackets.[4–5,18–20] One of the most significant healthcare disparities that exists in our nation today is the lack of trauma care and EMS system coverage throughout the United States.[5,20] This disparity in emergency and trauma care seems to be generalized among the more rural areas of the country.[5,20] Currently, only 35 states have formally designated trauma systems and recent reports suggest that comprehensive trauma care may be available to only 50% of the country.[4–5,18–19] Furthermore, it has been reported that 90% of the Level I and Level II trauma centers are disproportionately located within urban areas.[19]

In order to define the roles of trauma systems in a disaster or other public health emergency, we must first identify the role of the trauma system in the day-to-day operations of the healthcare delivery system. Planning and prevention, and the integration and coordination of trauma system preparedness and response, have all been cited frequently as the major roles of the trauma system. Among the major strengths of the nation's trauma systems are trauma care and the trauma system infrastructure. Additional strengths are the EMS system, partnerships in community planning, and disaster preparedness activities.[2,4–8,18–26] The most often-suggested enhancement of the trauma center and trauma system response to disasters is more integration and coordination with public health and community agencies in planning and prevention activities.

Structure and Essential Components of a Trauma System

A trauma system is defined as a comprehensive network of resources, integrated with the local public health system, that work together to coordinate and deliver optimal patient care to injured victims (Figure 3-1).[2,18] At the center of the trauma system is the trauma center. The trauma center is an acute care hospital that has been verified and/or designated by an independent entity, such as the ACS or a state health department, to provide specialty care to injured patients and victims of traumatic injury. Although the first trauma centers were established in urban areas in the early 1970s, a systems approach to trauma care and its impact was first described by West et al., in a landmark 1979 article *Systems of Trauma Care: A Study of Two Counties.*[27] This paper examined differences in preventable trauma mortality between a county with a trauma system and a county without a trauma system.[27] The authors reviewed cases of motor vehicle-related trauma in which the victims died after arrival at the hospital. They found that the county with a trauma system, where the victims were transported to a trauma center, had significantly less mortality than the county without any comprehensive system of trauma care.[27] The publication of this preliminary study influenced many subsequent studies on the benefit of trauma care and trauma systems. In 1990, Congress passed the Trauma Care Systems Planning and Development Act (PL 101-590), which allocated funding to states in order to develop regional trauma care systems.[28] As a result of this legislation, the Health Resources and Services Administration (HRSA) released the Model Trauma Care System Plan in 1992.[29] This plan outlined the fundamental components of a trauma system, emphasizing the need

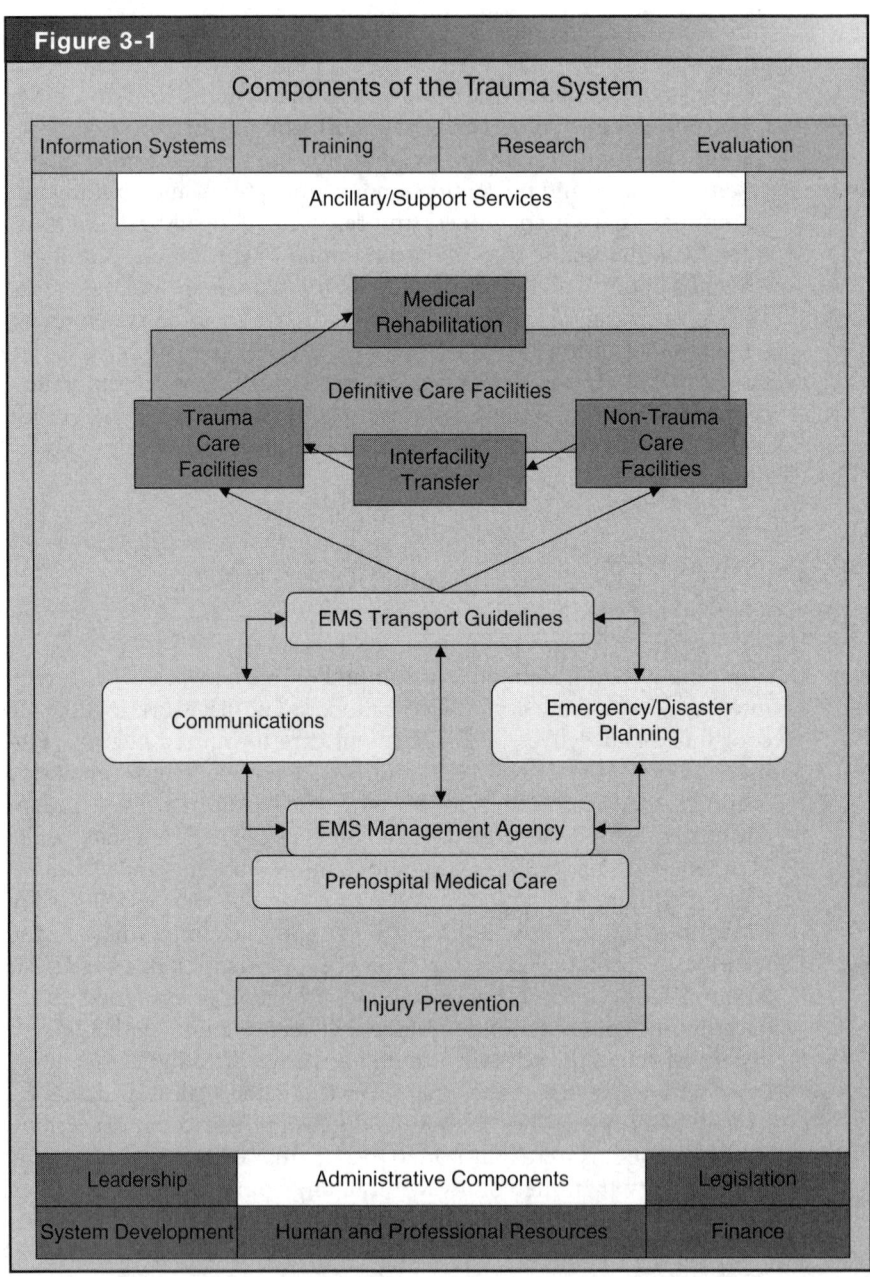

Figure 3-1

Components of the Trauma System

for integration of multiple agencies and institutions to fully meet the needs of injured patients.[2,29] At its core, the trauma system is organized around the following fundamental components: injury prevention; prehospital medical care (EMS system); acute care; post-inpatient care and rehabilitation; and system administration.[2,18]

The Emergency Medical Services (EMS) System

The emergency medical services (EMS) system was created in 1966, in response to the National Research Council's paper titled *Accidental Death and Disability: The Neglected Disease of Modern Society*.[30] This document listed trauma as the fourth leading cause of death in the United States, and the leading cause of death among people in the age group of 1–37 years.[30] One of the most shocking statements in the report was that the average U.S. citizen would have a greater chance of dying in their car on the highway than at war in Vietnam.[30] That same year, influenced in part by the National Research Council's report on motor vehicle-related trauma, the National Highway Safety Act (PL 89-564) was passed, creating the U.S. Department of Transportation.[31] This new cabinet-level agency was given oversight of the development of national EMS standards and curricula. As a result of this federal initiative, which provided federal money for the finance and improvement of EMS systems from 1968 to 1979, the first emergency medical technician (EMT) program was created, and in 1977 the first national education standards for the paramedic were established.[31] In 1973, the EMS Systems Act (PL 93-154) was passed to promote EMS planning, operations, research, and expansion.[32] This legislation was centered around a regional approach to EMS system management and emphasized a trauma focus.[32]

Today's trauma systems are designed to be seamlessly integrated into the EMS system, which acts as the critical point of entry into the healthcare system for injured patients. In 1988, the National Highway Traffic and Safety Administration listed 10 key components of an EMS system, as shown in Figure 3-2.[33] These 10 components still exist today and are used to evaluate the EMS systems in states across the United States. The modern EMS system operates on the principles of citizen awareness and activation of the EMS system, dispatch and communications, first responder care, advanced prehospital care, hospital care, and rehabilitation. This operational paradigm of the current EMS system is often referred to as the "chain of survival." The underlying principle is that each "link" in the chain must be present for the victim of an injury or acute illness to fully recover after the event.[34]

Prehospital care is a major portion of the response phase of any disaster or emergency plan. Prehospital responses to disasters will typically involve both a Basic Life Support (BLS) and an Advanced Life Support (ALS) component. The prehospital response to disasters utilizes the Incident Command System (ICS) with the major roles of the EMS response including triage, treatment, and transportation of victims. The EMS providers will typically interface with the hospital component of the trauma system at the emergency department of the receiving facility. Integrated into disaster and emergency response plans will often be a point-of-entry plan that will determine which facility will

Figure 3-2

Components of the Emergency Medical Services (EMS) System

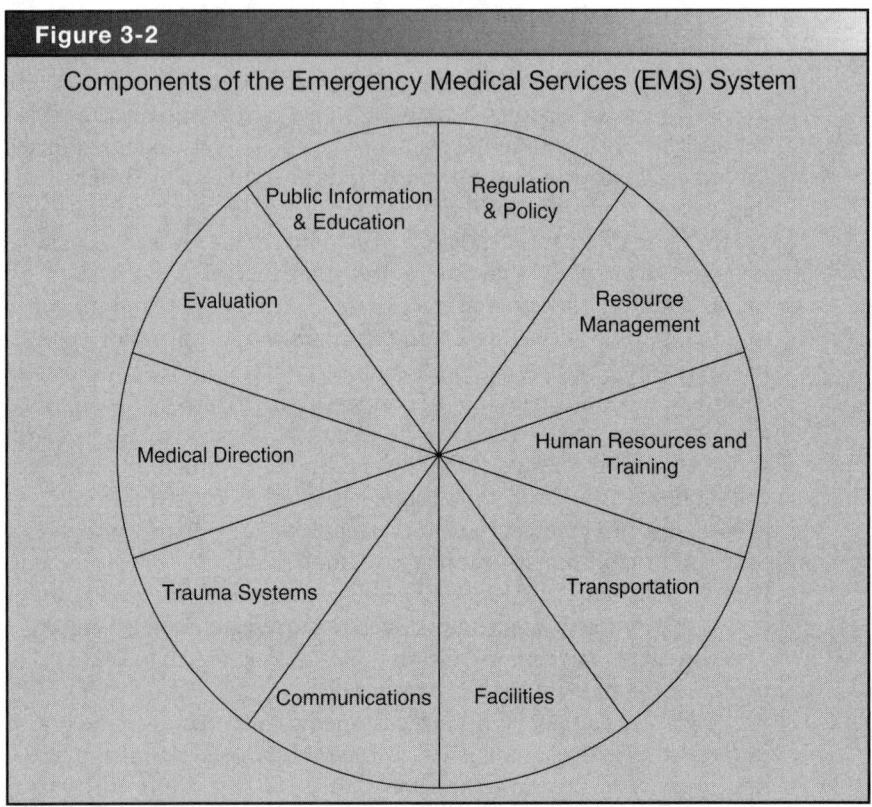

receive specific types of patients. Often point-of-entry plans will be determined based upon the capabilities and specialties of a particular facility (e.g., trauma center, burn center, pediatric hospital). In addition to point-of-entry protocols, transport decisions will be predetermined by the staging and/or transport officers at the incident, who will interface with the Emergency Operations Center (EOC) or the Central Medical Dispatch (C-MED) communications center, which will contact all the nearest receiving hospitals to determine how many patients of each severity (Priority I, II, III) they can handle from the scene. Without close contact with the communications center, the majority of EMS operations during a disaster or public health emergency would be ineffective.[35-36]

Communications systems are typically locally or regionally based and are integrated closely with all public safety providers and hospitals with emergency departments. The EMS system typically will be in contact with one or more dispatch centers at all times during field operations. Depending on the community, the EMS units will either communicate with the hospitals through a centralized dispatch center (i.e., C-MED) or initiate communications directly with the ED. The major role of communications as part of the EMS system during disaster and emergency response operations is to notify hospitals and trauma centers of the incident and maintain direct contact with online medical direction (an ED physician who coordinates EMS medical treatment).

Trauma Centers and Acute Care Hospitals

Acute care facilities include all levels of medical facilities that are capable of providing emergency medical care to ill or injured patients. Most acute care facilities will accept ambulance patients and have a designated emergency department (ED). The classification of these acute care facilities varies from state-to-state across the country.

TRAUMA CENTERS

The American College of Surgeons (ACS) has developed criteria for the verification of trauma centers at four levels, which are summarized in Figure 3-3.[2,19] ACS verification criteria examine the resources available within an acute care hospital to provide care to an injured patient. Acute care hospitals may be verified or designated as trauma centers, depending upon the local or regional trauma system, if one exists. Each state or region that has regulatory authority for trauma center designation determines which criteria it will use. Most use the ACS criteria, and consider verification by the ACS to be sufficient for designation. Other states may have alternative or additional requirements necessary for trauma center designation. Figure 3-4 depicts the national distribution of trauma centers in the United States.[19]

The role of the trauma center in disaster preparedness and response reflects upon the role of the trauma center during daily operations. The trauma center represents a definitive level of care for the injured patient. These facilities are equipped with numerous specialty services and unique resources that make them invaluable components of the medical response to a disaster. One notable difference in the typical trauma model is to marshal all available resources to the assessment and resuscitation of each patient. However, in times of disaster, as has been previously discussed in this text, the needs of patients may exceed available resources, forcing the hospital to shift from a single patient focus to a population-based focus. That being said, the core principles of triage, rapid assessment, and stabilization are still key to the prompt and efficient care of the disaster victim. It must also be recognized that while possessing significant resources for the disaster victim, the trauma

Figure 3-3

Summary of the (ACS) Criteria for Trauma Centers

LEVEL I TRAUMA CENTER

These facilities are typically located in urban areas or are located at the center of a trauma system. They provide leadership in teaching, research, and trauma system planning. A Level I facility is responsible for providing immediate in-house access to trauma surgery, anesthesia, multiple medical specialties, and trauma resuscitation. Level I trauma centers are required to treat at least 1200 admissions per year or 240 major trauma patients per year, approximately 35 major trauma cases per surgeon.

LEVEL II TRAUMA CENTER

Similar level of care as Level I, however, these facilities are usually located in less urban settings. Additionally, a Level II center does not have the performance requirements that a Level I has, and is not required to take part in research or education as part of its requirements.

LEVEL III TRAUMA CENTER

Level III facilities typically do not have the resources of Level I or II centers. They are often located in areas not immediately accessible to Level I or II centers. These facilities have the capability to perform emergency surgery, however, they will usually attempt to stabilize major trauma patients and transfer them to a Level I or II facility.

LEVEL IV TRAUMA CENTER

These facilities are minimally capable of providing trauma resuscitation and stabilization to trauma patients, and will arrange transfer of most patients to the most appropriate trauma center.

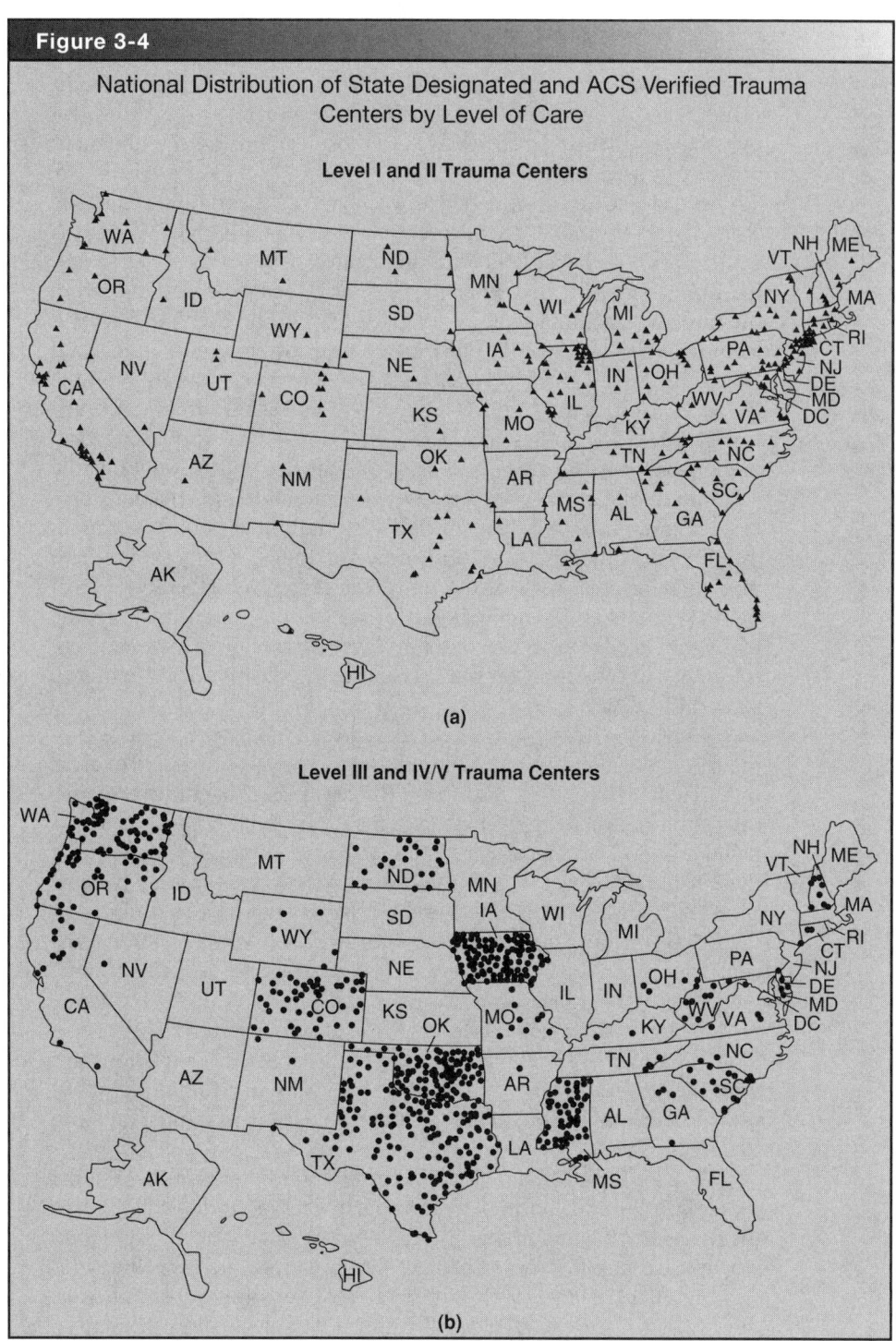

Figure 3-4

National Distribution of State Designated and ACS Verified Trauma Centers by Level of Care

Level I and II Trauma Centers

(a)

Level III and IV/V Trauma Centers

(b)

National Distribution of State Designated and ACS Verified Trauma Centers by Level of Care. Reprinted from MacKenzie, EJ, et al. "National Inventory of Hospital Trauma Centers." *JAMA*. 2003;289:1515–1522, p.1519. © 2003 American Medical Association.

center itself should be recognized as a scarce resource. Community emergency management plans and the actions of local incident commanders and/or healthcare system incident commanders must allow for the triaging of this scarce resource to those patients who will benefit most from its use.

In order to appropriately define the role of the trauma center, we should start by making a distinction between the Level I/II trauma centers and the Level III/IV trauma centers (Figure 3-3). Level I/II trauma centers will typically be the recognized acute care leaders within the trauma system and the community.[20–21] Both Level I and Level II facilities have the capability of treating critically injured patients and have subspecialty services available. Level I trauma centers are typically tertiary or academic medical centers that serve as resources to the entire trauma system. These facilities are responsible for providing comprehensive trauma care for all types of injuries and throughout the continuum of care; they also provide prevention through rehabilitation.[2] Level II trauma centers may also provide the initial definitive patient care for critically injured victims; however, they typically do not have immediate access to all of the resources of a Level I facility. Level II trauma centers are an integral part of the trauma system and provide leadership in certain aspects of trauma system activities. However, these facilities will often transfer patients exceeding their clinical abilities to a Level I facility.[2]

The Level III/IV trauma centers represent an important aspect of the trauma system, which is the ability to extend trauma care to areas that may not have other resources. The Level III/IV facilities are typically found in inclusive trauma systems where each hospital is designated at a level of trauma care as illustrated in Figure 3-3. The role of these facilities within the trauma system is to provide injured patients access to trauma care where a Level I/II facility may not be within reasonable proximity. The clinical resources available to the Level III trauma center are often limited; however, these facilities are required to provide access to surgical care.[2] Level IV facilities typically will provide resuscitation-based care consistent with advanced trauma life support (ATLS) standards.[2] These facilities require good working relationships with their system's Level I/II facilities to ensure that the services they provide allow patients to benefit from the extension of trauma care into the community.[2]

As a leader in the medical care of the injured patient, the trauma center is in a unique position to promote interventions that will result in the reduction of injury-related morbidity and mortality. Injury prevention may involve specific types of preventative initiatives, such as primary injury prevention geared towards prevention of a community-specific risk category, such as driving under the influence of alcohol or other drugs, or firearm-related suicide. Secondary and tertiary prevention activities are often more common in trauma centers, focusing on the response to an injury and dealing with its aftermath.

NON-TRAUMA CENTERS

Non-trauma centers include all acute care hospitals and inpatient facilities that have not been designated as trauma centers by their state or local authorities. This does not mean that some non-trauma designated acute care hospitals are not capable of providing some or all of the services rendered at designated trauma centers. In addition, 15 states do not designate trauma centers, in which case their trauma patients are frequently cared for in acute care hospitals.[19–20] Acute care hospitals normally have EDs that are staffed 24 hours a day, and are able to stabilize critically ill or injured patients. If a hospital lacks the resources necessary for treatment, it may transfer the patient to another facility for definitive care as required by the Emergency Medical Treatment and Active Labor Act (EMTALA).

Post-Inpatient Care Facilities

Rehabilitation hospitals and long-term care facilities are an integral part of the trauma system.[2] With the rise of managed care and third-party payers, there has been a national trend toward minimizing inpatient hospital stays to reduce overall health care costs. Rehabilitation hospitals and long-term care facilities provide less comprehensive, but often skilled, specialty services such as physical and occupational therapy, cardiac/neurologic/orthopedic rehabilitation, skilled nursing care, and physiatry. Studies have shown that by initiating a comprehensive patient-centered rehabilitation program that focuses on the patient's return to an independent baseline level of functioning, the costs associated with long-term care and rehospitalization are reduced by 90%.[37]

Administrative, Ancillary, and Support Components

Administrative, ancillary, and support (AAS) services provide the vital infrastructure upon which an effective trauma system can operate. AAS components (Figure 3-1) range from human and professional resources, system development, training, research, communication and information systems, quality improvement/quality assurance, and finance, to leadership and legislation. The AAS foundation is important in all components of the trauma system and must be supportive of the system's overall mission—to reduce morbidity and mortality resulting from injuries.

The Public Health Role in Trauma Systems and Hospital Preparedness

Although the public health infrastructure is not a recognized component of the trauma system, it does have a major role in the preparation, response, and recovery from disasters. Organizing and coordinating emergency health assistance involves collaboration with acute care facilities and other components of a trauma system. The critical roles of public health during the response phase of an emergency include: managing the overall medical response within the established incident command system (ICS); epidemiological response to incidents of bioterrorism; surveillance and contact tracing; environment monitoring; ensuring worker safety; emergency vaccination and prophylaxis; risk communication; and activation and deployment of the medical reserve corps.[22]

As traditional public safety and emergency response agencies are deescalating their operational roles in the postevent phase of a disaster, the public health community continues to maintain an active operational presence, assisting with health-related hazard remediation and recovery functions. Specific roles of the public health community during the postevent phase of a disaster include: restoration of the healthcare infrastructure, continued surveillance and follow-up, and evaluation of the overall medical and public health response to the incident.[22]

System Finance and Support—Barriers to Preparedness

A major challenge for trauma systems in the United States has been finding the financial means to support disaster and public health preparedness activities.[5,10,12,18] In HRSA's survey of state trauma systems, the most frequently cited weakness and threat to continued existence was the paucity of available funding to support system-related activities.[5] A national effort to strengthen trauma systems in ways that will access more of the population and provide better injury care to patients is needed. Funding these initiatives has not been a priority of the federal government. In the 2003 and 2004 executive budgets, HRSA's Division of Trauma and EMS was not funded.[38] Furthermore, in their report on the bioterrorism preparedness of hospitals in the United States, the GAO stated that hospital administrators were generally reluctant to spend their financial resources on preparedness initiatives that have little impact on daily hospital function and may never be utilized by the healthcare system.[6] There clearly is no current incentive for hospitals and trauma centers to spend critical funds on preparedness activities or surge capacities that will rarely be utilized in day-to-day operations or generate any revenue to offset their cost.[12]

Recommendations for Improvement

Trauma systems are an element of the nation's critical healthcare infrastructure that have the necessary framework on which to build a comprehensive "all-hazards" approach to hospital preparedness and public health emergency response. Studies have shown that regions with a comprehensive trauma system and a progressive approach to trauma care are more effective in managing disaster-related and mass casualty incidents, and report lower rates of overtriage, delays in access to trauma care, and an overall reduction in hospital mortality from trauma.[5,8,19] Although the non-trauma center may not be recognized for its ability to render specialized emergency medical care to injured victims, this does not mean that the non-trauma center will not be called upon in the event of a disaster or public health emergency to provide these services to patients. In many ways, non-trauma centers should invest more in preparedness than the trauma centers because they cannot easily call upon the medical and operational resources of the trauma center, and are more prolific throughout the United States. Non-trauma centers should seek guidance in disaster and public health response planning from their local academic medical centers, Centers for Public Health Preparedness (CPHP) and/or state public health agencies, and make the necessary partnerships necessary to provide the best medical response possible to their community.

The ATS/NHTSA *Trauma System Agenda for the Future* calls for an integrated systems approach toward developing disaster preparedness capacities.[18] The first step toward creating an integrated system for trauma care and disaster preparedness is to implement national standards and guidelines on trauma system organization. National standardization of trauma systems will lay the foundation on which trauma care and the integrated medical response to disasters and public health emergencies can be established.

Inclusive Systems Approach

The establishment of inclusive trauma care systems is based on the concept of integrated care, partnerships, and regionalization. In the inclusive trauma system model, all hospitals within the system whose EDs are staffed around the clock will have a trauma center designation from Level I to V. The notion of an inclusive trauma care system is based on the belief that Level I/II facilities are only one component of a multidisciplinary, integrated approach to trauma care.[2] Advantages to the inclusive system structure are that each hospital has established levels of competency for the treatment of injured patients, and trauma care is made more readily accessible to patients who may not have immediate access to a Level I/II trauma center. Understanding that during a disaster or public health emergency patients tend to go to the hospitals closest to them or the incident, this model allows the trauma resources to be extended across the system or region to provide patients with greater access to trauma care. Inclusive systems also capitalize on the relationships and partnerships that the trauma system has with community resources. Disadvantages associated with the inclusive system approach include the overall costs associated with the organization and integration of multiple trauma centers within a particular region or system. Additionally, logistic considerations tend to be considerable when the trauma system extends over a large geographic area or is incorporated into the statewide trauma system infrastructure. By participating in integrated planning activities and working toward an inclusive systems approach to trauma care and preparedness, trauma systems will become the standard of care among healthcare delivery systems and public health preparedness.[18]

Selective Trauma Systems

There are groups of physicians and surgeons who believe that Level I trauma centers should receive the majority of patients from a disaster or mass casualty incident and specifically all critical patients.[21] The idea behind this assertion is that Level I trauma centers have more experience dealing with critically injured trauma patients, and have more robust resources to offer than other trauma centers or community hospitals.[18-19,25] Therefore, trauma systems should be centered around the Level I or Level II trauma centers and all patients should be referred to those facilities. The vast majority (90%) of Level I trauma centers are located in urban areas and are often public nonprofit facilities that are larger and have more academic affiliations than other hospitals and trauma centers.[19] These facilities also have been shown to have more ED overcrowding, spend more time on diversion, and have a higher percentage of EMS overtriage than hospitals and trauma centers in suburban or rural communities.[18-26] The concern with a selective trauma system is that by limiting the number of Level I/II trauma centers and making verification and/or designation of all acute care hospitals voluntary, disparities in access to trauma care and enhancing the ability to deliver timely trauma care through the EMS system is undermined. Additionally, in developing a surge capacity for the trauma system, it may be more advantageous to the system to have more trauma care coverage, so field triage activities can be implemented that spread injured victims among the various levels of care within the trauma system, rather than overburden a few facilities with the majority of injured victims.

Not all trauma systems are the same, and perhaps one model of trauma system design is preferred in a particular community or region than another. This makes it difficult to generalize the "ideal" or "model" trauma system that excels in both trauma care and all-hazards disaster preparedness. Strategies in developing best practices for trauma system disaster preparedness should focus on developing partnerships with the public health departments, public safety agencies, and community resources to create an integrated, collaborative, and cooperative response effort that meets the specific needs of our region, based upon the elements identified during the initial vulnerability and hazard assessment.

Access to Trauma and EMS Systems—Addressing Gaps in Coverage

Among the areas of improvement cited to help correct these disparities are better evaluation tools and research to investigate the trauma system access issues, guidelines to measure the optimal number of Level I and Level II trauma centers, and more detailed guidance on the roles of Level III–V trauma centers in disaster preparedness and response activities.[19] In order to accurately address the nationwide gaps in trauma and EMS system coverage, trauma systems and EMS systems need to be organized and standardized at the federal level in order to minimize the widespread inconsistencies in quality of care, eliminate the gaps in coverage, and ensure that we are adequately prepared to respond to disasters and other public health emergencies.[2,4,18–20] A reasonable first step would be to implement trauma system coverage in the 15 states that currently lack any trauma system infrastructure.[5,20] It seems that although the majority of Level I/II trauma centers are located in urban areas, the Level III–V trauma facilities could be better utilized in those rural or suburban areas without the immediate availability of access to Level I/II care.[19] Another suggestion to improve access to care would be implementing national 911 system coverage and employing system status management of EMS units throughout rural areas in order to ensure a timely response to an emergency and attempt to provide coverage over large geographic areas.[4] Furthermore, by promoting inclusive trauma care systems with a regional focus, trauma and EMS services can be available to larger portions of the population through the integration of existing system resources.[18]

The American College of Surgeons and Hospital Disaster Preparedness

The ACS position on disasters, mass casualties, and unconventional acts of terrorism is simply that, in certain situations these events cause patients to suffer from a variety of disaster-related injuries, and that trauma centers and trauma surgeons will play a major role in the response to these disasters.[3,39–40] This is, for the most part, an accurate statement. Trauma centers and surgeons possess unique capabilities and resources for the management of patients who are victims of disaster-related trauma. Would it be prudent, however, for a surgeon to triage or be the treatment team leader for an event involving the dissemination of a biological agent or emerging infectious disease? Probably not. The ACS has made it fairly clear that when it comes to chemical, biological, and radiological agent exposures, surgeons require additional education and training on the identification and diagnosis of the exposure-related illnesses and their appropriate medical management. Additionally, surgeons have pointed out that a major advantage of a trauma center is its "highly competent" emergency department, and that ED staff are often "experts" in the medical management of chemical, biological, and radiological casualties.[20] Although the trauma literature suggests that the trauma surgeon would make the best hospital triage officer during a disaster with major injuries, the attending emergency medicine physician may be of particular assistance to the surgical staff in assessing and triaging injured victims, as well as providing primary triage for victims of other disaster etiology, such as chemical exposure, bioterrorism, infectious disease outbreaks, radiological emergencies, and certain natural disasters. By effectively and appropriately utilizing the ED's resources in a disaster or other public health emergency, surgical and other hospital resources and services can be focused on treating those victims requiring their sophisticated level of care.

It is also prudent to address the issue of whether trauma centers should be the designated receiving facilities for uninjured victims of chemical, biological, or radiological exposure. There is a concern that by transporting these patients to specialty care facilities, that if contamination of the ED or other portion of the facility should occur, the hospital would be forced to close and the trauma system would be unable to rely upon that particular facility's services. When it comes to the discussion of whether nuclear, biological, or chemical (NBC) patients should be treated at trauma centers or community hospitals, local hospital preparedness and emergency planners should develop protocols that best meet the anticipated needs of their community. Patients with contamination will inevitably arrive at all facilities, based on the proximity to the incident. Controlling access to hospitals; directing patients through the

ED; and having the appropriate training, equipment, and decontamination facilities to manage a percentage of patients who may arrive with contamination is the best strategy to take in preparing for hazmat and weapons of mass destruction (WMD)-related incidents.

The document, *Trauma System Agenda for the Future*, states that trauma care requires a multidisciplinary approach that involves all members of the trauma system staff in order to achieve an optimal patient outcome.[18] The ACS has supported the notion that surgeons may be the leaders in trauma and injury care, but should actively participate in a multidisciplinary, "all-hazards" approach to hospital and trauma system preparedness.[17]

Conclusions

It has been identified and is generally agreed upon throughout the literature that the implementation and development of trauma systems over the past 40 years has significantly decreased morbidity and mortality from injuries nationwide.[5,7] Trauma systems should be viewed by public health agencies and the emergency management community as a tangible asset in the public safety and medical response to disasters and public health emergencies. An important point to stress is the notion that disasters begin and end at the local level. Trauma systems should be integrated with the local and regional healthcare system by maintaining partnerships with public safety agencies and community resources that are focused on the common goals of injury prevention and delivering optimal patient care to the victims of trauma. In light of the current state of our nation's healthcare system and the related financial and administrative disincentives for preparedness activities, trauma systems have access to numerous systemwide resources that could be called upon during a public health crisis to help maintain the community's healthcare infrastructure and minimize morbidity and mortality in the first 24–48 hours of a disaster.[17]

Trauma systems can enhance the public health response to disasters by capitalizing on the multiagency relationships they maintain with members of the public safety community. Trauma systems have been successful in collaborating with emergency management agencies, public safety agencies, the EMS system, and the public health community to enhance their abilities to deliver effective trauma care. Utilizing these resources by directing response planning and incident management activities toward an all-hazards approach to emergency management will allow these resources to be utilized during the medical response to unconventional disasters and other public health emergencies.

Although there are numerous components of hospital and community disaster planning, one of the most important roles of the trauma center in disaster and public health preparedness is the ability of the trauma center to act as a model for critical patient care, disaster planning, resource management, and community partnerships, and to set the standard of care in hospital preparedness and disaster medical response.[2–4,18,21,25] The trauma system has at its disposal a unique and comprehensive infrastructure and a robust pool of resources, skills, and assets to draw upon during a public health emergency. Trauma systems and trauma centers should act as leaders among health systems and institutions, and be a resource to other hospitals and the public health community in developing emergency preparedness and response plans.[2–4,18,21,25]

References

1. Hadley J, Holahan J. *The Cost of Care for the Uninsured: What Do We Spend, Who Pays, and What Would Full Coverage Add to Medical Spending?* The Kaiser Commission on Medicaid and the Uninsured; 2004. http://www.kff.org/uninsured/upload/The-Cost-of-Care-for-the-Uninsured-What-Do-We-Spend-Who-Pays-and-What-Would-Full-Coverage-Add-to-Medical-Spending.pdf. Accessed January 5, 2010.

2. American College of Surgeons. *Resources for Optimal Care of the Injured Patient: 1999.* Chicago: American College of Surgeons; 1999.

3. American College of Surgeons. [ST-42] Statement on disaster and mass casualty management [by the American College of Surgeons]. American College of Surgeons Web site. http://www.facs.org/fellows_info/statements/st-42.html. Published 2003. Accessed January 5, 2010.

4. Peterson TD, Vaca F. Commentary: Trauma systems: a key factor in homeland preparedness. Ann Emerg Med. 2003;41(6):799–801.

5. U.S. Department of Health and Human Services, Health Resources and Services Administration. *A 2002 National Assessment of State Trauma System Development, Emergency Medical Services Resources, and Disaster Readiness for Mass Casualty Events.* Washington, DC: Health Resources and Services Administration; 2002.

6. U.S. General Accounting Office. *Hospital Preparedness: Most Urban Hospitals Have Emergency Plans but Lack Certain Capacities for Bioterrorism Response.* Washington, DC: U.s. General Accounting Office; August, 2003. Report GAO-03-924.

7. Mann NC, Mullins RJ, MacKenzie EJ, Jurkovich GJ, Mock CN. Systematic review of published evidence regarding trauma system effectiveness. J Trauma. 1999; 47(3):S25–S33.

8. May AK, McGwin G Jr, Lancaster LJ, et al. The April 8, 1998 tornado: assessment of the trauma system response and the resulting injuries. J Trauma. 2000; 48(4):666–672.

9. Roy MJ, ed. *Physician's Guide to Terrorist Attack.* Totowa, NJ: Humana Press, 2004.

10. Rubin JN. Recurring pitfalls in hospital preparedness and response. J Homeland Security. January, 2004. http://www.homelanddefense.org/journal/Articles/rubin.html. Accessed January 5, 2010.

11. Ghilarducci DP, Pirallo RG, Hegmann KT. Hazardous materials readiness of United States Level 1 trauma centers. *J Occup Environ Med.* 2000;42(7):683–692.

12. Barbera JA, Macintyre AG, DeAtley CA. Ambulances to nowhere: America's critical shortfall in medical preparedness for catastrophic terrorism. In: Howitt AM, Pangi RL, eds. *Countering Terrorism: Dimensions of Preparedness.* Cambridge, MA: MIT Press; 2003:283-297.

13. Hearing Before the Committee on Governmental Affairs, U. S. Senate (2001) (testimony of Henry L. Hinton, Jr., Managing Director, Defense Capabilities and Management. General Accounting Office).

14. Hogan DE, Burstein JL, eds. *Disaster Medicine.* Philadelphia: Lippincott Williams & Wilkins; 2002.

15. Cone DC, Weir SD, Bogucki S. Convergent volunteerism. Ann Emerg Med. 2003;41(4):457–462.

16. U.S. General Accounting Office. SARS Outbreak: *Improvements to Public Health Capacity Are Needed for Responding to Bioterrorism and Emerging Infectious Diseases.* Washington, DC: U.S. General Accounting Office; May 7, 2003. Publication GAO-03-769T.

17. Frykberg ER. Disaster and mass casualty management: a comment on the ACS position statement. *Bulletin of the American College of Surgeons.* 2003;88(8):12–13.

18. American Trauma Society and U.S. Department of Transportation, National Highway Traffic Safety Administration. *Trauma System Agenda for the Future.* National Highway Traffic Safety Administration; October 2002. Report #3P0138.

19. MacKenzie EJ, Hoyt DB, Sacra JC, et al. National inventory of hospital trauma centers. *JAMA.* 2003;289:1515–1522.

20. Trunkey DD. Trauma centers and trauma systems. *JAMA.* 2003;289:1566–1567.

21. Cushman JG, Pachter HL, Beaton HL. Two New York City hospitals' surgical response to the September 11, 2001, terrorist attack in New York City. *J Trauma.* 2003;54:147–155.

22. Landesman LY. *Public Health Management of Disasters: The Practice Guide.* Washington, DC: American Public Health Association; 2001.

23. White SR. Hospital and emergency department preparedness for biological, chemical, and nuclear terrorism. Clin Occup Environ Med. 2002;2(2):405–425.

24. Greenberg MI, Hendrickson RG. Report of the CIMERC/Drexel University Emergency Department Terrorism Preparedness Consensus Panel. *Acad Emerg Med.* 2003;10(7):783–788.

25. Jacobs LM, Burns KJ, Gross RI. Terrorism: A public health threat with a trauma system response. *J Trauma.* 2003;55(6):1014–1021.

26. Feliciano DV, Anderson GV Jr, Rozycki GS, et al. Management of casualties from the bombing at the Centennial Olympics. Am J Surg. 1998;176(6):538–543.

27. West JG, Trunkey DD, Lim RC. Systems of trauma care: a study of two counties. *Arch Surg.* 1979:114(4);455–460.

28. Trauma Care Systems Planning and Development Act of 1990, P L No. 101–590 (1990).

29. U.S. Department of Health and Human Services, Public Health Service, Health Resources and Services Administration, Bureau of Health Resources Development, Division of Trauma and Emergency Medical Systems. *Model Trauma Care System Plan.* Rockville, Maryland: Public Health Service, 1992.

30. Committee on Trauma and Committee on Shock, Division of Medical Sciences, National Academy of Sciences, National Research Council. *Accidental Death and*

Disability:The Neglected Disease of Modern Society. Washington, DC: National Academy of Sciences, 1966.

31. National Highway Safety Act of 1966, Pub L No. 89-564. 89 Stat. 3052 (1966).
32. Emergency Medical Services Systems Act of 1973, Pub L No. 93–154 (1973).
33. National Highway Traffic Safety Administration. *EMS System Development: Results of the Statewide EMS Technical Assessment Program.* Washington, DC: NHTSA; 1988.
34. American Red Cross. *Emergency Response.* Boston: StayWell; 2001.
35. Bledsoe BE, Porter RS, Cherry RA. Essentials of Paramedic Care. Upper Saddle River, New Jersey: Brady/Prentice Hall Health; 2003.
36. Maniscalco PM, Christen HT. *Understanding Terrorism and Managing the Consequences.* New Jersey: Brady/Prentice Hall Health; 2002.
37. Rehabilitation. In: Committee on Trauma Research, Commission on Life Sciences, National Research Council, Institute of Medicine, eds. *Injury in America: A Continuing Public Health Problem.* Washington, DC: National Academies Press; 1985:80–98.
38. Kellerman A. A hole in the homeland defense. *Modern Healthcare.* 2003;33(16):23.
39. American College of Surgeons. Disasters from biological and chemical terrorism—what should the individual surgeon do?: a report from the Committee on Trauma. American College of Surgeons Web site. http://www.facs.org/civiliandisasters/trauma.html. Accessed December 30, 2009.
40. American College of Surgeons. Statement on unconventional acts of civilian terrorism: a report from the Board of Governors. American College of Surgeons Web site. http://www.facs.org/civiliandisasters/statement.html. Accessed December 30, 2009.

Chapter **4**

Legal Issues and Regulatory Compliance

Doris R. Varlese, JD

Photo by Mark Wolfe/FEMA Photo

Learning Objectives

- Define a disaster declaration and describe its consequences.
- Identify patient privacy issues.
- Describe how workers can be protected.
- Explain the legal issues associated with volunteers.
- Identify the effects of the Emergency Medical Treatment and Active Labor Act (EMTALA).
- Describe altered standards of care that occur during a disaster.

Overview

Disasters often raise legal issues as well as issues relating to regulatory compliance. Most laws and regulations are written with "normal" operations in mind, not taking into account disasters, acts of terrorism, and public health emergencies that might severely stress systems. For example, the

September 11, 2001 disasters raised several issues with regard to laws and regulations pertaining to hospitals, workforce issues, and patient privacy. Using the September 11th event in New York City as an example, this chapter will describe the legal and regulatory issues raised in healthcare emergency management and how they might be addressed under current laws, regulations, and regulatory frameworks. This chapter will also describe issues discussed in the aftermath of September 11th or raised by other disasters. Specifically, this chapter will cover:

- disaster declarations and their consequences
- patient privacy issues as they relate to patient locator systems
- worker protection issues
- volunteer issues
- the Emergency Medical Treatment and Active Labor Act
- altered delivery of care and standards of care
- laws, regulations and accreditation standards and needs for disaster modification
- medical malpractice

This chapter is intended to provide a working knowledge of the many legal and regulatory issues that may arise during disasters, as well as an understanding of how emergency managers are attempting to resolve some of those issues beforehand.

Case Study

The September 11, 2001 World Trade Center attack highlighted several legal and regulatory issues that can occur during disasters. For example, medical providers rushed to the site, as well as to area hospitals to volunteer their services. As the towers burned, area hospitals became concerned about the air quality and feared it might be harming their employees and patients. A few hours later, when they had not heard from them, family members of those who visited or worked at the World Trade Center were very concerned about locating their loved ones and began posting signs with pictures all over Manhattan in an attempt to locate them. Family members began visiting and calling area hospitals to see if their family members were patients. President George W. Bush issued a disaster declaration which applied to the five boroughs of New York City. Anticipating a large influx of patients, hospitals activated their disaster plans, cancelled elective surgeries, and began discharging patients in order to create "surge capacity" (the ability to treat extra patients). In order to prepare to receive extra patients, some hospitals set up extra beds in areas not traditionally used for patient care. When hospitals became inundated with family members' inquiries, the Greater New York Hospital Association (GNYHA), along with the New York City Office of Emergency Management and the New York State Department of Health, began exploring the possibility of

Figure 4-1

Urban Search and Rescue at the Site of the World Trade Center

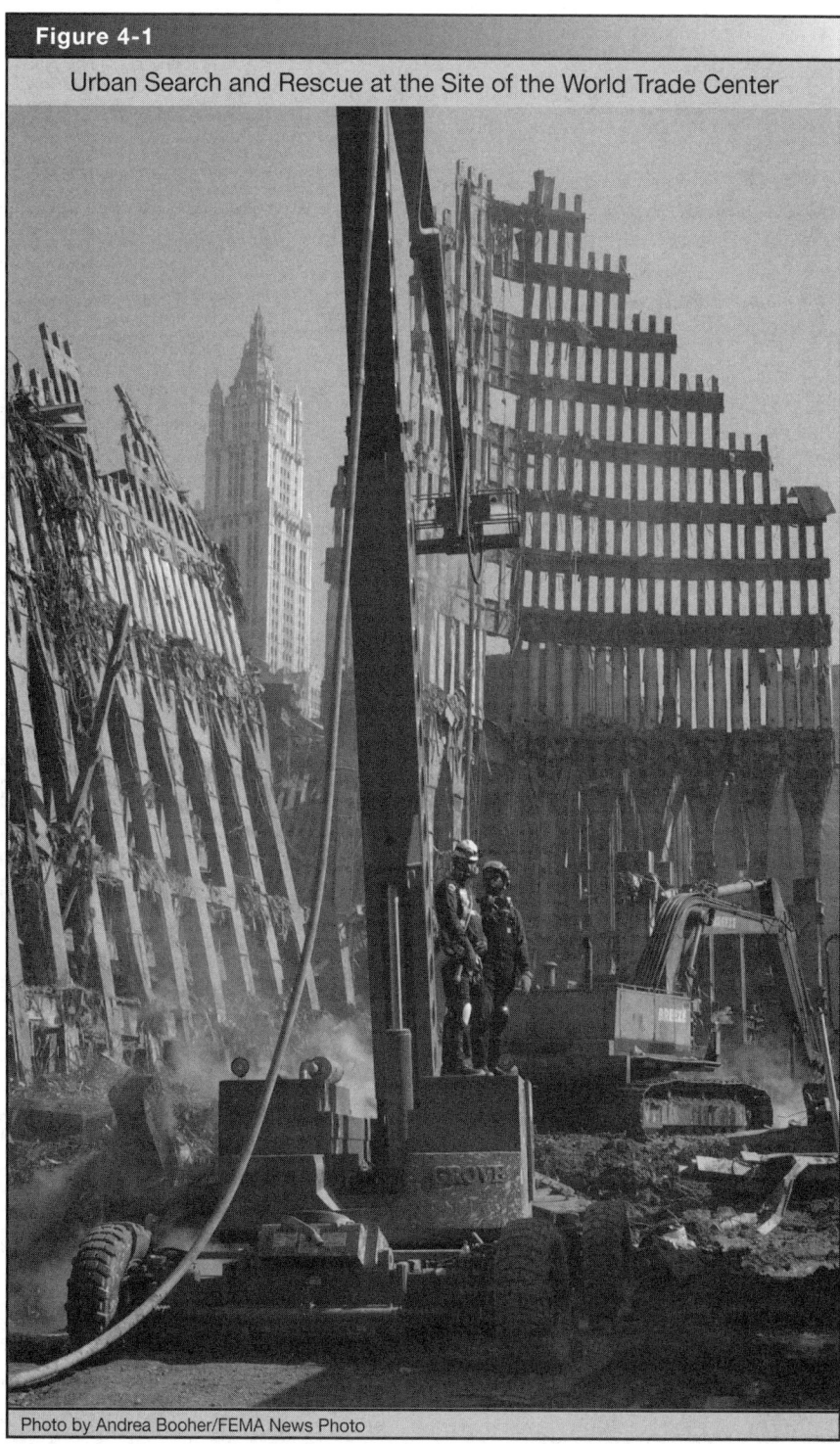

Photo by Andrea Booher/FEMA News Photo

setting up a publicly-accessible database where members of the public could conduct searches to see if individuals were being treated at local hospitals. A few days later, the "patient locator" system was up and running on the GNYHA and other publicly-available Web sites.

Figure 4-2

A FEMA Employee Views the Wall of People Still Missing from the World Trade Center Attacks

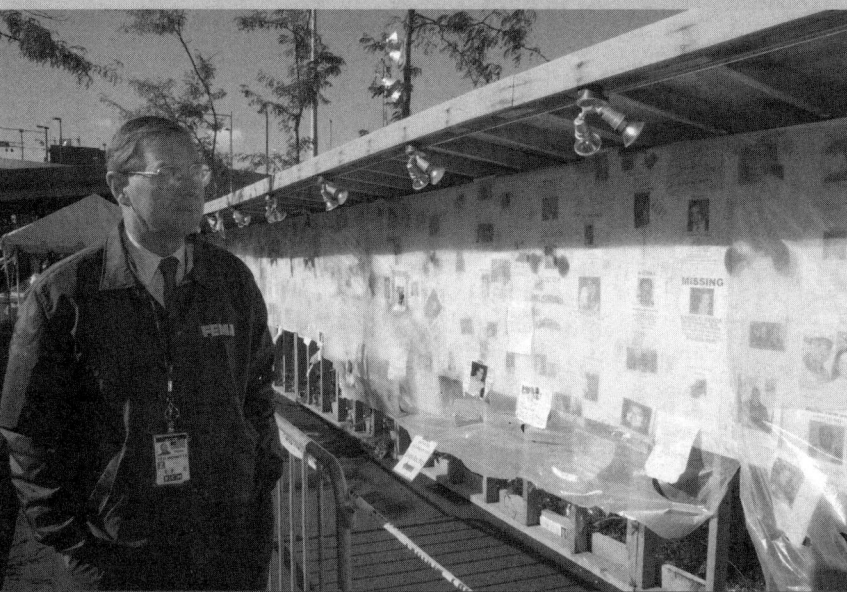

Photo by Andrea Booher/FEMA News Photo

Questions

Why was the declaration of a disaster important?

The declaration of a disaster was important because it triggered other actions by the government. Declarations of disaster can be at any level of government and in this case it was a federal declaration, which provided access to the resources of the federal government to support local resources. For example, as a result of President George W. Bush's declaration of a disaster, the Federal Emergency Management Agency (FEMA) was able to provide funding to New York City for recovery and cleanup efforts. The federal government was also able to provide resources needed for the response in New York City.

What legal and regulatory issues were raised by the patient locator system?

The federal Health Insurance Portability and Accountability Act of 1996 (HIPAA) Privacy Rule protects from disclosure individually identifiable protected health information (PHI) held by "covered entities." Covered entities include health plans and healthcare providers. The HIPAA Privacy Rule does, however, permit covered entities to disclose PHI under a variety of circumstances. Those circumstances include "to identify, locate, and notify family members, guardians, or anyone else responsible for the individual's care of the individual's location, general condition, or death."[1]

What legal and regulatory issues were raised by employees working at the World Trade Center site?

The Occupational Safety and Health Act of 1970 (OSH Act), which applies to most private sector employers, requires employers to provide a place of employment free from hazards likely to cause death or serious physical injury.[2] To the extent that employees were sent by their employers to the World Trade Center site to assist in the response and recovery efforts, their employers were required to ensure that they were operating in a safe environment.

Figure 4-3

Ground Zero Mourner Reflects on the Death of a Loved One During 9-11 Memorial Service

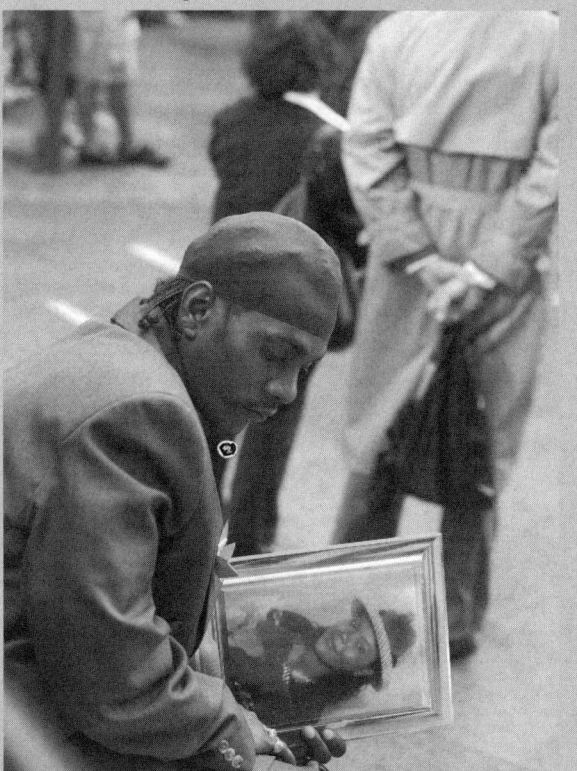

Photo by Andrea Booher/FEMA News Photo

What legal and regulatory issues were raised by "spontaneous volunteers" at area hospitals?

Before being provided with clinical privileges at hospitals, practitioners must undergo a process whereby their credentials are verified, so that the hospital can verify that the practitioner does have a valid license and appropriate education, training, and in some cases, board certification. During the September 11th event, several medical volunteers presented themselves at area hospitals, offering to volunteer their services. Those providers had not been credentialed prior to the event, and therefore, the hospitals did not know whether or not the providers had the appropriate credentials. In addition, the practitioners would likely not have been covered by the institutions' malpractice carriers had there been malpractice issues arising from the care rendered by the medical volunteers. This highlighted the need for a uniform, organized system of credentialing for medical volunteers.

Were there any laws or regulations that required approval for additional inpatient hospital beds if hospitals would have exceeded their licensed capacity?

Many states, including New York State, have laws and regulations that govern the process for approval of beds and services in hospitals, known

Figure 4-4

This Portion of Ground Zero of the World Trade Center Is Used as a Sorting Area to Sort Out the Thousands of Tons of Debris Still Left

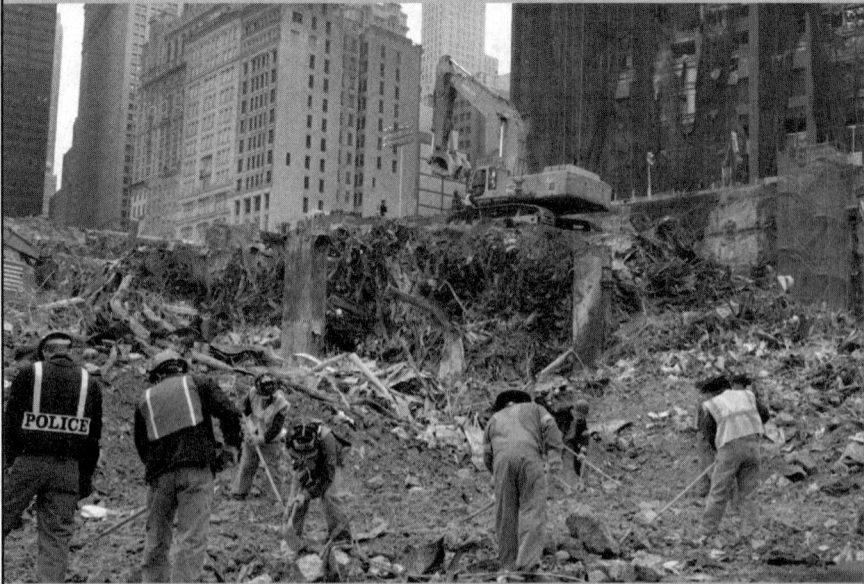

Photo by Larry Lerner/FEMA News Photo

as Certificate of Need (CON) laws and regulations. Included in those are the requirements that additional inpatient hospital beds be approved via the CON process. With regard to hospitals preparing to receive additional patients that would have caused the hospitals to exceed their licensed capacity, New York State regulations provide that a hospital "may temporarily exceed such capacity in an emergency."[3]

Disaster Declaration

A disaster declaration is a statement by a public official, with the authority to do so, recognizing that a disaster exists. Generally, emergencies are handled by the local jurisdiction, unless the emergency is so severe that the locality requires additional resources to respond. A disaster declaration may trigger certain powers not ordinarily available to government agencies. A disaster declaration may also trigger the activation of an individual facility's emergency response plan, if the plan is drafted to include that condition. Under federal law, the President has the authority to declare a disaster after being requested to do so by the governor of the affected state. The governor must have found that the emergency or disaster is so severe that it is beyond the capabilities of the affected state and local governments, and therefore they require assistance from the federal government.[4] On September 11, 2001, President George W. Bush issued a federal disaster declaration applicable to the five boroughs of New York City. This, in turn, permitted FEMA to provide funding for response and recovery efforts, including debris removal according to the provisions of the federal Robert T. Stafford Disaster Relief and Emergency Assistance Act.[5] The Stafford Act authorizes FEMA "to provide assistance essential to meeting immediate threats to life and property resulting from a major disaster."[6] The Stafford Act permits FEMA to provide funding or direct federal assistance in the form of equipment, personnel, supplies, food, and other resources.[7]

In response to the World Trade Center disaster, FEMA designated $20 billion to assist the New York City area.

[This] was the first time in which the amount of federal disaster assistance to be provided was set early in the response and recovery efforts and resulted in two major changes in the federal approach to this disaster. FEMA, in response to the designation of a specific level of funding, changed its traditional approach to administering disaster funds, and with congressional authorization, FEMA reimbursed the city and state for "associated costs" that it could not have otherwise funded within provisions of the Stafford Act to ensure that the entire amount of funds appropriated to FEMA for this disaster would be spent for the New York City area.[8]

The President's disaster declaration initially directed the federal government to pay 75% of the eligible costs for debris removal and repair and restoration of public facilities, with New York State and New York City paying the rest. However, under an order issued by President George W. Bush on September 18, 2001, the federal share was increased to 100% of those programs.[9]

In addition, under the Homeland Security Act, as amended by the Post-Katrina Emergency Management Reform Act of 2006, FEMA is responsible for leading and supporting a comprehensive emergency management system of preparedness, protection, response, recovery, and mitigation.[10]

It is significant to note that governors of affected states may also issue disaster declarations, and the powers that result vary by state law. For example, a state disaster declaration may result in permitting practitioners with out-of-state licenses to practice in the affected state. In addition, the ability to designate a disaster often also exists within all levels of government and rests with that level of government's executive. As the laws and regulations associated with disaster declarations vary from governmental entity to governmental entity, it is important for the emergency manager to be familiar with the various types of disaster declarations allowable at all levels of government in their area.

Patient Privacy Issues

The federal HIPAA Privacy Rule protects from disclosure individually identifiable protected health information (PHI) held by "covered entities." Covered entities include health plans and healthcare providers. The HIPAA Privacy Rule does, however, permit covered entities to disclose PHI under a variety of circumstances. Those circumstances include "to identify, locate, and notify family members, guardians, or anyone else responsible for the individual's care of the individual's location, general condition, or death."[11]

Thus, HIPAA provided authorization for the creation of the patient locator database. According to the U.S. Department of Health and Human Services (HHS), "when necessary, the hospital may notify the police, the press, or the public at large to the extent necessary to help locate, identify or otherwise notify family members and others as to the location and general condition of their loved ones."[12] Further, according to HHS, "when a health care provider is sharing information with disaster relief organizations that, like the American Red Cross, are authorized by law or by their charters to assist in disaster relief efforts, it is unnecessary to obtain a patient's permission to share the information if doing so would interfere with the organization's ability to respond to the emergency."[13]

OSHA and Other Worker Protection Laws

As described previously, OSHA applies to most private sector employers and requires those employers to provide a workplace free of hazards. To the extent that employees were sent by their employers to work at the World Trade Center site, employers were generally required by OSHA and other laws providing worker protections to provide a safe work environment. Unfortunately, because of the poor quality of the air at the site, workers participating in the response and recovery effort have complained about health effects from exposure to chemicals for extended periods of time. Some workers have sued New York City, alleging that the unsafe conditions caused illness. In addition, some families have sued, alleging that their loved ones have died because of contact with toxic chemicals at the World Trade Center site. However, in order to succeed with these lawsuits, the plaintiffs must prove that the death can directly be attributed to work at the World Trade Center site.

The recent case of New York City Police Officer James Zadroga highlights the complicated issues involved in these cases. Detective Zadroga died in 2006 and the medical examiner of Ocean County New Jersey attributed Detective Zadroga's death to conditions at the World Trade Center site. However, after his review, New York City's chief medical examiner determined "'with certainty beyond doubt,' that the material in Detective Zadroga's lungs was not dust from the Trade Center but ground up pills he had injected into his veins."[14] The cause of death is important because that determination has implications for liability, disability pensions, and inclusion in the September 11th Victim Compensation Fund, which could result in substantial monetary awards.

Volunteer Issues

As indicated during the World Trade Center disaster in 2001 and Hurricane Katrina in 2005, hospitals and public health agencies may need to supplement their workforces in order to care for patients. Healthcare facilities and public health agencies must ensure that volunteer staff are licensed and appropriately credentialed prior to granting privileges to them to practice clinically. Licensing is conducted on the state level. A governor in an affected state may have the power to waive licensure requirements during a disaster or confer liability protection for volunteers under state law, if none exists. Credentialing (whether a practitioner has the education and training to appropriately treat patients) is done on an institutional basis. When volunteering to assist during emergencies, medical personnel are often concerned about the liability protection that they might receive in the event that they are sued as a result of care rendered during the disaster. Volunteer systems are premised on the belief that a pre-arranged process for credentialing and privileging is preferable to a system that utilizes "spontaneous volunteers."

NATIONAL SYSTEMS

During Hurricane Katrina, the solution to the legal concern regarding potential liability was that the federal government appointed the medical personnel as unpaid temporary federal employees, thereby providing them with legal protections in the form of tort liability coverage under the Federal Tort Claims Act.[15] That meant that the volunteer would not be held individually liable for actions taken within the scope of the assignment. It also meant that they would be provided with benefits under the Federal Employees' Compensation Act if they were injured while engaged in their volunteer assignments.[16]

In response to issues relating to privileging and credentialing, HHS is requiring all states to implement programs for credentialing volunteers. The program must be consistent with HHS' Emergency System for the Advanced Registration of Volunteer Health Professionals (ESAR-VHP) compliance requirements. Under the guidelines, states are required to assign different levels to the volunteers based upon the information that the system is able to verify. (The highest level is "hospital ready.")

In addition, the Emergency Management Assistance Compact (EMAC), an organization ratified by the United States Congress, provides structure for aid between states during disasters.[17] Through EMAC, which is a form of mutual aid, a state impacted by a disaster can request and receive assistance from other member states. This assistance may include medical personnel. Under this compact, the recipient state recognizes the professional license of volunteers dispatched via the sending state's system. In New York State, volunteers dispatched via EMAC will be granted the civil liability and any workers' compensation protections afforded to New York State workers (as described later).[18] EMAC is administered by NEMA, the National Emergency Management Association. The only requirement for a state to join is for a state legislature to ratify the language of the compact; states are not required to assist other states in emergencies unless they are able to.[19] All 50 states, Puerto Rico, the United States Virgin Islands, and the District of Columbia have ratified EMAC.[20] Under EMAC, states requesting assistance must reimburse the states that provide assistance.[21] Figure 4-5 provides a diagram regarding how EMAC works.

STATE SYSTEMS

Several states, including the state of Connecticut, for example, have already implemented programs consistent with the ESAR-VHP require-

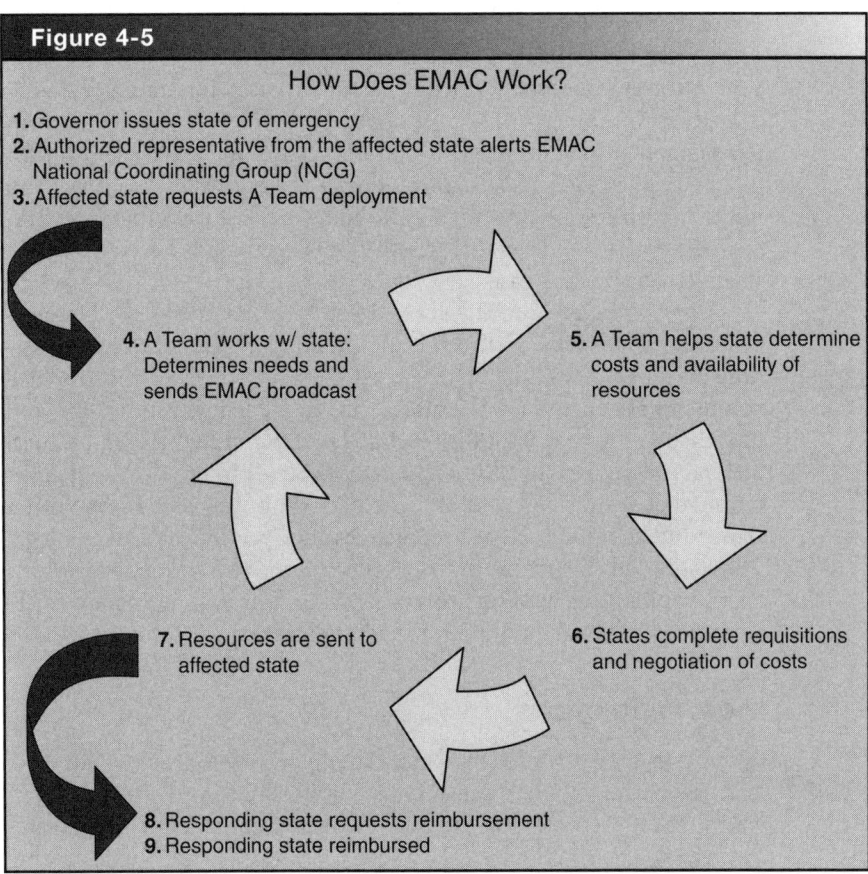

Figure 4-5

How Does EMAC Work?

1. Governor issues state of emergency
2. Authorized representative from the affected state alerts EMAC National Coordinating Group (NCG)
3. Affected state requests A Team deployment

4. A Team works w/ state: Determines needs and sends EMAC broadcast

5. A Team helps state determine costs and availability of resources

7. Resources are sent to affected state

6. States complete requisitions and negotiation of costs

8. Responding state requests reimbursement
9. Responding state reimbursed

Courtesy of FEMA and EMAC

ments. All of Connecticut's acute care hospitals have agreed to participate in the program, which utilizes a Web-based system for managing volunteer enrollment, credential verification, communication, and training. Volunteers in the Connecticut system are required to complete training courses and participate in drills and exercises. The program is activated by the governor of the state of Connecticut in response to a local, state, or regional request. Each receiving hospital must conduct primary source verification of each volunteer's professional credentials as soon as it is feasible. Each hospital is also responsible for providing privileges to volunteers. Volunteers deployed through the Connecticut system are provided with state-sponsored liability and workers' compensation coverage when enrolled in the program prior to volunteer service and when other conditions are met.

In addition, in some states, such as New York State, when volunteers are activated and deployed by the New York State Department of Health, they are treated as "employees" for purposes of the New York State

Public Officers Law and receive protections in the form of defense (e.g., a defense attorney) and indemnification through the New York State Attorney General's Office if personally sued for actions taken as a medical volunteer.[22] Though deployed by New York State, volunteers may be controlled by the local requesting agency. This legal protection applies to all professional volunteers (e.g., MDs and RNs), but not to nonprofessional volunteers. Volunteers may be eligible for workers' compensation coverage; whether it is available is based upon the specific facts of each case.

Currently, New York State laws do not provide defense and indemnification to hospitals that might be sued as a result of receiving volunteers during disasters. Thus, hospitals that are receiving medical volunteers are encouraged to discuss any possible indemnification and malpractice coverage with the sending hospitals and with their medical malpractice carriers. In addition, New York State protectors do not cover criminal actions. Therefore, if a medical volunteer is charged with a crime and acquitted, New York State cannot pay the volunteer's legal fees. While this New York example is one approach to medical volunteers' liability and workers' protection, healthcare emergency managers need to check how their state handles medical volunteers.

LOCAL PROTECTIONS

In addition, local jurisdictions, such as those in New York State, may enact local laws or provide insurance for medical volunteers. For example, in New York City, according to the New York City Department of Health and Mental Hygiene (NYC-DOHMH), New York City's General Municipal Law provides that Medical Reserve Corps volunteers are considered an extension of the NYC-DOHMH workforce when deployed and therefore receive certain legal protections.[23]

As the protections and authorizations for local volunteers, if any, may vary considerably between local jurisdictions, it is important for the healthcare emergency manager to understand their regional and local governmental volunteer medical system and any existing laws and regulations.

JOINT COMMISSION STANDARDS

The Joint Commission is an accrediting body for hospitals and other facilities (e.g., nursing homes). Accreditation is voluntary, and hospitals and other facilities that wish to be accredited by The Joint Commission are required to adhere to a comprehensive set of standards. Those include standards with regard to privileging during disasters. The standards do not require that an accredited hospital grant disaster privileges, but provide a process for doing so if the hospital so chooses. The standards provide processes for both licensed independent practitioners (LIPs) (e.g., physicians) as well as providers who are not licensed independent practitioners.[24] Before a volunteer practitioner is eligible to function as a LIP, the hospital must obtain a valid government-issued photo identification and a least one of several items on a list (e.g., a picture identification card from a healthcare organization, a current license to practice).[25] With regard to providers who are not licensed independent practitioners, but who are required by law and regulation to have a license certification or registration (e.g., RNs), the hospital must also obtain a valid government-issued photo identification as well as another document on the list.[26] The standards also require that "the medical staff oversees the performance of each volunteer licensed independent practitioner" and there is similar language with regard to volunteers who are not licensed independent practitioners.[27] Under both sets of standards, the hospital's Emergency Operations Plan must have been activated and within 72 hours of the practitioner's arrival, the hospital must determine if the disaster privileges that have been granted should continue.[28]

Emergency Medical Treatment and Active Labor Act

The Emergency Medical Treatment and Active Labor Act (EMTALA), which applies to all hospitals with emergency departments that participate in the federal Medicare program, requires hospitals to provide a medical screening exam, stabilize, and transfer or treat all patients presenting to emergency departments.[29] The statute also applies when a patient is on hospital property or in a hospital-owned ambulance. In 2002, legislation was enacted authorizing the Secretary of the U.S. Department of Health and Human Services to waive sanctions for EMTALA violations when the violation arises from a transfer of an unstable patient during a public health emergency.[30] In addition, EMTALA regulations provide that sanctions for inappropriate transfer during a national emergency do not apply to a hospital with a dedicated emergency department that is located in an emergency area, as defined in the Social Security Act.[31] After Hurricane Katrina, the federal centers for Medicare and Medicaid services, which enforces EMTALA, published additional guidance, stating:

> [The] Center for Medicare and Medicaid Services (CMS) will not impose sanctions on a hospital located within the jurisdiction of the public health emergency declaration if the hospital redirects or relocates an individual to another location to receive a medical screening examination pursuant to a state emergency preparedness plan or transfers an individual who has not been stabilized if the transfer is necessitated by the circumstances of the declared emergency within a limited period

of time after implementation of the hospital's disaster protocol. This waiver, however, is not effective with respect to any action taken that discriminates among individuals on the basis of their source of payment or their ability to pay.[32]

Further clarification of EMTALA and possible waivers regarding disaster operations were provided during the 2009–2010 H1N1 influenza pandemic. This provided one of the first times when EMTALA requirements and the need for modification were clarified in an actual event by CMS. CMS provided two approaches to EMTALA during the pandemic: those which required no waiver and those which required a waiver.

Box 4-1

CMS Fact Sheet

Options for Managing Extraordinary ED Surges Under Existing EMTALA Requirements (No Waiver Required)

Hospitals may set up alternative screening sites on campus.

- The medical screening exam (MSE) does not have to take place in the ED. A hospital may set up alternative sites on its campus to perform MSEs.
  - Individuals may be redirected to these sites after being logged in. The redirection and logging can even take place outside the entrance to the ED.
  - The person doing the directing should be qualified (e.g., an RN) to recognize individuals who are obviously in need of immediate treatment in the ED.
- The content of the MSE varies according to the individual's presenting signs and symptoms. It can be as simple or as complex, as needed, to determine if an emergency medical condition (EMC) exists.
- MSEs must be conducted by qualified personnel, which may include physicians, nurse practitioners, physician's assistants, or RNs trained to perform MSEs and acting within the scope of their State Practice Act.
- The hospital must provide stabilizing treatment (or appropriate transfer) to individuals found to have an EMC, including moving them as needed from the alternative site to another on-campus department.

Hospitals may set up screening at off-campus, hospital-controlled sites.

- Hospitals and community officials may encourage the public to go to these sites instead of the hospital for screening for influenza-like illness (ILI). However, a hospital may not tell individuals who have already come to its ED to go to the off-site location for the MSE.

- Unless the off-campus site is already a dedicated ED (DED) of the hospital, as defined under EMTALA regulations, EMTALA requirements do not apply.
- The hospital should not hold the site out to the public as a place that provides care for EMCs in general on an urgent, un-scheduled basis. They can hold it out as an ILI screening center.
- The off-campus site should be staffed with medical personnel trained to evaluate individuals with ILIs.
- If an individual needs additional medical attention on an emergent basis, the hospital is required, under the Medicare Conditions of Participation, to arrange referral/transfer. Prior coordination with local emergency medical services (EMS) is advised to develop transport arrangements.

Communities may set up screening clinics at sites not under the control of a hospital.

- There is no EMTALA obligation at these sites.
- Hospitals and community officials may encourage the public to go to these sites instead of the hospital for screening for ILI. However, a hospital may not tell individuals who have already come to its ED to go to the off-site location for the MSE.
- Communities are encouraged to staff the sites with medical personnel trained to evaluate individuals with ILIs.
- In preparation for a pandemic, the community, its local hospitals, and EMS are encouraged to plan for referral and transport of individuals needing additional medical attention on an emergent basis.

EMTALA Waivers

- An EMTALA waiver allows hospitals to:
  - Direct or relocate individuals who come to the ED to an alternative off-campus site, in accordance with a State emergency or pandemic preparedness plan, for the MSE.
  - Effect transfers normally prohibited under EMTALA of individuals with unstable EMCs, so long as the transfer is necessitated by the circumstances of the declared emergency.
- By law, the EMTALA MSE and stabilization requirements can be waived for a hospital **only if**:
  - The president has declared an emergency or disaster under the Stafford Act or the National Emergencies Act; **and**

- The secretary of HHS has declared a Public Health Emergency; **and**
- The secretary invokes her/his waiver authority (which may be retroactive), including notifying Congress at least 48 hours in advance; **and**
- The waiver includes waiver of EMTALA requirements and the hospital is covered by the waiver.
- CMS will provide notice of an EMTALA waiver to covered hospitals through its Regional Offices and/or State Survey Agencies.
- Duration of an EMTALA waiver:
  - In the case of a public health emergency involving pandemic infectious disease, until the termination of the declaration of the public health emergency; **otherwise**
  - In all other cases, 72 hours after the hospital has activated its disaster plan.
  - In no case does an EMTALA waiver start before the waiver's effective date, which is usually the effective date of the public health emergency declaration.

Source: CMS Fact Sheet. Emergency Medical Treatment and Labor Act (EMTALA) & Surges in Demand for Emergency Department (ED) Services During a Pandemic, Ref: S&C-09-52. August 14, 2009.

Altered Standards of Care and Medical Malpractice

Medical malpractice is a civil claim that arises when a plaintiff claims that a healthcare institution and/or provider have not met the provider's duty to provide the generally accepted standard of medical care. The plaintiff must demonstrate damages as a result of the provider's care. There is no federal medical malpractice law; state laws set forth circumstances that determine medical malpractice.

During disasters that involve large numbers of patients, despite the best efforts of hospitals and providers, systems may become overwhelmed. Providers or regulators may determine that in order to save the greatest numbers of patients, the usual standard of care must be altered. For example, the New York State Department of Health recently released a set of guidelines regarding allocation of ventilators during a pandemic. The document was developed by the New York State Workgroup on Ventilator Allocation. It provides suggested guidelines for allocating ventilators during a severe pandemic, when despite advance planning, ventilator stockpiling, and centralized management of resources, there are not enough ventilators for the number of people who need them.[33] The document calls for clinicians to evaluate patients based on objective medical criteria and proposed a system with several components for allocating ventilators, including limiting the noncritical use of ventilators as the pandemic spreads, guidelines for allocating ventilators among all patients in acute care facilities (not only those affected by pandemic influenza), and an appeals process so that physicians and patients may request a review of triage decisions with which they disagree.[34] While the guidelines do not have the force of law or regulation, if a provider undertook to utilize the guidelines under the circumstances specified in them and were then sued for medical malpractice, a court would be unlikely to assign civil liability to a provider who followed the guidelines promulgated by the New York State Department of Health, which regulates hospitals.

A case that arose during Hurricane Katrina illustrates how physicians may face criminal liability as a result of actions taken during a disaster. Dr. Anna Pou was arrested and accused of second-degree murder for allegedly administering lethal doses of painkillers to nine patients after Hurricane Katrina, when the hospital in which she was working, Memorial Medical Center, was awaiting assistance to be evacuated. Three nurses were arrested as well. The charges were ultimately dropped when a grand jury failed to indict her and the three nurses.[35] However, she may still face civil liability because she is being sued by the families of the nine patients for wrongful death. Because the burden of proof in civil lawsuits is generally lower than the burden of proof necessary to find criminal liability, it is possible that Dr. Pou can be found liable in the civil lawsuits. In addition, Dr. Pou is suing the State of Louisiana and its attorney general in order to obtain a legal counsel to defend herself against the lawsuits filed against her by the families of the patients.[36]

Mutual Aid Agreements

Some entities, such as hospitals and agencies that provide ambulance services, have entered into written agreements to share resources during emergencies or disasters, termed "mutual aid agreements." The agreements generally do not obligate entities to assist each other, but provide a mechanism to notify others of the disaster and request assistance. The agreements are important in emergency planning because they evidence a prearranged agreement for entities to contact each other and request aid. For example, in New York City, in the event of a major emergency, the New York City Fire Department or the New York City Office of Emergency Management may request additional ambulance units from hospital ambulance services, volunteer ambulance services, and proprietary ambulance services. Hospital mutual aid agreements typically contain provisions to share staff or equipment during disasters.

Model State Emergency Health Powers Act

This model act was drafted by the Centers for Law and the Public's Health, a joint venture of Georgetown University and Johns Hopkins University. The federal Centers for Disease Control and Prevention had commissioned the Centers for Law and the Public's Health to produce the Model State Emergency Health Powers Act.[37] The Model Act would revise some laws currently addressed by existing public health laws, such as communicable disease reporting and quarantine. For example, the Act would require healthcare workers, pharmacists, veterinarians, laboratories, and others to report suspected illnesses or conditions to the local public health authority to detect a serious threat to the public's health.[38] The Act would also allow a public health authority to perform physical examinations as necessary for the diagnosis or treatment of individuals during an emergency and provides that persons who refuse may be isolated or quarantined.[39] The Act would also provide general immunity for the governor, public health agency, and other state agencies for their actions during a public health emergency.[40] As of July 15, 2006, 38 states have passed "bills or resolutions that include provisions from or closely related to the Act. The extent to which the Act's provisions are incorporated into each state's laws varies."[41] The Model Act has been criticized for providing greatly expanded powers to local public health agencies and one critic has said that the Model Act would "eliminate our freedom to choose our medical care and health treatment and potentially eliminate a broader range of our basic civil liberties."[42]

Other Legal and Regulatory Issues

CONSENT TO TREATMENT

Informed consent to health care is generally required in all treatment settings and failure to obtain informed consent may result in malpractice claims. Generally, exceptions to informed consent requirements recognize that care in an emergency may be rendered when the patient is unable to consent, no surrogate decision maker is available (e.g., a healthcare proxy or other individual authorized by state law to provide consent), and a delay in treatment could result in serious harm.

EVACUATION

The Joint Commission requires that hospitals include evacuation procedures in their Emergency Operations Plans.[43] However, total evacuation of a facility is a complex undertaking and is generally considered a last resort after all other options have been considered (e.g., moving patients to other floors).

Hospitals are generally licensed and regulated by their state departments of health and, generally, those entities must provide permission for hospital closures. When considering whether or not to evacuate during a disaster, hospital administrators should ideally consult with the licensing entity to obtain permission. However, it might not be possible to do so during a disaster when communication may be impossible. A hospital's evacuation plan should be developed in coordination with local emergency management and regulatory authorities so that all parties understand the circumstances under which an evacuation might be necessary and how it might be achieved. Hospitals should have transfer/evacuation agreements with other facilities or include provisions relating to transfers of patients in mutual aid agreements, which would evidence prearranged agreements to receive patients in the event of an evacuation.

SCOPE OF PRACTICE

It may be necessary to utilize providers during a disaster to undertake tasks that are outside the usual scope of practice for the provider. For example, although they might not be permitted to do so on a daily basis, during a pandemic, a facility might want to utilize a pharmacist to administer vaccines. Or a facility might want to utilize a paramedic to provide in-hospital care. State statutes relating to scope of practice may, however, prohibit such providers from learning or practicing those skills during emergency preparedness exercises. Therefore, in those cases, during a disaster "just in time" training will need to be provided. In addition, some facilities are reluctant to document in their written Emergency Operations Plans that such providers might act outside their scope of practice during a disaster. It may be prudent to include plans to utilize those providers outside their scope of practice, but note that the facility will only do so after obtaining permission from the appropriate regulatory authority.

Conclusion

The September 11, 2001 events and subsequent disasters, such as Hurricane Katrina, raised many issues including: disaster declarations and their consequences, patient privacy issues as they relate to patient locator systems, worker protection issues, volunteer issues, the Emergency Medical Treatment and Active Labor Act, altered standards of care, and medical malpractice. Since the September 11, 2001 events, many of the issues previously described have been analyzed in light of what occurred, as well as what might occur in future disasters. If similar issues arise in future disasters, the preceding discussion provides a framework for how they may be addressed. However, it is likely that many unanticipated issues may arise as well. Hospital, public health, and other emergency managers should, to the extent possible, engage in discussions to resolve those issues when they arise so that they are not barriers to care. Ideally, if planning has occurred with appropriate regulatory authorities and emergency managers, providers will know whom to contact during the disaster. If it is not possible to engage in those discussions during the disaster, providers should engage in actions that are prudent under the circumstances in order to render the best patient care possible.

References

1.   U.S. Department of Health and Human Services, HIPAA Frequent Questions. Available at: http://www.hhs.gov/hipaafaq/permitted/emergency/960.html. Accessed October 7, 2008.
2.   29 U.S.C. Section 654(a).
3.   10 New York Code of Rules and Regulations, Section 401.2(a).
4.   42 United States Code Sections 5170, 5191 (a), 44 Code of Federal Regulations Section 206.48.
5.   Stafford Act Public Law 93-288, 88 Stat 143 (1974), as amended; 42 U.S.C. 5121–5201.
6.   Stafford Act, Section 403(a).
7.   Ibid.
8.   United States General Accounting Office Report. September 11 Overview of Federal Disaster Assistance to the New York City Area. October 2003.
9.   White House Press Release, September 18, 2001.
10. Public Law No. 107-26. As amended Public Law No. 109–25.
11. U.S. Department of Health and Human Services, HIPAA Frequent Questions. Available at: http://www.hhs.gov/hipaafaq/permitted/emergency/960.html. Accessed October 7, 2008.
12. Ibid.
13. Ibid.
14. DePalma, Anthony. Medical Examiner, Differing on Ground Zero Case, Stands His Ground. *The New York Times*. November 25, 2007.
15. 42 United States Code Sections 1291, 1346, 1402, 2671–2680 (2000).
16. Greater New York Hospital Association Memorandum. Legal Protections Provided to Medical Volunteers in Relief Efforts. September 21, 2005.
17. Public Law No. 104–321 (1996).
18. GNYHA Memorandum.
19. EMAC FAQ. Available at: http://www.emacweb.org/. Accessed November 3, 2008.
20. Ibid.
21. Ibid.
22. New York State Public Officers Law, Section 17.
23. New York City General Municipal Law Section 50-k.

24. 2009 Joint Commission Hospital Standards, EM. 02.02.13, EM. 02.02.15.
25. 2009 Joint Commission Hospital Standards EM. 02.02.13.
26. 2009 Joint Commission Hospital Standards EM. 02.02.15.
27. 2009 Joint Commission Hospital Standards EM. 02.02.14, EM. 02.02.15.
28. Ibid.
29. 42 United States Code Section 1395dd.
30. Public Health Security and Bioterrorism Preparedness and Response Act of 2002, Public Law No. 107–188.
31. 42 C.F.R. Section 489.24(a)(2); 42 C.F.R. Section 1320b-5(g)(1).
32. CMS, Frequently Asked Questions. Available at: cms.gov.
33. New York State Department of Health Allocation of Ventilators in an Influenza Pandemic: Planning Document. Available at: http://www.health.state.ny.us/diseases/communicable/influenza/pandemic/ventilators/. Accessed November 10, 2008.
34. Ibid.
35. *The Times-Picayune*, July 25, 2007.
36. Ibid.
37. Hodge JG, Jr., Lawrence, GO. The Model State Emergency Health Powers Act—A Brief Commentary January 2002, page 3. Available at: http://www.publichealthlaw.net/MSEHPA/Center%20MSEHPA%20Commentary.pdf.
38. Ibid., at 14.
39. Ibid., at 16.
40. Ibid., at 17.
41. Center for Law & the Public's Health. Available at: http://www.publichealthlaw.net/ModelLaws/MSEHPA.php. Accessed November 25, 2008.
42. The Heritage Foundation. Available at: http://www.heritage.org/Research/HomelandSecurity/HL748.cfm. Accessed November 25, 2008.
43. 2009 Joint Commission Hospital Standards, EM. February 1, 2001.

Chapter 5

Developing the Hospital Emergency Management Plan

Nicholas V. Cagliuso, Sr., MPH; Nicole E. Leahy, RN, MPH;

and Marcelo Sandoval, MD

Dedicated to the memory of Neill S. Oster, MD—Physician, Humanitarian, Friend

Photo by Robert Kaufmann/FEMA Photo

Learning Objectives

- Describe the key elements of a hospital emergency management plan.
- Describe how to conduct a hazard vulnerability analysis.
- Describe how to test a hospital emergency management plan.

Introduction

The notion of planning is an elusive, yet necessary, topic for healthcare emergency managers. From a regulatory and accreditation perspective, healthcare institutions must craft documents to ensure compliance with the myriad standards that demonstrate an all-hazards approach to "preparedness." From a practical point of view, healthcare emergency managers work to develop and revise these documents to ensure accuracy. However, many often cite these voluminous plans as the mere "papering" of a process that could be significantly more concise if we expect them to be effective. Somewhere in the middle of this conundrum lies the optimal hospital emergency management plan that satisfies regulatory and accreditation requirements while serving to accurately represent the mitigation, preparedness, response, and recovery efforts of the institution.

The importance therefore of developing a hospital emergency management plan will, by the end of this chapter, become self-evident. As the pivot point upon which all other emergency management efforts rely, the emergency management plan (EMP) serves a number of purposes:

1. Maximize the hospital's ability to provide and sustain core services in a safe environment for all staff, patients, visitors, and the community.
2. Achieve expected actions by key stakeholders (e.g., staff) before, during, and after emergency incidents.
3. Provide explicit guidance for key stakeholders to follow before, during, and after an emergency incident.

Ultimately, a hospital emergency management plan is a concise, timely set of documents that provide both macro- and micro-level information on the institution's efforts before, during, and after incidents that affect it, regardless of intensity, scope, or duration. Its value lies not only in its comprehensiveness, but also in its flexibility and scalability.

Hazard Vulnerability Analysis

In today's resource-constrained healthcare environment, it is not realistic to plan for every conceivable hazard or eventuality that might befall the institution.[1] As such, hospital emergency managers must use the scarce resources available to them to prioritize their efforts to manage hazards and their associated risks.

In its most basic form, a hazard vulnerability analysis (HVA) is a tool that emergency managers employ to screen for risk and plan for the strategic use of limited resources.[1] Healthcare institutions' complex combinations of equipment and hazardous materials, along with an ever-changing population within, including visitors and patients in varied conditions of physical and mental health, make these sites more susceptible to untoward events.[2]

The first step in conducting an HVA is the identification of potential hazards. This process, which is a field of expertise unto itself, is a logical starting point. Doing so offers hospital emergency managers the chance to identify those hazards that are most likely to occur and that will have the greatest impact, in terms of life and economic costs, should they take place. As the realities of resource limitations (e.g., time, money, and personnel) exist, an HVA helps entities focus their work on those hazards that would be likely to yield the maximum adverse consequences.

Developing the list of potential hazards is best managed through the surveying of key hospital stakeholders. One method is to distribute, via mail or email, a blank HVA table and ask respondents to list all hazards that could impact the hospital. To assist, the hospital emergency manager can suggest that these be divided between natural (e.g., earthquakes, floods), technological (e.g., rail accidents and power failures), and intentional hazards (e.g., terrorism).

Keep in mind that no definitive literature exists as to the optimal manner in which to perform this. A common method is to list various types of emergencies and assign scoring values to each one that reflect its likelihood, its impact, and the institution's readiness for the emergency. For instance, a pandemic avian flu outbreak may be scored as very high impact, low likelihood, and intermediate readiness score. A summation or product of the values then assigns a total score to the hazard (pandemic flu). Other hazards on the HVA will also be scored in a similar manner. This allows numeric comparisons between hazards. As can be surmised, this is a rather arbitrary method that allows much subjectivity in terms of the actual numeric ratings and the validity of the comparisons. However, the strength of this concept is that it does create an organized framework to direct where an institution's emergency management committee's energy and efforts should go. An HVA then lists the mitigation, preparedness, response, and recovery activities necessary for each hazard, with the resultant measures taken to manage each hazard varying for each.

Preparedness Efforts

To effectively manage the full spectrum of emergency incidents that a hospital may face, hospital emergency managers—in collaboration with the institution's emergency management committee (which this chapter discusses later) comprises members of every clinical, operational, and financial department—must develop and maintain a comprehensive, effective emergency management plan.

Hospital emergency preparedness efforts are, by their nature, often contrary to the daily realities of hospital operations. Whereas most hospitals operate on stringent budgets and seek to minimize financial losses on unfilled beds, storing unnecessary perishables (e.g., medications, food, and supplies), and reducing unnecessary staffing in excess of providing essential services, emergency management efforts require just the opposite—an increase in many or all of these limited, often taken-for-granted resources. And given the fact that emergency incidents occur with modest frequency, regardless of scope, intensity, or duration, comprehensive emergency planning is necessary despite the fact that many deem it to draw from, rather than add to, the bottom line.

Some emergency managers erroneously anticipate that in the event of an emergency incident, federal, state, and local resources will be activated to supplement the hospital's ability to respond. As seen time and time again with various incidents, most notably Hurricane Katrina, these outside resources are often significantly delayed and may be too unreliable to effectively be counted upon in emergency planning. While potentially overwhelming to local resources, some incidents may not be large enough to warrant mobilization of resources beyond the immediate response area. The notion that "all disasters are local" can be vouched for by many hospital emergency managers.

The emergency management plan is the core of the hospital's emergency preparedness activities, which the hospital assumes to bolster its capacity and categorize resources that it may employ before, during, and after an emergency incident. Preparedness efforts range from developing a resource inventory and conducting institutionwide emergency management training, drills, and exercises, to leading a hospital emergency management committee.

The Hospital Emergency Management Committee

The hospital's emergency management committee should consist of membership reflective of a broad cross-section of hospital departments, including those clinical, support, operational, and financial units. Qualifications of the committee chairperson should include significant fluency in emergency management principles and practices, familiarity with the ever changing regulatory and accreditation requirements of this complex aspect of healthcare, and organizationally empowered to enact the hospital emergency management plan and recommendations of the committee. Members should represent all hospital areas, including, at a minimum, senior leadership, legal, environmental health, security, laboratory, emergency department, chaplaincy, public affairs, clinical and academic affairs, human resources, occupational health, infection control, engineering, life safety, and housekeeping. Though there is no literature that outlines the optimal makeup of an emergency management committee, inclusion of clinicians from departments such as emergency medicine, surgery, medicine, pediatrics, infectious diseases, and employee health should be strongly considered, given the expertise they can offer. Additionally, members from nursing departments should also sit on this committee to provide their unique views on the challenges they face and potential solutions. Administrative leaders such as the chief executive, medical officers, operating officers, and other senior vice presidents will also provide leadership to the committee and are important to ensure buy-in and support. The importance of their presence is immeasurable and sends a significant message to the entire institution that emergency management is a key facet of the hospitals' daily operations.

The committee should also interface with representatives from local, state, and federal agencies involved in emergency management and public health and become familiar with the plans made by these agencies. Many hospitals will find it imperative to build alliances with local community groups, nongovernment organizations, and other grassroots efforts that are the foundation of neighborhood cohesiveness.

Key responsibilities of the hospital emergency management committee include overseeing and guiding the hospital's mitigation, preparedness, response, and recovery efforts. It is also responsible for carrying out planned drills and exercises that test the hospital's resource and response capabilities. From there, the committee should collaborate to develop and review after-action reports that the institution can use to adjust and improve the emergency management plan. This is similar to the continuous quality improvement (CQI) processes familiar to most administrators. Meetings are held as needed by the institution; however, monthly meetings should be considered feasible and adequate to ensure that changes to the institution's capabilities can be addressed.

Given the limitations of all emergency management plans, the committee should also become familiar with the practical challenges these efforts face and ways to continue operations even if the planning by external agencies falls short or fails. This is not only a sound practice, but it is required by accreditation bodies such as The Joint Commission.

Alliance Building

Collaborative emergency management planning between hospitals and their communities is imperative to ensure that all stakeholders, internal and external to the institution, are aware of and familiar with the hospital's emergency management measures. Examples of entities that hospitals should approach for collaborative planning are local and state departments of health, government emergency management offices, Centers for Disease Control and Prevention (CDC), Federal Emergency Management Agency (FEMA), and the Department of Health and Human Services (HHS).

Most nongovernment community groups have periodic forums that welcome hospital participation and presentations on emergency management and bolster dialogue in areas such as prioritizing local emergencies and response efforts. Often, these forums offer opportunities for various healthcare institutions (primary, acute, and long-term care facilities), government agencies, community organizations, and others to discuss emergency management topics and plans. This may be especially true when planning for large-scale incidents such as tornadoes, earthquakes, and hurricanes, and can prove to be invaluable during training, drills, and exercises. Active participation in these local and regional committees is an essential preparedness function for hospitals.

Integration with the Hospital Incident Command System (HICS)

A key element of a hospital's emergency management efforts is its training in and use of the Incident Command System (ICS). Initially created for use at emergency scenes, ICS has become a model tool for command, control, and coordination of effective emergency response.[3] Although its organization arrangement was originally developed exclusively for fire response, the initial version has been adapted for application to a broad spectrum of incidents that vary in type, size, and complexity, and include natural disasters, hazardous materials incidents, mass gatherings, and terrorist incidents.[4] Specific to hospitals and healthcare organizations, the Hospital Incident Command System (HICS) provides a manageable scope of supervision for all personnel[5] and has been adapted by more than 75% of hospitals surveyed in 2003–2004.[6] Through HICS, a predictable chain of command is established, which although structured, is flexible and adaptable to meet the incident at hand as it evolves, changes scope, and eventually devolves to a state of "normalcy."[5]

In following the principles of HICS, hospital staff is pre-assigned to specific job positions analogous to those of nonhospital-based emergency responders (e.g., police, fire, military agencies). This allows common terminology during interaction with these agencies during incidents. Additionally, there are individual Job Action Sheets for each of the essential leadership positions that detail actions to be taken throughout the phases of the event.

Adopting HICS can be a rather complex undertaking because of the need for staff education on its structure, unfamiliarity with the HICS job titles and roles, and the fact that some job functions are difficult to fill with existing hospital staff. However, adoption of HICS offers numerous benefits that include compliance with regulatory and accreditation requirements, and more importantly, enhancing the ability of individuals to perform essential activities during incidents.

The hospital emergency management plan, therefore, should include all aspects of its flexible, clear, and integrated incident command structure, including relevant organization charts and Job Action Sheets.

Mitigation Measures

As the cornerstone of the healthcare system, the hospital receives the injured, infected, and ill during a major incident.[7] During incidents, healthcare leaders must impart judgment based on the best available data, which is often incomplete, incorrect, or both; remain cognizant of the time-sensitive nature of the issue at hand; and ensure that a well-defined command structure is initiated and remains intact throughout the duration of the incident.[5]

To that end, hospitals must take actions to attempt to lessen the likelihood and impact of hazards. These sustained efforts may be either structural or nonstructural in nature.

Structural efforts include those that the hospital performs through the construction or alteration of the physical environment through engineered solutions. Examples include employing disaster resistant construction, structural modifications (e.g., "hardening"), and detection systems (e.g., radiation monitors at the hospital's portals).

Nonstructural mitigation measures are those that the hospital undertakes by modifying human behaviors or processes. This may include regulatory measures, staff awareness, and education programs.

Typically, mitigation activities are based on a cost-benefit analysis that assesses the costs of both the losses and the necessary action for mitigation against the likelihood of the incident.[8]

The emergency management plan must specify the institution's mitigation efforts and ensure that these elements meld into the other phases of the plan (preparedness, response, and recovery) to ensure a seamless approach.

The Response Phase

Oftentimes, the most visible and well-supported of the emergency management plans' activities are those that fall under the response phase. Despite the significant time and effort that hospitals put into attempting to mitigate and prepare for emergency incidents, reducing the likelihood and consequences of the countless hazards hospitals may face to zero is simply not possible. Consequently, as part of their all-hazards approach to emergency management, hospital emergency managers must spend considerable time strengthening their organization's response capacities.

Efforts here are those taken when an emergency incident occurs and may include providing care to patients, staff, and visitors. The goal is to limit injuries, loss of life, and damage to the physical environment. Regardless of the scale of the incident, the impact on the institution in terms of physical damage, and the volume of patients it may receive, the public's expectations are that hospitals remain safe havens for all. This rather unrealistic expectation yields challenges for all involved in the hospital's emergency management work and is the reason that the concept of surge (either capacity or demand as discussed later in this chapter) remains an important challenge to stakeholders.

Because the response phase is said to commence as soon as the incident is apparent and conclude when leadership declares it over, it is often the most comprehensive of the emergency management plans sections.

Hospital emergency managers must remain mindful of the fact that emergency incidents generate patients with both physical and behavioral effects whose first impulse is to go to the location in their community that relentlessly dedicates itself to helping those in need: the hospital.

Effective information and coordination are key to the response phase, yet are often the weakest aspects of an emergency management plan. The diverse elements that comprise an incident shape the capacity to obtain and disseminate information, which is needed to coordinate response actions.

Thanks to the widespread availability of information via television and the Internet, response is the most visible emergency management function, which helps to bolster support for the work done in this area. However, hospital emergency managers must not rest on these laurels because response remains the only phase other than recovery that we hope to never require. Hopes aside, the ability for stakeholders to perform fundamental response functions will likely be the leading factor that determines the severity of the incident and how quickly those affected can recover.

The Recovery Function

The primary goal of recovery efforts is to restore core service and normal operations. From a hospital planning perspective, the institution's recovery actions and implementation activities for its core financial, human resources, and support services should also be addressed.

Given the significant costs associated with incidents that directly impact hospitals, the recovery section of the emergency management plan should also detail its insurance coverage and include copies of the actual insurance certificates, key contact information for agents, and mechanisms to rapidly access funding.

Because emergency incidents often disrupt vital supply chain processes, it is imperative that alternative means for purchasing goods and services to support the hospital's core services be thoroughly outlined, again, with key contact information readily available. Ultimately, the institution's ability to recover from any incident, be it small or large, internal or external, will be based in large part on the recovery planning steps it has in place and activates postincident.

Surge

U.S. hospitals, and emergency departments in particular, continue to experience increased demand for their services, pushing many to the breaking point, as outlined by the Institute of Medicines' report on the future of emergency care.[9] Because many facilities operate at or beyond maximum capacity on a regular basis, bed capacity must be addressed and surge capacity may be required to accommodate victims of emergency incidents.[10]

While many cite 9/11 as the turning point in hospital emergency management, it is important to point out that the shaping efforts in this field prior to that day continue to have long-standing impacts on hospitals' approaches to surge capacity.[5,11] The goal of hospital surge capacity planning relates back to basic economic principles, namely resource allocation.[5] To that end, emergency managers develop a series of prepositioned processes to ensure the delivery of appropriate care with appropriate resources in a graded, phased response.[11]

Important scarce resources that emergency managers work to identify to assist in managing hospital surge are alternative care facilities, which include "locations, preexisting or created, that serve to expand the capacity of a hospital or community to accommodate or care for the patients or to protect the general population from infected individuals during mass casualty events."[12]

Further, to ensure compliance with The Joint Commission emergency management standards, hospitals must demonstrate the ability to handle scheduling, triage, assessment, treatment, admission, transfer, discharge, and evacuation elements for both incoming patients and those that are already in the hospital. The activities associated with planning for a large, unexpected influx of patients involve two main components: rapid patient discharge and increasing inpatient bed capacity.

To ensure that the hospital can safely and rapidly discharge patients to make way for those with more urgent clinical needs, the hospital emergency management plan should include a section on rapid patient discharge. In it, the hospital outlines its system for the rapid discharge of stable patients and includes a real-time assessment of individual patients by the clinical staff present in the hospital. This may serve as a departure from usual operating procedures that may require that the patient's private physician provide discharge approval. During emergency incidents however, rapid patient discharge plans would allow those physicians already present in the hospital to discharge patients. Nursing and social work departments would partner with the physician staff to assess the patient's psychosocial status to determine if discharge is safe, adequate, and appropriate. The participating departments would then contact families, significant others, and appropriate medical and/or community agencies to ensure a safe discharge and procurement of follow-up care as necessary.

While there are significant benefits to employing a rapid patient discharge process, numerous pitfalls exist as well. Central to the success of any such measures is that the hospital's emergency management committee thoroughly outlines, trains, tests, and exercises with relevant staff the elements of performing a rapid patient discharge and that the institution's emergency management plan documents necessary components.

The second element of managing hospital surge is increasing inpatient bed capacity. Attempts to do so are crucial to a hospital's ability to manage an emergency incident and emergency management plans should specify the actions necessary to cancel elective surgeries and admission to the hospital. While often a difficult decision given the ensuing loss of revenue, hospital leadership must remain aware that their entity's primary mission is to provide care to the most gravely sick and that ethical, not financial, decisions must drive their choices, especially during crises.

Other strategies to increase bed capacity involve converting those rooms that are holding one or two patients into areas that can accommodate three or four patients. The creation of such surge beds can be accomplished by converting ambulatory patient care areas (e.g., presurgical holding areas) to inpatient care areas, and nonpatient care areas into triage or holding areas. Closed units should be opened and those areas that the hospital decants because of cancellations of aforementioned elective procedures and admissions (e.g., cardiac catheterization holding areas, ambulatory surgery recovery rooms) can be utilized for incoming patients.

Further, the hospital emergency management plan should list nontraditional spaces (e.g., hallways, auditoriums, solariums, visitor waiting areas) and the mechanisms necessary to convert such areas for patient care use.

Finding dormant space contiguous with the hospital for use during an emergency incident may be challenging for many hospitals, given that many institutions battle spatial limitations during day-to-day operations. Consideration should be given to utilization of outpatient clinics, specialty care hospitals/practices, and nearby physician's offices as emergency department-like space for less severely ill or injured victims. Planning for this may include converting specialty institutions (e.g., cardiac, ophthalmology, orthopedic institutes) into space for treatment of emergency incident victims and would often require written agreements (e.g., memoranda of understanding) that detail the specifics of such arrangements.

Other off-site facilities may include skilled nursing/chronic care/inpatient rehabilitation facilities, religious/community/recreation centers, public buildings, schools/education complexes, hotels/motels, and ambulatory care sites.[10] Coordination of such resources requires pre-planning by both the hospitals and the partnering sites and includes elements such as community and public health system coordination to address logistics of patient awareness of facilities, transportation to and from, staffing, supply availability, and regulatory requirements. Further, emergency managers should consider the creation of mutual aid agreements between the hospital and these facilities to specify the details of the arrangement.

Regardless of the strategy the hospital employs, it is important to ensure that processes for triage account for limitations that these ad hoc spaces may have in terms of allowing care for more seriously ill patients. These spaces may not have sufficient oxygen/medical gas systems, electrical power, lighting, cooling, sanitation, or water systems as usual hospital spaces and the hospital emergency management plan should make note of such realities.

Staffing

The current state of the U.S. healthcare system, with its widespread staffing shortages, namely in the field of nursing, negatively impacts hospital emergency management efforts.[5] Moreover, the supply of healthcare professionals does not meet the demand for even basic healthcare services, so the idea of surge capacity, particularly in light of nursing resources, may be challenging to address.[5] With decreasing rates of experienced staff and increasing turnover, the seasoned clinicians that we have come to rely upon as our first line of care, particularly during emergency incidents, are nonexistent.[5] Alternatively, healthcare providers may also act in dual public safety capacities within the community (e.g., hospital-based first responders may also be volunteer firefighters within the community), thus limiting these staff's abilities to respond in both capacities simultaneously. Consequently, emergency managers responsible for developing their institution's emergency management plan must ensure that issues of staff availability be paramount and accurately reflect the true capabilities of their resources.

Compounding these already weighty challenges, emergency incidents will affect many hospital staff members' willingness to remain at and report for work. During these times, concerns for themselves, their families, and the confidence they have in their own abilities to provide care during times of crisis pervade.[5] Emergency incidents may also hamper staff's abilities to physically report to their hospital, given impacts on transportation systems and personal obligations such as caring for children, elders, and pets.[5] Institutions must realize that employees prepared on the individual level are better able to help themselves, and therefore, others.[5] Hospital emergency managers, with support of senior leaders, should encourage the utilization of personal preparedness resources that include checklists for food, water, medications, and financial records, and suggestions for pediatric and geriatric preparedness. These valuable resources will assist healthcare leaders in ensuring that the notion of emergency management takes roots at home.[5]

It is imperative, therefore, that the hospital emergency management plan addresses the challenges of staffing during crises and that the emergency management committee collaborate with staff to ensure the highest levels of service provision throughout the duration of any incident.

STAFF ROLES AND RESPONSIBILITIES

Because many hospital leaders are members of or represented on the emergency management committee, they will often be well-versed in emergency procedures. However, it is possible that some may be thrust into the role of leading an essential aspect of the emergency incident without having sufficient training or practical experience. This is most likely to occur when leadership staff may be at home and managers with less emergency management experience may be on duty. Ideally, emergency managers should work to ensure that staff members who could potentially undertake a HICS role are trained in advance and familiar with the relevant Job Action Sheets.

CREDENTIALING

It has been shown that well-meaning volunteers will come to hospitals during crises to offer assistance. Hospital emergency management plans must address the means to screen and place volunteers. Some plans may call for volunteers to register in advance, so that in case of an emergency incident, they will already be conversant with the facility's emergency management plan.

To address the accreditation issues in this area, The Joint Commission requires that hospitals have procedures in place to rapidly credential volunteer health personnel. Some states issue healthcare provider identification cards that verify an individual's professional status. However, this does not ensure that a presenting volunteer provider maintains the required license and insurance to practice nor is familiar with the basic elements of emergency management.

Stockpiling and Logistics

The ability for a healthcare institution to remain self-sufficient to provide and sustain core services without the support of external assistance for at least 96 hours from the inception of an incident, with a goal of seven days, remains a vexing problem for healthcare leaders.[5]

Unfortunately, the stark realities of lean organizations and just-in-time inventory management are directly counter to effective hospital emergency management planning. While these efforts seek to reduce costs and waste through the delivery of products on an as-needed basis, thin supply chains can lead to shortages of critical material resources such as pharmaceuticals, blood products, oxygen masks, disposables, and ventilators when demand for these goods rises sharply.[5] A simple rule of thumb when developing the stockpiling and logistics section of the hospital emergency management plan is, "If a resource is not accessible by foot, it does not exist."[5]

RESOURCE INVENTORIES

Hospital emergency management plans must include documentation and tracking of equipment, supplies, and resources. These inventories should include medical, nonmedical (e.g., food, linen, water, fuel for generators, and transportation vehicles), personal protective equipment, and pharmaceutical supplies. The emergency management plan must detail means for replenishing these critical assets and most hospitals will find Memoranda of Understanding (MOU) with their supply vendors for use during emergency incidents to be invaluable.

The challenge, however, is that in densely populated areas, a relatively small pool of vendors will have such agreements with a disproportionately large number of hospitals. Though this may work if an emergency incident is localized to a small geographic area and affects only a handful of hospitals, larger incidents would make these agreements likely to fail as a result of the overwhelming demand on the vendors. The same is true of agreements with transportation and ambulance companies. Additionally, vendors who are geographically removed from the site of an incident may not be able to get supplies to the beleaguered institutions because of impacted transportation infrastructure.

Emergency managers must be aware of these limitations to the MOUs. In large-scale events, it is likely that regional or state authorities will take over the distribution of supplies and vehicles. Regardless, alternative MOUs with local suppliers who may not be the usual vendor to a hospital would be a wise move.

Many different methods exist as to what and how to track hospital resources, and such methods should be a core component of the hospital's standard operating procedures. During emergency incidents, tracking the usage and arrival of items becomes challenging. Standard tracking may not be done in real time, but at periodic intervals based on projected and historical usage patterns. Automated real-time computer bar code scanning systems are superior and helpful as long as power and computer infrastructure remain intact. If not, manual systems need to be in place to track adjustments in usage based on the emergency. Regardless of the means the hospital uses to carry out these functions, the emergency management plan should detail the options available to ensure that resource inventories remain accurate.

Another source of resources is neighboring or affiliated hospitals, or hospitals distant from the affected area. Again, MOUs set up in advance give hospitals an advantage in situations where they may be challenged to maintain adequate supplies. These MOUs should also establish methods and timetables for repayment after the emergency incident has been secured.

In the case of pharmaceuticals, some hospitals choose to keep stockpiled caches of commonly used drugs for use in certain emergency incidents. Antibiotics such as ciprofloxacin, doxycycline, bronchodilator drugs, anticholinergic, and cyanide poisoning antidotes may be kept in reserve and used for nonemergency indications before they expire, as long as they are replaced by newer stock when consumed. The hospital emergency management plan should contain a section on pharmaceutical stockpiles and the emergency management committee must have regular, engaged participation by pharmacy leadership to ensure accuracy.

INSTITUTION SELF-SUSTAINABILITY

From an accreditation standpoint, The Joint Commission requires hospitals to be able to plan for events that require it to remain self-sufficient for at least 96 hours. Doing so requires these institutions' key stakeholders to understand and recognize the limitations of its resources, assets, utility systems, and supply chain. Emergency managers must document these assessments and methods in the emergency management plan to describe the means for rationing limited resources to decrease usage in emergency incidents.

Accreditation Issues—The Joint Commission

The Joint Commission is the primary credentialing group for hospitals in the United States and directly addresses emergency management in its accreditation processes. While accreditation programs can improve overall quality, the costs involved in seeking accreditation may overshadow the increases in revenues. Consequently, emergency management activities often compete for resources, making their implementation even less likely.[5] However, The Joint Commission created a separate chapter on emergency management effective January, 2009, so hospital leaders are now facing the need to address emergency management issues in the same light as other, more traditional healthcare activities, such as hand hygiene. The hope is that this increasing attention will move emergency management to the forefront of healthcare leaders' daily agendas to the point where emergency management truly becomes an expansion of day-to-day operations and covers the gamut of potential hazards that institutions may face.

Regardless, hospitals seeking The Joint Commission accreditation would do well to frame their entire emergency management program, particularly the development of the emergency management plan, around The Joint Commission's standards. While complex, the standards offer a comprehensive framework to build an emergency management plan and details individual elements of performance.

NOTIFICATIONS AND COMMUNICATIONS

Notification and communications are typically the first and most significant aspect of emergency management efforts to suffer during emergency incidents. Following Hurricane Katrina, communication between institutions was severed, leading to days on end when individual hospitals could not ascertain whether nearby institutions were functional or engage in dialogue about sharing resources. The most common daily communication systems, telephone land lines and cellular communications, are frequently incapacitated in the early phases of an emergency incident. Therefore, robust and redundant alternative communication systems are desirable and the hospital emergency management plan must address the resources available to support these systems and the plans for enacting them.

Moreover, interoperability with systems used by other hospitals and community agencies should be considered as the elemental form of communicating. Of course, coordinating such systems requires advance dialogue with the relevant external community emergency management agencies and, oftentimes, shared funding responsibilities. Technologies that may be used include two way radios and base stations, SMS (text messaging) systems, satellite phone systems, and Internet platforms such as email and chat rooms. The funds required for this would most likely be considered as a capital investment that hospitals would be wise to make in regards to planning. Here, the endorsement of hospital senior leadership, the hospital emergency management committee, and communications experts is vital to ensuring that adequate, appropriately suited systems are used. Again, whatever decisions are made, the emergency management plan should serve as the primary reference source for information.

UTILITIES

Given the expectation that hospitals will provide services to those in need regardless of the impact an incident has on the facility's utility systems, the hospital emergency management plan must outline alternative means of providing for the myriad utilities required to operate the institution.

Ensuring that basic electric services are provided is often best handled through the use of emergency generators. The specifics of these devices, which vary in size, capability, and cost, will often be outlined by local building codes and regulations, which can be invaluable to hospitals. However, with their functionality come significant support requirements. The hospital emergency management plan must detail the specifics of the generator's monthly maintenance activities, locations, specifications, capacities, and possibility most importantly, sources for fuel. Emergency managers should take note of the generator's physical location, particularly during weather or geographic emergencies that can compromise their function (e.g., flooding if in basements, extreme heat or cold, or high winds if on rooftops).

Water needed for consumption and essential care activities is a taken-for-granted resource, the consumption volumes of which, when calculated, are staggering. Many hospitals maintain a cache of bottled water for consumption using the baseline metric of three bottles per person per day. Water needed for equipment and sanitary purposes presents additional challenges. The hospital emergency management plan should assist by providing the limits of the facility's water storage tanks. Emergency managers should prepare by limiting the usage of water-consuming equipment, noting that air conditioning and refrigeration chillers require most of this. Sanitary needs may in large part be satisfied by judicious use of cloth wipes, alcohol gels, or sponge bathing when water is necessary, and use of bedpans and urinals instead of toilets for human waste. Again, the emergency management plan should contain sections on means to provide these services, either with limited water supplies or significant restrictions on the use of water.

FACILITY EVACUATION

Evacuating a hospital is an extremely complex action that requires much advance planning. Because it is so difficult, it should be reserved for the direst circumstances when the hospital environment cannot support basic care services. Immediate evacuation, such as in a fire, will usually involve a relatively limited number of the hospital patients and staff, and transfers to specific units. Staff on individual units should be aware of fire escape routes. All staff, clinical and nonclinical alike, must be trained in the principles of evacuation. In an incident where time is limited, ambulatory patients should be moved first with minimal guidance from staff. The greatest efforts should be directed to rapid transport of patients who must remain prone and life-support dependent patients. Several commercially available evacuation aids, such as Skeds, stair chairs, infant carriers, and Evacusleds, are available and should be kept for such occasions. However, common hospital resources such as wheelchairs, stretchers, blankets, and isolettes should also be considered for use during rapid evacuations. The hospital emergency management plan should list the methods used to evacuate people and inventories of the resources and related equipment and supplies also needed to be evacuated.

When time is less pressing, but evacuation is still necessary, hospitals may be required to transport not only the patients, but also the patient's related, relevant medical information and necessary supportive equipment. If evacuation to a distant alternative care site is warranted, hospital staff may be required to accompany patients to the new site and aid in their care.

Triage systems that are usually used for influx will be reversed for evacuation. The least sick will likely move first, and those who need the most care will likely move later. Staging areas should be developed ahead of time to house the patients awaiting vehicles for transportation to an alternative facility. Ambulatory patients may wait in large spaces, such as those atriums, cafeterias, and auditoriums designated as emergency alternative care sites. Sicker patients would have to be transported to a staging area on the ground floor that has the capability to supply care to the critically ill. In most hospitals this means the emergency room.

SAFETY AND SECURITY

Maintaining order is a significant challenge during emergency incidents. Most hospitals do not have enough security staff to handle the chaos and uncertainty that even a moderately sized emergency incident would bring to patients, staff, visitors, and the community. Large natural disasters, such as Hurricane Katrina, demonstrate the potential to break down societal law and order, with few hospital security staff being appropriately trained and equipped to handle such incidents.

Because hospitals are responsible for controlling traffic accessing their facility during emergency incidents, establishing physical barriers becomes even more important. Strategically placed barriers may be more effective than a score of security staff and less labor intensive. Measures such as this would free up security personnel to enforce gatekeeping entrance points and monitor the movements of individuals within the facility itself. Visitor policies would be more strictly enforced and names of visitors should be recorded. Even hospital employee movements may have to be restricted.

Hospital security leadership, as members of the emergency management committee, need to have an ongoing relationship with community security agencies (e.g., police, sheriff, and National Guard). Some community law enforcement agencies will hold periodic meetings with hospital security representatives in order to prepare for potential incidents.

Some hospital emergency management plans allow only certain staff in possession of readily identifiable items such as vests, armbands, and hats access to restricted patient care areas. The specifics should be discussed during the emergency management committee meetings, vetted with appropriate stakeholders, including local law enforcement entities, and be an integral part of the emergency management plan.

CLINICAL AND SUPPORT ACTIVITIES

Because emergency incidents often create patients that bypass on-site triage, prehospital care, and decontamination stations, proceeding directly to hospitals, hospital emergency management plans must address the core clinical and support activities that provide for the emergent care of ambulatory patients.

Moreover, because many patients arrive at hospitals by a variety of nonambulance vehicles (e.g., private cars, police vehicles, buses, taxis, or even on foot), hospital notification of an emergency incident may be from the first arriving patients or the news media, rather than from authorities on the scene. As such, information and updates about incoming casualties are imperfect and incomplete, with the least serious, rather than the most critically injured patients arriving first.

For these reasons, the hospital emergency management plan must delineate processes to manage the vulnerable populations served by the institution, including patients who are pediatric, geriatric, disabled, or have serious chronic conditions. Mental health services should be anticipated as well, with emergency management committees being mindful that up to 80% of patients presenting from emergency incidents, especially intentional terror-related incidents, are psychological casualties.

While many hospitals have sufficient resources to manage a variety of small-scale incidents, many large-scale events will generate patient counts and fatalities that exceed both individual institution and municipal mortuary capacity. Hospitals will need guidance from local health departments in such incidents (e.g., pandemic flu in which hundreds of people may die each day). In particular, victims' bodies will require storage until families can identify and claim the decedents. Plans may include keeping bodies in unused cold rooms, such as operating rooms, or in isolated empty patient care units.

While electronic patient record charting is becoming more and more common and has many advantages, some institutions may prefer to document emergency incidents' charts on paper when patient volume is overwhelming.

UTILIZATION OF OUTPATIENT RESOURCES

Primary care providers will play significant roles in a communitywide emergency incident. These providers are often the first to screen, diagnose, and manage physical and mental health conditions of the "walking wounded" who present or are triaged to community clinics or primary care sites following disasters. These providers also respond to continuing primary care needs of the community. Not only do these providers respond to acute injuries and problems, but they also address chronic conditions and medically unexplained physical symptoms.

Hospitals can facilitate these resources by engaging practitioners in emergency management, specifically by determining how these practitioners can be incorporated into the institution's response.

Community-Based Emergency Management Approach

While all emergency incidents may commence locally, the field of disaster research provides vivid examples of the concentric circles that emanate from the epicenter of an incident location.[5] Moreover, during events of this sort, resources are quickly overcome, making collaboration with internal and external stakeholders (e.g., public health, police, fire, and emergency medical services) likely to take many forms.[5] While many institutions maintain transfer agreements to approve the routine transfer of patients between healthcare facilities during nonemergency times, mutual aid agreements take these alliances a step further, documenting the agreement that institutions have to share resources (e.g., clinicians and supplies) during emergent incidents. The key to success often lies in the intentional vagueness of these documents, so there is significant interpretive latitude with regard to the volume of goods and services that institutions will share, acknowledging that participants will take care of their own needs first and then use any surplus to assist mutual aid partners.[5]

The scope of a hospital's emergency management program depends in part on how likely its leadership believes it will face one,[13] paired with the recognition that emergency incidents repeatedly cut across functional and jurisdictional boundaries, and consequently, require multiorganizational cooperation.[14]

Conclusion

Developing the hospital emergency management plan is an essential element of a hospital's overall, comprehensive emergency management program. The plans should adopt an all-hazards approach to all emergency incidents based upon the institution's hazard vulnerability analysis, from which the emergency management committee can collaborate to develop a core plan. From the core plan, key stakeholders must ensure that hazard-specific annexes and appendices reflect the unique hazards, which are preferably divided into natural, technological, and intentional categories.

After it is developed, the plan must serve as a constant work in progress; a document or collection thereof, of guidance, policies, procedures, and related information that the institution routinely examines for timeliness and accuracy. Key to this is ensuring that the plan serves as the nucleus around which all emergency management training, drills, and exercises revolve.

Prevention, preparedness, and public health are vital to the well-being of families and communities.[15] Through collaborative efforts to develop the hospital emergency management plan, our nation's healthcare system can ensure its readiness and resiliency to address the stark realities we must face.

References

1. Chang JC, Gluckman W, Weinstein ES. Health care facility hazard and vulnerability analysis. In: Ciottone G, Anderson PD, Auf der Heide E, et al, eds. *Disaster Medicine*. 3rd ed. Philadelphia, PA: Mosby Elsevier; 2006:117–123.
2. Pan American Health Organization. *Principles of Disaster Mitigation in Health Facilities*. Washington, DC: Pan American Health Organization; 2000:14–17.
3. Sutingco N. The incident command system. In: Ciottone G, Anderson PD, Auf der Heide E, et al, eds. *Disaster Medicine*. 3rd ed. Philadelphia, PA: Mosby Elsevier; 2006:208–214.
4. Federal Emergency Management Agency. *Emergency Management Institute: Basic Incident Command System Independent Study*, Washington, DC: U.S. Government Printing Office; 2000.
5. Cagliuso NV Sr, Lazar EJ, Lazar AN, Berger LJ. Hospital emergency Preparedness.

In: Pinkowski J, ed. *Disaster Management Handbook*. Boca Raton, FL: CRC Press; 2008:369–385.

6. Niska RW, Burt CW. Training for terrorism-related conditions in hospitals: United States, 2003-04. *Adv Data*. 2006;380:1–8.

7. Chaffee MW, Oster NS. The role of hospitals in disaster. In: Ciottone G, Anderson PD, Auf der Heide E, et al, eds. *Disaster Medicine*. 3rd ed. Philadelphia, PA: Mosby Elsevier; 2006:34–42.

8. Halpern S, Goldberg-Alberts A. Keeping damages to a minimum. *Provider*. 1999;25(7):71–73.

9. Committee on the Future of Emergency Care in the United States Health System, Board on Health Care Services, Institute of Medicine of the National Academies. *Hospital Based Emergency Care: At the Breaking Point*. Washington, DC: The National Academies Press; 2006.

10. Hick JL, Hanfling D, Burstein JL, DeAtley C, Barbisch D, et al. Health care facility and community strategies for patient care surge capacity. *Ann Emerg Med*. 2004;44(3):253–261.

11. Casani JAP, Romanosky, AJ. Surge capacity. In: Ciottone G, Anderson PD, Auf der Heide E, et al, eds. *Disaster Medicine*. 3rd ed. Philadelphia, PA: Mosby Elsevier; 2006:193–202.

12. Lam C, Waldhorn R, Toner E, Inglesby TV, O'Toole T. The prospect of using alternative medical care facilities in an influenza pandemic. *Biosecur Bioterror*. 2006;4(4):384–390.

13. Sternberg, E. Planning for resilience in hospital internal disaster. *Prehosp Disast Med*. 2003;18(4):291–300.

14. Auf der Heide E. *Disaster Response: Principles of Preparation and Coordination*. St. Louis, MO: Mosby; 1989:34–25.

15. Blueprint for a Healthier America: Modernizing the Federal Public Health System to Focus on Prevention and Preparedness. Trust for America's Health, October, 2008.

Chapter 6

Introduction to Exercise Design and Evaluation

Garrett T. Doering, MS, EMT-P, CEM, MEP

Photo by Michael J. Reilly

Learning Objectives

- Describe the process of planning a hospital-based drill or exercise.
- List the eight exercise design steps.
- Discuss how to effectively evaluate a drill or exercise.
- Discuss how a properly executed drill or exercise can assist in the evaluation of a preparedness training program.
- Compare and contrast the different types of drills and/or exercises.
- Discuss the requirements that mandate that hospitals and medical centers conduct drills and exercises.
- Describe the after-action reporting and improvement planning process.

Introduction

Exercises are the most effective means to examine how our institutions would respond to unique, infrequent, but high-impact events. An exercise is used to determine if the plans we have put in place will work. Well-constructed, thought-out plans are the beginning, and include collaboration with all departments and agencies that have a role within the plans. Sharing those plans with appropriate partners is the next step. A thorough hazard vulnerability analysis (HVA), as discussed in Chapter 5, will provide the target types of events and circumstances that our institutions will focus on for exercise efforts. The HVA provides not only the topic of the exercise, but should also provide guidance on how much time and resources should be dedicated to preparing for certain events. In a perfect world with unlimited resources, we would be fully prepared for every conceivable event. Because this is not reality, we must carefully consider those events that are most plausible and concentrate our efforts on our planning process, not on the written plan.

Exercises should be developed in such a fashion that they reinforce the concept that true disasters are both quantitatively and qualitatively different from normal operations. Exercise development **must** focus on the development of general principles and not specific details, because the details will **always** be different between events and exercises. Effective exercise design incorporates the latest social science knowledge that currently moves us away from the command and control models to a much more dispersed decision and action model.

In the aftermath of a real event or a simulated event, when we hear "everything went according to plan" we tend to assume that means everything done during the response was as good as it could have been. That may or may not be a good assumption to make. The assumption does not suggest that the plan was very well written; it suggests that the plan was able to predict the numerous details and the subsequent responses to those details. A difficult task indeed! In this chapter, we are going to discuss how exercises are used to evaluate the assumptions and the plans we make in response to events that have not occurred. Good exercise design, conduct, and evaluation are invaluable components to effective preparedness efforts.

Preparedness efforts need to become an integral part of the hospital culture, much like quality has become part of the culture over the past twenty years. Preparedness and quality have much in common: often talked about, acknowledged as very important, and very difficult to measure. One distinguishing characteristic is that quality efforts in healthcare have a track record going back many years. Initial efforts at creating "quality" benchmarks were met with skepticism, much like preparedness efforts are today.

Background, History, and Current State of the Art

Preparation for emergencies encompasses several key components. The first component is the ability to envision what may occur and the impact that the event will have on your facility and your organization. The typical approach has been to conduct a hazard vulnerability assessment. Hazard vulnerability assessments are discussed in depth in Chapter 5, but it is important to recognize how important HVAs are in the development of exercises. Exercises will be utilized to test the plans, procedures, and resources anticipated in response to those potential scenarios. The mere consideration that an event may occur is the first step in preparation. The consideration will trigger some initial consequence management strategies as well as preparing our minds to accept it as a possibility. We cannot solve problems that we have not accepted as possible. It is also important to consider the potential warning signs that may be associated with particular events.

Scenarios for exercises are generally created from our HVA, in response to an actual incident, or from a preestablished, common platform, such as the California Emergency Medical Services Authority Hospital Incident Command System (HICS). If you are starting a new exercise program, a good source for generating objectives comes from the Universal Task List (UTL) and the Target Capabilities List (TCL). Most objectives are

---

Exhibit 6-1

Universal Exercise Scenarios for Hospitals

External Scenarios

- nuclear detonation—10-kiloton improvised nuclear device
- biological attack—aerosol anthrax
- biological disease outbreak—pandemic influenza
- biological disease outbreak—plague
- chemical attack—blister agent
- chemical attack—toxic industrial chemicals
- chemical attack—nerve agent
- chemical attack—chlorine tank explosion
- natural disaster—major earthquake
- natural disaster—major hurricane
- radiological attack—radiological dispersal device
- explosives attack—improvised explosive device
- biological attack—food contamination
- cyber attack

Internal Scenarios
- bomb threat
- evacuation, complete or partial facility
- fire
- hazardous material spill
- hospital overload
- hostage/barricade
- infant/child abduction
- internal flooding
- loss of heating/ventilation/air conditioning (HVAC)
- loss of power
- loss of water
- severe weather
- work stoppage

FEMA

going to be generated internally. The purchase of new equipment, the integration of new staff, the after-action reports (AARs) from previous exercises, and improvement plans from actual events all provide a rich source of fertile ground for developing scenarios. Exhibit 6-1 lists several universal exercise scenarios for hospitals.

Exercises are also developed to evaluate new resources and equipment, new plans, or new procedures.

Hospitals and healthcare institutions have been conducting various forms of exercises for many years. Fire drills, generator testing, and mass casualty incident preparation are all forms of exercise. The quality of exercises, our expectations from these exercises, the investment we make in exercises, and the results from exercises continue to change and increase.

Exercise designers and planners need to recognize that there is a constant struggle to make disaster and emergency response conform to the plans that we have invested much time and effort in crafting. The true art of exercise design is appreciating the social science aspect of disasters that has repeatedly found that disaster response requires significant creativity and role improvising. Because of the different forms an exercise can take, it can introduce a random, unpredictable element into the response milieu that varies with the magnitude of the event, and it can lead to tensions within organizations that vary with the timeframe over which decisions must be made. Volunteers and others who converge to a disaster site also exhibit creativity in the pursuit of their objectives, which can present both benefits and challenges to emergency managers. This creativity is difficult to measure, and thus is often neglected in exercise development.

Why Exercise?

Organizations conduct exercises to accomplish two very broad goals. Exercising enables staff to learn and practice the roles they are expected to fill during an emergency. Exercising also improves the organization's ability to resolve the emergency. It is important to realize that exercising alone does **not** provide the full range of potential benefits, but benefits are also gained by carefully designing the exercise, evaluating the exercise, and then making changes in response to the exercise findings.

The Federal Emergency Management Agency (FEMA) provides the following reasons to exercise:

- Test and evaluate plans, policies, and procedures.
- Reveal planning weaknesses.
- Reveal gaps in resources.
- Improve organizational coordination and communications.
- Clarify roles and responsibilities.
- Train staff in their anticipated roles and responsibilities.
- Improve individual performance.
- Gain program recognition and support from senior leadership.
- Satisfy regulatory requirements.

The goal is to find and eliminate as many problems as possible prior to an actual event. Planning over time, with due consideration to all reasonable factors, without the stress of an actual emergency will provide a better outcome. It is important to recognize that even with prior planning, not all problems can be eliminated. Acknowledgment and awareness of those challenges is also very important in creating alternate strategies in mitigation and response efforts.

Exercises validate policies, plans, and procedures. Exercises may also be utilized to assess facilities and equipment, training effectiveness, and how well the people perform to expectations.

JOINT COMMISSION REQUIREMENTS

In addition to the preceding reasons, hospitals and healthcare organizations accredited by The Joint Commission must meet various elements of performance for drills and exercises. These are frequently subject to change, so it is important that hospital emergency managers frequently review the emergency preparedness standards and elements of performance established by The Joint Commission. FEMA and Joint Commission requirements focus on learning the plans and enhancing our communication and coordination. What is missing is an emphasis on improving our staff's ability to recognize the most important problems facing them, how to rapidly identify needed information, critically analyze the data, and then collaboratively and effectively utilize the limited resources they have available to them to solve the problem. Gary Klein, in his book *The Power of Intuition*, suggests that challenging a person to make tough judgments, honestly appraising those judgments to learn from the consequences, and actively building up an experience base will lead to better decisions. For example, hospital leaders are very accustomed to trying to make the very best decision possible. They often take in a vast amount of data, analyze it from different perspectives, and then get feedback on the different potential options. In emergencies, we need to think differently. We don't need the best option—we need to quickly identify an acceptable option. There might be a better one, but if it takes hours to find and evaluate, then there is no practical benefit from searching for the optimal course of action. Exercises can help us develop decision-making models that are suitable during an emergency.

Exercise Types

There are two broad categories of exercises: discussion-based and operations-based. As the titles imply, discussion-based exercises require thought, analysis of data, critical decision making, and following policies and procedures, but no movement of staff, supplies, or equipment. Operations-based exercises require people to perform and execute tasks. Exercise design will often bridge the formal recognized exercise types and create hybrids. The exercise type is driven by several factors: time to plan, conduct, and evaluate the exercise; where the organization is in their comprehensive exercise planning cycle; the expertise available to the organization to design the exercises; and a host of other relevant factors we will discuss.

Discussion-based exercises rarely involve "real-time" play; whereas operational exercises often require real-time sequencing. The scope of each category can be a single department within a larger organization or multiple agencies across vast geographic distances. The duration of each category can also be very short (an hour or less) to very long (weeks in duration).

There are simple discussion-based exercises and simple operational exercises, as well as very complex discussion- and operations-based exercises. Generally speaking, discussion-based exercises are simpler to design, conduct, and evaluate. They are also generally less expensive to conduct.

SEMINARS/ORIENTATION

The most common reasons to provide a seminar/orientation exercise are to introduce plans, policies, programs, operating procedures, authorities, response resources, and annexes to new staff. Existing staff may require a seminar/orientation to review changes and the impact of those changes from the aforementioned list. Initial introduction to new equipment and organizations; reviewing roles and responsibilities; building the base for future exercises; and when possible, to motivate people to participate in subsequent exercises are all additional reasons to conduct this type of exercise.

A seminar/orientation often breaks down a strategy or procedure into very easy-to-understand steps. The seminar/orientation will often provide the rationale behind the policy and the procedure that is often lost when reading a new policy or plan for the first time. The rationale will also help to get "buy-in" from the staff impacted by the changes. The facilitator should allow discussion and questions at each discreet step or level and provide clarification.

A seminar or orientation exercise can take several forms. The primary purpose and feature of an orientation is to relay information to a group of participants. A seminar/orientation should be a low-stress event. It resembles a lecture, with one distinguishing characteristic— the participants are encouraged to ask questions and fully comprehend the material. The material presented during these seminars is often the foundation for each of the subsequent types of exercises we are going to discuss. No previous exercise experience or emergency management response function is required to participate.

Seminars and orientation exercises can also be presented in a panel or forum setting. In this format, the moderator or facilitator would guide the discussion points and direct questions from the audience to the appropriate panel member. Each panel member typically has a distinct expertise or role in the material being presented; the panel as a whole supports the objectives of the exercise. A less formal, and sometimes more practical form of seminar, is to conduct the exercise much like a meeting.

Regardless of the format chosen, seminars and orientations are appropriate for all levels of personnel within your organization. However, you will want to choose the format that fits your intended audience the best. For example, providing a lecture to senior hospital administrators may not be as effective as a meeting format. The meeting format can be smaller and can keep them directly engaged in the topic at hand without giving them the opportunity to keep glancing at their Blackberries.

A classroom orientation may be a more appropriate fit if you are trying to provide an orientation to every new employee during their new employee orientation.

The potential impact of the information you are presenting should also be considered when deciding on the format that will be most effective. Is the information "nice to know" and required by some regulatory requirement, but may have little or no impact on the employee's ability to respond appropriately? Or, is the information more important, so it must be understood and retained?

The typical duration for a seminar/orientation is 60 minutes to 3 hours. Accordingly, the amount of staff time required to conduct a seminar is minimal. The typical orientation/seminar requires very little in terms of equipment required. The average seminar requires a conference room with tables and chairs, an LCD projector, a screen, and perhaps a sound system if it is a large room. The amount of preparation required is "minimal," as it relates to the other exercise types, and is led by a presenter or facilitator.

There is no formal evaluation of exercise participants or response in a seminar/orientation. However, there should be a simple and easily completed evaluation of the presenter and the method of delivery for the information. The information presented is not the object of this evaluation. This particular feedback will be utilized to promote better delivery of the material presented. The objective of the seminar/orientation is to relay information to the participant in a fashion the participant finds useful.

Review the following example of a hospital-based orientation/seminar: The Joint Commission has just published the final version of changes to its Emergency Management Survey guidelines and Elements of Performance. It is expected that all participants on the hospital's disaster committee be reasonably aware of what all the elements are, even if they are not directly responsible for all of them. The chair of the committee may want to provide a brief didactic orientation and answer questions clarifying the standards. This would be a good use of an orientation/seminar exercise.

WORKSHOPS

Workshops are often considered the second step in a comprehensive exercise program. This is only partially true as it relates to the exercise program. The primary objective while conducting a workshop is to produce a product. The product is often a draft policy or procedure. During exercise development, the goal of a workshop is to produce exercise objectives, develop scenarios, and define evaluation criteria. A workshop is typically focused on a very narrow topic and the outcome of the workshop must be clearly defined. This is a working meeting.

The individuals selected to attend the meeting should be carefully considered. The number of people in the room should not exceed 10 participants. The experience and background of the participants is very important to consider. You need to develop plans or strategies that will be acceptable to your organization in terms of cost, resource allocation, etc. The participants must have a working knowledge of the topic, and the authority to implement the resulting plans and procedures.

There is no sense in developing "perfect" plans that cannot be implemented because the resources are not there to support them.

A workshop needs a facilitator to be effective. The facilitator can be a member of the team or an outsider. An outside person brings some advantages. We have all been in meetings and workgroups where one or two people dominate the discussion. The challenge is to get input and collaboration from the other eight people, whom you selected based on their expertise. Prior to the workshop, an agenda needs to be circulated to all participants. The ground rules need to be established for the meeting and any reference material that is appropriate to the meeting's objective should be distributed to all participants in sufficient time for them to review the material prior to the workshop.

The cost of conducting a workshop is primarily driven by the cost of the salaries of the people you invited to participate. Otherwise, the only costs are the incidentals of meeting supplies. One note to consider: interactive whiteboards are a valuable asset in this setting. As the group brainstorms, ideas are written on the whiteboard for all to see, discuss, and dissect. All too often, the material is erased or forgotten to make room for additional conversation. The interactive whiteboard technology enables you to print what is on the board and to save a "photocopy" image of the whiteboard to a computer file for later distribution. All participants can focus on the content of the conversation while the facilitator takes the notes, and no one needs to worry about missing what was written on the board.

An example of a hospital-based workshop would be how a facility could maximize its generator capacity during an electric utility failure. For the sake of illustration, imagine a hospital that is fully supported by generators. Under normal circumstances, the facility operates the same on generator power as it does on utility power. The on-site fuel tanks have enough capacity to support the generators running at full capacity for 48 hours. The purpose of this workshop is to determine how to extend the operating life of the generators for essential services to 96 hours **without** increasing fuel storage capacity.

The initial participants would be the plant operators and electricians. However, when their discussions turn to "shedding load," it will have a direct impact on operations. The first targets of shedding will be elevators, air conditioners, CT scans, etc. How can operations change to meet the stated goal of providing essential services for 96 hours while on generator power? All major departments within the facility will need to participate at some point, but not necessarily all at the same time. For example, if it is decided that elevator usage will be reduced from five to three hours of dedicated time, what is the impact on diagnostic testing, food services, housekeeping, etc? The desired product at the end of this exercise is a draft procedure that has been reviewed and vetted by appropriate key staff.

TABLETOP EXERCISES

Tabletop exercises (TTXs) are the most common exercises in use today. They are discussion-based exercises that are designed to place little or no stress on the participants, including time pressures. They are designed to evaluate existing or potential Emergency Operations Plans and procedures based on a hypothetical scenario in an informal setting. They can also be utilized to clarify roles, responsibilities, coordination, and integration. The typical participants include policy-level and management personnel, who simulate discussion and decisions based on a presented scenario. Often, TTXs include representatives from multiple agencies and/or jurisdictions who do not work together very often, or the TTXs examine a particular scenario that may expect the participants to interact. TTXs are an excellent modality to facilitate understanding of concepts, strengths, and shortfalls, and achieving a change in approach to a particular situation.

The informal, comfortable environment is conducive to discussing complex issues in depth and to developing or reinforcing key decisions in a slow-paced collegial atmosphere rather then the very hasty, stressful, and spontaneous decision making that is bound to occur during a real event. Tabletop exercises can range from fairly simple to challenging. In all cases, a facilitator introduces the group to the scenario through a combination of means—PowerPoint presentations, video clips, audio recordings, etc. The scenario presented by the facilitator "sets the stage" and gives all the participants the relevant facts they need to get started. An effective strategy to employ when developing a TTX is to present a case study that may have happened to a similar institution in the past. This has two benefits—it takes away the "that will never happen" philosophy that some participants may want to express, and it provides some actual feedback on decisions made and outcomes achieved.

The facilitator ends his presentation of the scenario with a problem to be addressed by the group. In a simple TTX, the group applies their collective skills and experience to the problem. It is typically conducted in one large room and all participants partake in the same problem at the same time. There are no small group discussions. The facilitator summarizes the solutions presented.

The more complex TTXs involve the delivery of injects to participants. The injects are messages designed to elicit a specific response that was designed into the exercise during the formation of the exercise objectives. The injects are useful to keep the group focused on the exercise while new challenges are presented to them. The best injects are those that anticipate the group's decisions and provide feedback on the group's earlier decisions. The injects are a stimulus and the group's decision is the response.

Another common feature of a more complex tabletop exercise is to divide the group into functional areas of responsibility. Injects are presented to the smaller groups for them to discuss and to solve. At predetermined intervals, each group reports their progress and their decisions to the larger group. The decisions of the smaller groups can then be used by the other small groups to continue "working the problem."

Tabletop exercises work very well to determine how effectively the group is applying established plans and policies to the scenario, how well the participants share information, how the group solves problems as a team, how well interagency/interdepartment participants coordinate, and how familiar senior officials are with their responsibilities.

One key aspect of tabletop exercises is to determine how different people in the group use different perspectives to interpret the same message. One example of the same message being interpreted in two very different ways is evident in the following example that is more urban legend then real event (at least I hope so). The story goes like this. During a recent large-scale disaster, the local law enforcement officers requested assistance from a U.S. Army National Guard unit. The scenario was that a wanted fugitive was hiding out in an abandoned house. The local law enforcement officers planned to approach the house very quietly, burst through the door, and apprehend the suspected criminal during the confusion. The National Guard unit was assigned the mission of providing perimeter security, to ensure that no one entered a potentially dangerous area and no one escaped out the doors and windows while the police were going in the front door. Just as the police squad's commanding officer was about to commence his stealth approach to the house, he requested the commanding officer of the National Guard unit to "cover me." The difference in the meaning "cover me" became evident very quickly.

In the world of law enforcement, "cover me" means personnel should take a protected position and be ready to return hostile fire if needed. In the military world, "cover me" means to begin heavy firing in the direction of the enemy, so the enemy keeps his head down and does not have the ability to aim his weapon and shoot at you. Fortunately, no harm came to anyone in this event.

There are several advantages to conducting tabletop exercises over other types of exercises. A TTX requires only a modest commitment in terms of time, cost, and resources. It is effective in reviewing plans, policies, and procedures. The disadvantages are that there is no sense of realism, and the review of plans and policies is superficial. The skill and expertise of the facilitator is the single most important component to a successful tabletop exercise. The facilitator must be familiar with the agency's policies and procedures as well as have the ability to ask relevant questions to the group. An entry-level employee is not likely to succeed in this position because senior officials have to be asked questions they may not be at ease answering in a fashion that does not make anyone uncomfortable. It is a difficult skill.

The success of a tabletop exercise is determined by the feedback from participants and the impact the feedback has on the evaluation and revision of existing plans and procedures. The participants in a tabletop exercise are rarely the ones who draft the plans and policies, but are the ones responsible for approving them or making sure they are implemented. At the end of the TTX, all participants should know if the plan makes sense. Will we follow the plan given this scenario? What do we have to change?

The best location to conduct a tabletop exercise is in the same room where your organization would be addressing the problem presented in the scenario. The setting provides a more realistic feel and any needed supporting material or data should be readily accessible to the participants. If this option is not available, any conference room where the tables can be rearranged into a U-shaped layout is acceptable. Materials that will be needed to make appropriate decisions should be made readily available—maps, plans, reference books, etc.

Tabletop exercises are the first in the exercise sequence that may begin to serve a duel role—testing and educating simultaneously. Individuals are not tested during a TTX, but plans and policies certainly are. Individuals will learn several key lessons during an exercise such as how well they understand the plan being tested, how other individuals they interact with will react during a given scenario, and lastly, what those same individuals will expect of that participant given a similar scenario.

DECISION MAKING EXERCISES

A decision making exercise (DMX) does not fit with the traditional exercise format. Rather than focus training on the specifications and capabilities of new plans, policies, and technologies, a DMX provides participants with scenarios that force them to resolve ambiguous or contradictory information from multiple sources, fuse disparate sources of information, filter information, and manage limited resources.

The participant must make a series of decisions that ultimately affect how the story plays out. The consequences and feedback are predicated not just on the alternative chosen, but on the information sources used to make the decision. Thus, emphasis is placed on the student's ability to collect and use information.

Decision making exercises should be easy to play, technologically easy, simple, flexible, and adaptable. They should be able to be played in the lunchroom, in the backseat of a car, or even on a plane ride. Generally, each exercise will have a name, some detailed background information, and a scenario that combine to create a compelling story that builds to a climax and a dilemma.

The dilemma must place the participant into a position where the participant knows he or she has to make a decision. The crux of developing a DMX is finding a scenario that has more than one right answer, because then the motivation is to find the "right" answer. This is the key difference between a TTX and a DMX—a TTX prompts the participants to react according to a plan. A DMX prompts the participant to evaluate the information and make a decision with less-than-perfect information—the goal is to trigger the decision-making process. This process will be described in greater detail later in this chapter.

In this example of a DMX, you are the senior hospital administrator on duty during an unusually heavy rain event. The river near your hospital has crested its banks. After several hours of sandbagging efforts, the river overtops the sandbags and begins to flood the hospital basement, which contains all the typical mechanical equipment and a generator. The National Weather Service anticipates continued rain for the next several hours. The local emergency management officials supplement your sump pumps with two heavy-duty pumps. The water continues to rise for the next hour. The water level is just below the point where you must disconnect from both utility and generator power, and the hospital will be totally without power of any kind. You have already requested that EMS not bring any additional patients to your hospital. You have stabilized all critical patients and no surgeries are expected. Here is your dilemma—if the water continues to rise another few inches, you will be forced to evacuate your hospital in the dark with no elevators. If you evacuate now, you have lights, elevators, printers, fax machines, and information services available to you. What do you do?

GAMES

Games are the newest type of exercise to enter the realm of preparedness efforts. Games often involve multiple teams trying to "win." The competitive nature of games stimulates a small degree of stress in the participants. The competition can be between networked teams competing against each other at the same time, or two teams competing against each other by trying to achieve the highest score. Technology has enabled the game designer to provide realistic settings, customize rules and procedures, identify resources that may be available, and determine realistic time estimates on how to acquire those resources.

The amount of effort required to build an effective game is very high. The number of times it can be played is limitless and subtle changes can keep the variety of the decisions to be made very realistic. Games can provide instant feedback on the quality of decisions that are made. It is also fairly easy to demonstrate a player's improvement over time. Like all exercises, the quality of the game is dependent on the exercise design team and how well they approximate real-life circumstances.

DRILLS

Prior to providing the formal definition of what constitutes a drill, it is important to clarify one important fact: a drill is a type of an exercise, but not all exercises are drills. For many years, these two terms have been used interchangeably, and both terms are sometimes still used today. They are closely related, but they are not synonymous.

A drill is the simplest of the operations-based exercises. It is a demonstration of a single operation or procedure in a supervised setting. It provides the opportunity for the participants to demonstrate their performance of a skill in an isolated environment. A drill should be designed so that the evaluator can provide immediate feedback to the participants, so that it is also a teaching and learning opportunity. A drill is limited to occurring within a single department or agency.

Drills can occur at any time, with little preparation required, in almost any location, and can be very simple. Drills are appropriate to all levels of staff and are typically low-cost events. Some drills can be spontaneous—a unit manager may request a staff member to demonstrate the proper use of an evacuation chair immediately following a false fire alarm. Doffing and donning appropriate personal protective equipment is a single operation that, in real life, would be part of a much larger mass patient decontamination event. This may seem like a simple exercise, but the amount of time, the amount of space, the little things required, and the extra staff required to be on hand cannot be fully understood by all participants until practiced.

Another example of a hospital drill would be to activate the off-duty emergency notification process. Every hospital has some process to notify off-duty staff of an event that requires their participation. A communication notification drill would be a test to evaluate if everyone who is designated to be notified receives a message and how long it takes to accomplish the task. These are also good exercises to demonstrate performance improvements in emergency management.

FUNCTIONAL EXERCISES

A functional exercise is an interactive scenario-based execution of specific tasks or more complex activity within a functional area of an Emergency

Operations Plan. Functional exercises are typically conducted with increasing levels of stress and constraints that are designed to improve realism. Participants must complete expected tasks, especially communication skills that require collaboration, cooperation, and interactive decision making. A functional exercise will clearly demonstrate the effectiveness of interdepartment or interjurisdiction relationships and how well communication crosses those perceived boundaries.

The target audience for the typical functional exercise is the personnel that would staff an emergency operations center or other central coordinating point that requires receiving and soliciting information from different sources utilizing different modes (dispatch center, command center, incident command post, etc.). The common staffing models for these areas usually involve a combination of policy-level staff and senior operations officials. Within an Incident Command System, the staffs of the direction and control branches are well suited for functional exercises.

A functional exercise can be utilized to evaluate an individual's competencies, but is much better suited to evaluate system performance. It is the sum of all the parts, the interactions, the collaboration, the sharing of information, or the absence of such, that often drives the success or failure of real and simulated events. Every organization has strong and weak players. The successful teams recognize this and develop strategies to compensate for this normal occurrence. The successful resolution to a disaster is a team effort, and should be evaluated as such.

A functional exercise is often considered the most difficult to design and conduct from an exercise design team's perspective. The exercise is typically lengthy and challenging, and requires careful scripting and detailed planning. The design team must anticipate and become everyone the participants would normally interact with in their scenarios. A functional exercise is also very difficult to evaluate for the very same reasons. It requires multiple evaluators, who also must talk to each other to understand the dynamics of the event.

A functional exercise requires much more time and effort to produce. It requires the use of controllers, players, simulators, and evaluators. Each of these categories requires some specific level of training to fulfill the desired role. Players respond to a series of realistic messages given to them by the simulators. The messages reflect a series of ongoing events and challenges. The players' decisions are made in real time and generate additional responses from the other players and simulators. There is no actual movement of personnel or equipment during a functional exercise. There are a lot of phone calls, radio traffic, breaking news television reports, intense conversations, and noise.

FULL-SCALE EXERCISES

A full-scale exercise (FSX) is the apex of the exercise cycle. It is the dress rehearsal for the real event. An FSX is the most complex type of exercise because it is interactive, and it will involve multiple agencies, multiple departments within each agency, and multiple jurisdictions. The objective of the FSX is to validate the plans, procedures, and most importantly, the cooperative agreements and communications between agencies that do not work together on a daily basis. A full-scale exercise should integrate the products and lessons produced or learned during the previous discussion- and operations-based exercises. It is the coordinated effort we hope to see during a real event.

A full-scale exercise should produce the highest level of stress in the participants. It must be designed to require rapid decision making to resolve complex and realistic problems. The injects presented must allow the participants to adhere to their response doctrine as it currently exists. An FSX achieves realism through the utilization of moulage applied to actors, who have been coached to act their parts; the participants' equipment; and communication devices. The scene should be staged to look and feel like a real event. An FSX involves players from all levels of the organization, playing the roles they would likely fill. The single most important aspect of any FSX is the critical analysis of community linkages.

The level of expertise to design, conduct, and evaluate a full-scale exercise is very high. It is very common to conduct a full-scale field-based exercise with a command-based functional exercise. This permits all elements to interact as they would during a real event. Exercise events occur in real time, and most response functions occur in real time. Participant safety must be everyone's priority. An FSX permits you the ability to promote your preparedness efforts to many people in and out of the organization and promotes awareness that the participating organizations are proactive to potential crisis.

The most common hospital full-scale exercise is the multiple casualty incident, or MCI. This type of event is practiced by all hospitals, regardless of size or trauma designation. There are a few obvious items to consider: How is the hospital notified? How does the hospital activate its internal MCI or surge plan? How well does the hospital notify its on-duty and off-duty staff that an event has occurred? From housekeeping to operating staff to senior administrators, do **all** departments in the hospital understand their roles and responsibilities during such an event? Because there are so many possible things to focus on during an FSX, it is important to appreciate those things that do **not** need to be tested. For example, EMS agencies from multiple jurisdictions routinely speak to the regional trauma center emergency department. There would be no need to test this component during an FSX.

Developing a Comprehensive Exercise Program Plan

ESTABLISH THE FOUNDATION

To achieve the most out of each exercise, exercises need to be part of a larger, more comprehensive progressive exercise program with widely-known accepted goals and objectives to be achieved. The program needs to have established long-term goals that integrate into progressively more challenging exercises. The goals need to be accepted by the organization as a whole, and not just the individual or department responsible for emergency management within the organization. This is a critical factor. Because effective exercises require the commitment of time, money, and effort across the organization, it is imperative that all departments understand it is the organization's mission, and not just that of one department. The length of an exercise program is typically from two to five years in duration. An endeavor such as this should not attempt to define every potential exercise over the course of five years, but rather provide the backbone to an overall preparedness effort.

A comprehensive exercise program will require the commitment of senior-level executives from the onset and is very similar to the more commonly recognized strategic planning process. The program will provide continued familiarity with exercise participation by all involved parties as well as continuous reinforcement that preparedness efforts are important to the organization. The process supplies opportunities to provide step-by-step confidence building as well as opportunities to motivate participants. Players will begin to anticipate and look forward to the next exercise.

Needs Assessment

The first step in developing a comprehensive exercise program is to examine how well the current exercise schedule meets the needs of your organization. Is there a current exercise schedule or do you hurriedly throw an exercise together to meet a deadline? Joint Commission hospitals are required to participate in at least two exercises per year. Actual events may be substituted for exercises, so facilities have been known to wait until it is near the end of the year to plan an exercise, with a twisted hope that there could be a real event they can substitute for the exercise requirement. Do your exercises build on one another to achieve overarching goals? Do all of the right participants fill their anticipated roles? Do you take your lessons learned and incorporate them into your next exercise? Do you have an integral exercise development team, a consultant, or one overworked employee with multiple other responsibilities? Is the current exercise program a function of a multidisciplinary committee? Do all the major clinical and support departments participate in the development and execution? Do all of your objectives focus on the emergency department or command staff? Do the "lessons learned" from your exercises become part of the facilitywide quality improvement process, or do they sit unattended until the next event? Analysis of your current capabilities is an important component. Through previous exercises and actual events, you probably have a good understanding of your institution's current capabilities. Do you have sufficient material and human resources to meet your current expectations? A thorough review of the current Emergency Operations Plan is the fundamental starting point for creating an exercise program. The same needs assessment will be utilized as the first step in a specific exercise design.

An often overlooked component of a needs assessment is the training and experience to design, conduct, and evaluate exercises. FEMA has created the National Standard Exercise Curriculum (see Figure 6-1). The curriculum provides a list of detailed training courses that exercise design team participants should complete. It does not include any practical experience in the curriculum, which is a significant shortfall to widespread acceptance.

Who Participates?

Participants need to learn and understand their roles and responsibilities as they pertain to disaster response. Is the employee's role going to be any different during a crisis than it is during normal operations? The vast majority of employees in a hospital or healthcare facility will continue to do the job they do every day. The exercise program does not want to focus on those employees, but rather on those supervisors, managers, and senior leaders whose roles will change significantly. A staff nurse in the emergency department will most likely continue to provide the clinical care he or she provides every day. The volume may change, the conditions may change, the resources available to do the job may change, but the essential provision of clinical care will not change in a significant fashion. The nurse supervisor/manager of the emergency department will have to change his or her role significantly in response to a disaster. The exercises need to focus on those changes and the competencies required to effectively perform those roles.

There are few obvious exceptions to the new roles categories. The most obvious exceptions are members of the hospital decontamination team. The majority of hospitals that may perform mass patient hazardous material decontamination utilize a variety of staff from multiple disciplines from within the facility. None of those disciplines spend any significant part of their normal workday performing decontamination. In a disaster, you will expect the members of the decontamination team to perform duties they do not normally perform. The only way that expectation could possibly meet with success is to

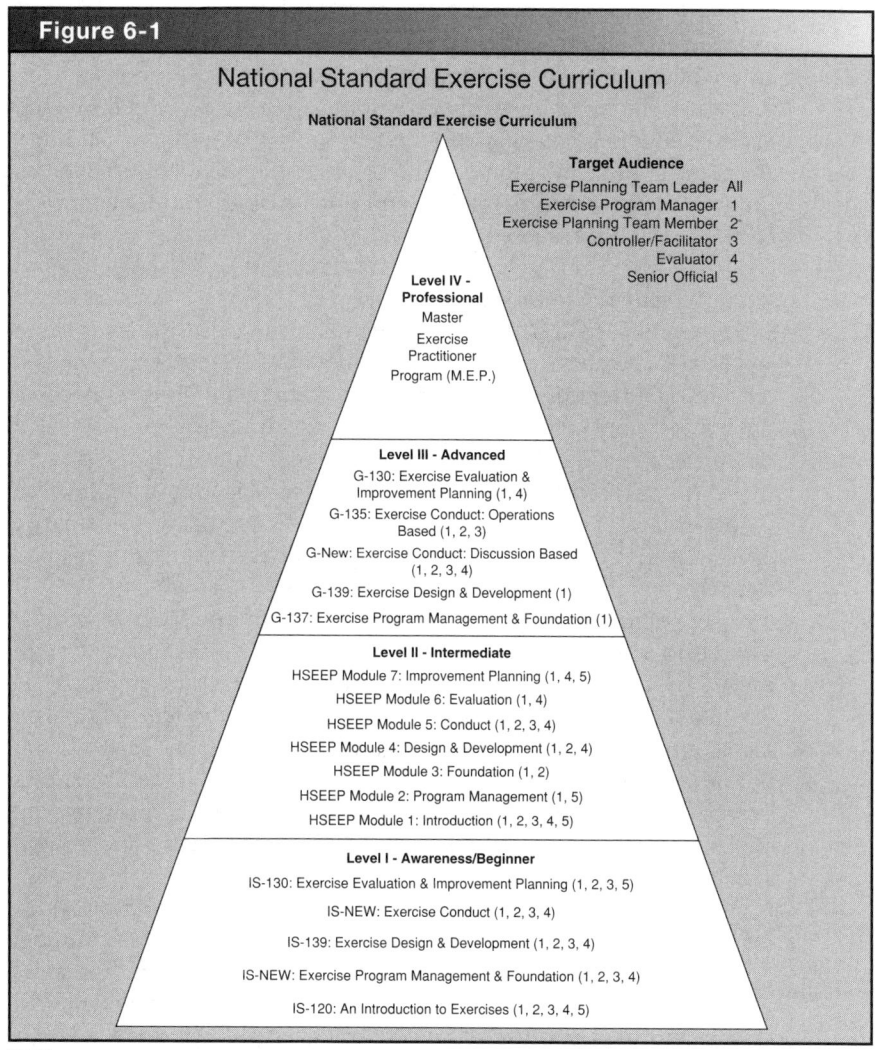

Figure 6-1

National Standard Exercise Curriculum

National Standard Exercise Curriculum

Target Audience

Exercise Planning Team Leader	All
Exercise Program Manager	1
Exercise Planning Team Member	2
Controller/Facilitator	3
Evaluator	4
Senior Official	5

Level IV - Professional

Master Exercise Practitioner Program (M.E.P.)

Level III - Advanced

G-130: Exercise Evaluation & Improvement Planning (1, 4)

G-135: Exercise Conduct: Operations Based (1, 2, 3)

G-New: Exercise Conduct: Discussion Based (1, 2, 3, 4)

G-139: Exercise Design & Development (1)

G-137: Exercise Program Management & Foundation (1)

Level II - Intermediate

HSEEP Module 7: Improvement Planning (1, 4, 5)

HSEEP Module 6: Evaluation (1, 4)

HSEEP Module 5: Conduct (1, 2, 3, 4)

HSEEP Module 4: Design & Development (1, 2, 4)

HSEEP Module 3: Foundation (1, 2)

HSEEP Module 2: Program Management (1, 5)

HSEEP Module 1: Introduction (1, 2, 3, 4, 5)

Level I - Awareness/Beginner

IS-130: Exercise Evaluation & Improvement Planning (1, 2, 3, 5)

IS-NEW: Exercise Conduct (1, 2, 3, 4)

IS-139: Exercise Design & Development (1, 2, 3, 4)

IS-NEW: Exercise Program Management & Foundation (1, 2, 3, 4)

IS-120: An Introduction to Exercises (1, 2, 3, 4, 5)

FEMA

provide regular training sessions with ample training exercises. Besides being the "right thing to do," the Occupational Safety and Health Administration (OSHA) requires it with a thorough explanation published in the *OSHA First Receivers Document.*

The Joint Commission Emergency Management Standards for 2009 require hospital leaders, including medical staff, to participate in planning activities. It seems reasonable that participation in the development exercise program would contribute to meeting this element of performance. The other Joint Commission Emergency Management

Standards requirement that suggests who should be involved in the exercise program is EM.03.01.03 (13), which states that "the hospital evaluates all emergency response exercises and all responses to actual emergencies using a multidisciplinary process (which includes licensed independent practitioners)." It only makes sense that if you are expected to evaluate the success of an exercise, you understand how the exercise was developed and how various components were, or were not, incorporated into the design.

What Activities Are Included?

A common shortfall of exercise programs is the exclusive focus on response. This is certainly understandable, but not desirable. A successful exercise program needs to include recovery components in their exercises. The recovery portion of real events often takes more time and money to complete, and is much more complex then the initial response phase. It is also more difficult to get active exercise participation from involved parties. It is not the adrenaline-producing response that gets people excited; it is the complex and often daunting tasks of getting things back to normal.

Let's examine one potential scenario from this perspective. Imagine a scenario where there is a fire in your facility's kitchen late at night caused by an electrical malfunction. The fire alarms are sounded, the doors close, and patients even have to be laterally evacuated to avoid some light smoke conditions. Your nursing, security, and facilities staff performed very well in their response to the event. We typically end our exercises at the point where the fire is extinguished, and patients and staff are accounted for. In this example, this is where we are going to **start** the scenario.

The fire has done significant damage to your kitchen and it is clear that you will be unable to use your kitchen for some period of time to provide meals to your patients. Let's assume it is 2 AM and breakfast is normally served in a few hours. All the food that was in your refrigerators and freezer, on your shelves, or anywhere near the kitchen, is no longer viable because it suffered either smoke or water damage. What do you do now? The short answer is you will be doing many, many things. Arranging for an alternative source for meals is just one of the many items. Contacting insurance companies, the health department, contractors, employees, vendors, etc., is just the beginning. It is not hard to see how the recovery from an event such as this can easily be more complex and time-consuming than the immediate response. The response phase of this event would be over in one or two hours. The recovery phase will take months.

There are several valuable resources when you are beginning to develop a comprehensive exercise program. The initial starting point is to evaluate the institution's internal capabilities and compare them to your recent HVA. If fire ranks high on your HVA, but you perform quarterly drills, monthly inspections, initial orientation, and annual refreshers, you may not feel the need to conduct a fire-focused exercise.

In December, 2003, the President issued Homeland Security Presidential Directive 8 (HSPD 8) to establish a national policy to strengthen the preparedness of the United States to prevent, protect against, respond to, and recover from terrorist attacks, major disasters, and other emergencies. HSPD 8 required the development of the National Preparedness Guidelines (the Guidelines). The Guidelines define what it means for the nation to be prepared by providing a vision for preparedness, establishing national priorities, and identifying target capabilities. The Guidelines adopt a Capabilities-Based Planning process supported by three planning tools: the National Planning Scenarios, Target Capabilities List (TCL), and Universal Task List (UTL). They can be viewed online at https://www.llis.dhs.gov.

There are several capabilities focused on hospitals. The first series of desired capabilities is communication. One example is: "Communications interoperability is the ability of public safety agencies (police, fire, EMS) and service agencies (public works, transportation, hospitals, etc.) to talk within and across agencies and jurisdictions via radio and associated communications systems, exchanging voice, data, and/or video with one another on demand, in real time, when needed and when authorized. It is essential that public safety has the intra-agency operability it needs, and that it builds its systems toward interoperability." A hospital may choose to include some or all of these national preparedness goals in its exercise program.

There are several valuable Web sites that assist you in developing both an exercise program and the individual exercises. The first Web site is the Homeland Security Exercise and Evaluation Program (HSEEP) at https://hseep.dhs.gov. The Homeland Security Exercise and Evaluation Program is a capabilities- and performance-based exercise program that provides a standardized methodology and terminology for exercise design, development, conduct, evaluation, and improvement planning. The Homeland Security Exercise and Evaluation Program constitutes a national standard for all exercises. Through exercises, the National Exercise Program helps organizations to achieve objective assessments of their capabilities so that strengths and areas for improvement are identified, corrected, and shared as appropriate prior to a real incident. The HSEEP is maintained by the Federal Emergency Management Agency's National Preparedness Directorate, Department of Homeland Security. The most useful component of this Web site is the HSEEP Toolkit that provides step-by-step guidance on exercise development. It is important to note that many federal and state grants that relate to hospital preparedness now require the utilization of the

HSEEP templates if you want to utilize grant funds to support the exercise.

The Homeland Security Digital Library (HSDL) at https://www.hsdl.org is the nation's premier collection of documents related to homeland security policy, strategy, and organization management. The HSDL is sponsored by the U.S. Department of Homeland Security's National Preparedness Directorate, FEMA, and the Naval Postgraduate School Center for Homeland Defense and Security. Their mission is to strengthen the national security of the United States by supporting federal, state, local, and tribal analysis, debate, and decision-making needs and to assist academics of all disciplines in homeland defense and security-related research. The Homeland Security Digital Library is composed of homeland security-related documents collected from a wide variety of sources. These include federal, state, tribal, and local government agencies, professional organizations, think tanks, academic institutions, and international governing bodies. Resources are carefully selected and evaluated by a team of librarians and subject-matter specialists. There are many hospital-related documents available for your review.

To see an extensive collection of after-action reports, visit the national network of Lessons Learned Information Sharing (LLIS) Web site at https://www.llis.dhs.gov. It is designed for emergency response providers and homeland security officials, but also has numerous health-related documents. The mission is to provide a secure, restricted-access portal for information that is designed to facilitate efforts to prevent, prepare for, and respond to acts of terrorism and other incidents across all disciplines and communities throughout the United States. LLIS is an encrypted system and all users are verified emergency response providers and homeland security officials. It provides peer-validated content by homeland security professionals. The Web site houses an extensive catalog of AARs as well as an updated list of homeland security documents from Department of Homeland Security, and other federal, state, and local organizations.

Design and Development

A program that starts with the basics and builds in both complexity and scope will provide the best opportunity for improvement. Seminars/orientations and drills are the fundamental building blocks of a comprehensive exercise program. They should be conducted frequently on different topics. They should also be easy to conduct, require few resources to plan and conduct, and ideally, be done during a normal workday. Taking 10–15 minutes to demonstrate the use of an evacuation chair to your nursing, security, and engineering staff is a good example of integrating simple drills into everyday life without a big commitment of time or resources. Smaller, more frequent, dispersed exercises will provide more people with the opportunity to learn important skills than one "big" exercise provides.

Utilizing communication devices that will be used during a disaster should occur on a regular basis. For example, many facilities have a backup telephone system in place, often called the "red phones." Is it possible to utilize this backup system on a regular schedule? Can the facility function the first Sunday night of each month using the backup communication systems? Because most backup systems do not have the same capacity as their primary system, an exercise such as this should occur during hours of decreased demand. If the backup system is too small for that, the phones do not have the capacity, or the phones are in the wrong locations, you may need to consider other options. If the entire facility cannot switch to the backup system, perhaps a specific department, floor(s), or buildings can participate in the exercise and rotate the exercise among participants. The goal is to get all the staff that you would expect to use the "red phone" comfortable utilizing the system, and to ensure you have a thorough understanding of capacity and utilization issues.

A corresponding clinical drill that is commonly performed is "Triage Tuesdays." This drill requires all EMS providers to triage each of their patients on Tuesdays as if their patient was part of a mass casualty event. The emergency department staff gets experience reading triage tags and re-evaluating and re-triaging the very same patients. The amount of effort required for an exercise such as this is minimal and the benefits can be very high. If we want our triage efforts to be effective during very rare and very stressful events, we must build our skills during times of routine, when we can learn, adjust, and build our level of competence.

Tabletop exercises should also be done frequently, but with a different target audience. The TTX is aimed at managers and department heads. Frequently, TTXs can be performed monthly over an extended lunch period. The culmination of a progressive exercise program is the full-scale exercise that encompasses an entire region. The results of the exercise will not only provide feedback on the plans and procedures, but on how well the exercise program readied the participants.

The scope of the exercises also needs to change from single entity or facility to multiple jurisdictions or regional. Hospitals must exercise their plans and procedures in response to both catastrophes and disasters. It is important to remember that disasters and catastrophes are very different, and the plans and exercises should reflect those differences. For example, in a catastrophe, most or all of the community-built structure is heavily impacted. This means that the community is unable to help itself. For example, in hurricanes and earthquakes, many survivors find immediate assistance (food, shelter) with family and friends in areas near the disaster. In a catastrophe, that is not an option. The community may also lose the buildings that contain political offices, police, fire, and EMS as well as hospitals. In a disaster, local officials can perform in their expected roles—signing disaster declarations, requesting assistance from outside communities, providing direction to the community at large, etc. Following a catastrophe, they will not be able to perform those essential tasks. Most if not all of the everyday community functions are sharply and simultaneously interrupted. In a catastrophe, most if not all places of work, recreation, worship, and education, such as schools, totally shut down and the lifeline infrastructure is so badly disrupted that there will be stoppages or extensive shortages of electricity, water, mail, or phone services as well as other means of communication and transportation. Even in major disasters, there is no such massive across-the-board disruption of community life, even if particular neighborhoods may be devastated. Finally, help from nearby communities cannot be provided. In many catastrophes, not only are all or most of the residents in a community directly affected, but often those in nearby localities will be similarly stricken. In short, catastrophes tend to affect multiple communities and often have a regional character. This, for instance, can and does affect the massive convergence that typically descends upon any stricken community after a disaster. In a disaster, there is usually only one target for the convergence, whereas in a catastrophe not only can nearby communities not contribute to the inflow, but they themselves often become competing sources for an eventual unequal inflow of goods, personnel, supplies, and communication.[2] It is easy to see how exercising for a disaster will be vastly different than exercising for a catastrophe.

THE EIGHT EXERCISE DESIGN STEPS

The next portion of this chapter will discuss the established steps in creating larger, operational-based exercises. The reader can certainly delete steps for smaller, less complex exercises. There are many ways and formats used to design exercises, but as discussed previously, many facilities are switching to the HSEEP model to ensure funding. The HSEEP Design and Development System is divided into 5 major portions, 16 intermediate steps, and 96 detailed steps.

Needs Assessment

The needs assessment that was conducted in creating the overall comprehensive exercise program provides most of the information required when starting to design specific, focused exercises. The specific items that still need to be addressed for each exercise are funding, available resources, and potential conflicts. For example, a hospital may not want to plan an evacuation exercise that occurs simultaneously with a regional or statewide exercise. In some instances, you may want to coordinate a local exercise to integrate into a much larger exercise.

During the needs assessment, the exercise design team members are identified and overall responsibilities are assigned. A very general timeline is agreed upon, and usually an exact date for the exercise is set.

Scope

The scope of the exercise is comprised of six elements. First, the scope of the exercise must define activities or procedures you want to evaluate. As an example of a scope statement:

> "This exercise will evaluate the facilities to assemble the equipment and staff to utilize all available operating rooms."

Second, the scope needs to detail the departments and agencies participating in the exercise. Will the mass casualty exercise require local EMS support or will the design assume the patients have already arrived at the emergency department? The third component of the scope needs to identify exercise participants and exercise design team members by position, title, or name. The fourth item to include in the scope is the hazard to be addressed by the exercise. Is it an internal flood from a broken water main or a hurricane? The geographic area the exercise will involve is the fifth item. Is this a department-specific event, a facilitywide event, a community event, or a regional event? More often than not, the boundaries are not so clear or easy to define. Lastly, what is the degree of realism you expect from the exercise? Will all actors have moulage applied and be coached to represent their symptoms in a realistic manner? Or will a simple, completed triage tag meet your needs?

Purpose Statement

The purpose statement defines the intent of the exercise and clearly states, in a concise manner, what you hope to achieve during this exercise. It is important to note that a purpose statement and objectives are not the same thing and serve two very different purposes. An example of a purpose statement might read as follows:

> The purpose of the radiation decontamination exercise at Community Hospital is to test the following emergency operations: notification of ED staff from EMS; the ability of the ED staff to ready the trauma room to accept a potentially radioactively contaminated patient; utilizing the hospital radiation decontamination procedures; and to demonstrate appropriate treatment of the patient for his presenting medical or traumatic injuries while not cross-contaminating other areas of the

hospital. The exercise will involve Community General Hospital (Emergency Department, Radiation Safety Office, Environmental Services, and facilities), Community EMS, and Community Office of Emergency Management in a full-scale exercise

Objectives

Objectives will specifically define the parameters of the exercise and provide measurable standards for the exercise to be evaluated. The objectives identify the functions that will be tested. Objectives are generated by reviewing the needs assessment, the scope, and the purpose alongside the current Emergency Operations Plan. The objectives will specify exactly what has to be accomplished and the actions that are expected from the participants. Objectives must be clear, concise, and provide the backbone for exercise design and evaluation. Each objective must state who should do what, under what conditions, and according to which policy or procedure.

Formation of the objectives and how the exercise will be evaluated occur in parallel. Exercise objectives should be "SMART." The acronym has the following meaning:

S – Simple

M – Measurable

A – Attainable

R – Results-oriented

T – Time-sensitive

This is a critical step in exercise design. For example, many hospital exercise objectives are stated as: "Rapidly deploy decon shelter." This statement is fine as a goal, but how do you define success or failure if you are the evaluator? The objective can easily be refined to state: "The decon unit leader will assemble the initial six-person team and provide decontamination to ambulatory patients in Level B suites in 25 minutes." This SMART objective then drives the rest of the exercise design process and is an integral part of the evaluation criteria. Objectives can be drawn from several different locations. Improvement plans and after-action reports are the most common source of objectives.

The lead planner and/or planning team schedules a "Concepts & Objectives" (C&O) conference to accomplish the three preceding detailed items. They should create a draft of the exercise purpose and a list of participating agencies for planners to discuss and agree upon. The C&O meeting is often viewed as the official starting point of the exercise design process. It should involve representatives of the sponsoring agency or department, the lead exercise planner, senior officials from each participating agency, and any other stakeholders in the exercise.

Participants should seek agreement on the proposed exercise purpose, scenario, type, participating agencies, funding, location, and date.

To make the most out of this meeting, provide background material for the C&O attendees that they will need to reach consensus on the exercise's purpose and scope. The information should include proposed agenda items, purpose, scope, timeline, task lists, relevant background information (e. g., previous after-action reports). This material should also convey the importance of the exercise.

Narrative

The narrative is used to "set the stage" for the exercise. You will describe the time and date the participants are "playing." It describes the hazard and existing conditions, along with identifying the known problems. It should stimulate the players into action. The narrative must also include sufficient background information to be realistic. It prepares the participants for the exercise.

Major and Minor Events

Major events updates are added to the narrative and provided to the participants as the exercise progresses. Based on the narrative and related to the exercise objectives, events move the exercise along. They are bits of information that cause players to respond. Major events are created as a result of the scenario, not the players' actions. Major events are the foundation for message development.

Detailed events are the injects that prompt players to perform expected actions. The detailed events create the opportunity for the players to meet the objectives. For example, if you are interested in testing how well the hospital activates its mass casualty notification plan, the detailed event may be the following example: "EMS has just called the emergency department and confirmed that they will be bringing X patients to our facility in 15 minutes." In many institutions, such an event would be followed by a predetermined notification process.

Detailed events also provide the design team with an opportunity to pull the participants back to common ground. For example, an often-used inject is: "The CEO's office just called and she wants an update from all departments in 5 minutes." This forces the various participants of the exercise to focus on what they have accomplished and then to share that information with the other groups in the exercise.

Expected Actions

Expected actions are also closely tied to the exercise objectives. They are the actions or decisions that the design team expects the players to make in response to messages. Expected actions can take a variety of forms. Making decisions, implementing policies, executing procedures, establishing priorities, and discussing and evaluating information lead to negotiation and building a consensus for the best course of action.

Expected actions are important because they keep the exercise focused on the objectives. By focusing on the objectives, the evaluators and the players can easily understand if their response was appropriate.

For example, hospitals utilize expected actions routinely. When the fire alarm system is activated, there are several expected actions that should occur. The hallway fire doors are automatically released and the floor staff closes each patient room door. The expected action is clear and easy to observe.

Messages

Messages are how the information is delivered to the players. The purpose is to motivate action. It is the means of transmitting the design details to the exercise participants. The messages can take almost any form of communication, but are traditionally transmitted via telephone or radio. Messages are best generated by the design team prior to the exercise, but experienced controllers can sometimes create "spontaneous" messages to redirect the exercise if it appears to be going off course. The use of spontaneous messages must still be tied to the objectives and should be limited because it is difficult to notify all controllers and evaluators of the unexpected inject.

All messages are placed on a Master Scenario Events List (MSEL)[a], which should include the inject time, the major and detailed event numbers, message number, the actual message to be delivered, the recipient, the sender, and finally the mode of transmission.

If there are going to be any exercise enhancements, this is the point in the process that they are developed. Mock breaking news segments and utilization of journalism students to portray the news media are two examples of enhancements that are readily available.

At the conclusion of the design process, but prior to the exercise, the evaluation criteria need to be developed and distributed to all evaluators.

At the conclusion of the exercise design process, the team will have developed several exercise-related documents: the exercise plan, the Master Scenario Events List, and Evaluation Plans.

The exercise plan (ExPlan) is the foundation planning document from which all other plans and exercise documentation are developed. This plan will be viewed by key leadership and stakeholders as well as the exercise design team.

The Master Scenario Events List moves an exercise forward from the starting scenario, creating realism and challenges for exercise

---

[a] The MSEL is a chronological timeline of expected actions and scripted events to be injected into exercise play by *controllers* to generate or prompt *player* activity. It ensures necessary events happen

participants by adding new twists to the basic exercise plot. The MSEL is a chronological listing of the events and injects that drive exercise play. It links simulation to action by the orderly infusion of an event or message that will prompt players to implement a policy or take an action. Development of the MSEL should be started as early as possible.

Evaluation Plans (EvalPlans) provide guidance and instruction regarding assessing exercise performance. An EvalPlan may include observation methodology to be used as well as essential materials required to execute their specific functions (e.g., evaluation forms for specific functions). The EvalPlan is included in the *Controller and Evaluator (C/E) Handbook*.[b] The C/E Handbook contains detailed information about the exercise scenario, and describes the roles and responsibilities of individual controllers and evaluators. It should be distributed to only specifically designated individuals. It contains detailed scenario information (including agent fact sheets), roles and responsibilities of a functional area or individual controllers and evaluators, an exercise safety plan, a controller communications plan, and an Exercise Evaluation Guide (EEG).[c] However, during larger, more complex exercises, planners may develop a separate EvalPlan.

Selection, recruitment, and assignment of controllers and evaluators are crucial components of exercise design. Controllers should be

---

so that all *objectives* are met. Larger, more complex exercises may also employ a *Procedural Flow* (*ProFlow*), which differs from the MSEL in that it only contains expected player actions or *events*.

The MSEL links simulation to action, enhances exercise experience for players, and reflects an incident or activity meant to prompt *players* to action. Each MSEL record contains a designated *scenario* time, an *event* synopsis, the name of the *controller* responsible for delivering the inject; and, if applicable, special delivery instructions, the *task* and *objective* to be demonstrated, the expected action, the intended player, and a note-taking section.

[b] The C/E Handbook is an exercise overview and instructional manual for *controllers* and *evaluators*. A supplement to the ExPlan, it contains more detailed information about the *scenario*, and describes controllers' and evaluators' roles and responsibilities. Because the C/E Handbook contains information on the scenario and exercise administration, it should be distributed only to those individuals specifically designated as controllers or evaluators. Larger, more complex exercises may use a separate Control Staff Instructions (COSIN) and EvalPlan in place of the C/E Handbook.

[c] EEGs are HSEEP documents that support the exercise *evaluation* process by providing evaluators with consistent standards for observation, analysis, and *AAR* development. Each EEG is linked to a target capability and provides standard activities, performance measures, and tasks to be evaluated based on the exercise *objectives*. Additionally, an EEG contains a Capability Narrative section, in which evaluators provide a general chronological narrative of exercise events associated with the capability; and an Evaluator Observations section in which evaluators provide specific strengths and areas of improvement linked to the capability.

The consistent guidelines provided in EEGs facilitate creation of After Action Report/Improvement Plan (AAR/IPs) resulting in actionable IPs that target specific personnel, planning, organization, equipment, and training needs within capabilities.

familiar with agency/jurisdiction operations and procedures. This will ensure that agency Emergency Operations Plans (EOPs) and Standard Operating Procedures (SOPs) are understood by all controllers. It is beneficial to use local evaluators who are familiar with the functional area where they will be assigned. The lead evaluator should be a senior-level person familiar with emergency response functional areas as well as regional/local plans, policies, and procedures.

Packets should be developed for controllers and evaluators, players, media, actors, and very important persons (VIPs). These materials should be placed in a packet (e.g., folder, notebook) and distributed ahead of the exercise. The controller and evaluator (C/E) packet should contain the *C/E Handbook*, Master Scenario Events List, and Exercise Evaluation Guides.

A simulation cell (SimCell)[d] is used to generate injects and receive player responses to nonparticipating agencies. It includes both the physical location and the personnel who operate it. SimCell staff portray nonparticipating organizations, agencies, and individuals who would likely participate in response to an actual event. Depending on the type of exercise, the SimCell may require a phone, fax machine, computer, email account, or other means of communication.

After the exercise is designed, there are still a number of items that need to be addressed, including site considerations, safety, videotaping, press releases, etc. For a complete list of tasks, see the HSEEP Toolkit Web site, https://hseep.dhs.gov.

Conduct the Exercise

The final phase of the exercise is the evaluation of the response to the simulated events. The development of the evaluation plan occurs in parallel to the design process. After the exercise, a few items still need to occur. Immediately following the conclusion of the exercise, the players should participate in a facilitated discussion called a *hot wash*. The hot wash needs to be brief and concise to collect the participants' immediate feedback. The feedback should focus on what procedures worked well, what procedures did not work as anticipated, equipment feedback, etc. It is important to stress that the hot wash must be billed as a "no blame" event. The focus of this meeting is not on people.

[d] The SimCell is an exercise area where *controllers* generate and deliver *injects*, and receive player responses to non-participating organizations, agencies, and individuals who would likely participate actively in an actual incident. Physically, the SimCell is a working location for a number of qualified professionals who portray representatives of non-participating organizations, agencies, and individuals who would likely participate during an actual incident.

Feedback on the effectiveness of the exercise design and execution needs to be collected at this time. Participants' will have definite opinions on how they felt the exercise was conducted and it is equally important to improve the quality of the exercise as it is to improve the quality of participant response—they are inseparable.

Collection of evaluator and observer comments should occur immediately following the exercise. The evaluators will be the ones that comment on individual responses to messages. The data will be collected, analyzed, and summarized in report form. The standard template utilized by HSEEP can be found at https://hseep.dhs.gov.

After the data has been collected and analyzed, it is advisable to circulate a draft report among the evaluators to ensure that their observations and comments were incorporated to reflect their findings. Once the report it is finalized, it is submitted to the responsible executive with an improvement plan to meet any identified gaps.

References

1. Kendra K, Wachtendorf T. *Creativity in Emergency Response After the World Trade Center Attack.* University of Delaware Web site. http://dspace.udel.edu:8080/dspace/handle/19716/733. Published 2002. Accessed 2009.
2. Quarantelli EL. *Emergencies, Disasters and Catastrophes Are Different Phenomena.* University of Delaware Web site. http://dspace.udel.edu:8080/dspace/handle/19716/674. Issued 2000. Accessed 2009.

Chapter 7

Integration with Local and Community Resources

Isaac B. Weisfuse, MD, MPH

Learning Objectives

- Understand the National Response Framework, and more specifically, Emergency Support Function #8 in responding to health emergencies.
- Explain the host of U.S. government resources that may be mobilized during an emergency.
- Understand how healthcare institutions and their state and local health departments, first responder agencies, and non-government organizations should work together to prepare for and respond to disasters.
- Understand the role of partnerships for addressing the needs of vulnerable populations.
- Describe how collaborations may work for specific emergencies, such as pandemic influenza or a power outage.

Overview

Healthcare institutions are dependent on federal, state, and local governments as well as nongovernment organizations and private entities in responding to disasters. The resources that these groups supply are critical to the health and well-being of affected populations. In order for this to happen, all parties need to become familiar with the capabilities each possesses during the preparedness phase that is prior to emergency disaster, and important relationships need to be developed.

This chapter will review the United States government's planning efforts, federal emergency resources, the role of state and local health departments, as well as other key response partners such as emergency management organizations, and police and fire departments. The role of key nongovernment organizations, as well as local and community resource integration as it relates to "vulnerable" populations, will be reviewed. Finally, key partnerships in several different types of emer-

Case Study
Case Study: The Response to Hurricane Katrina

Figure 7-1
At Dobbins AFB, this New Orleans Katrina evacuee is at the Yellow Triage Center for assessment and possible medical service. Dr. Steedman Sarbah (Augusta, GA, VA Hospital), and assistants are about to determine if this woman is critically ill.

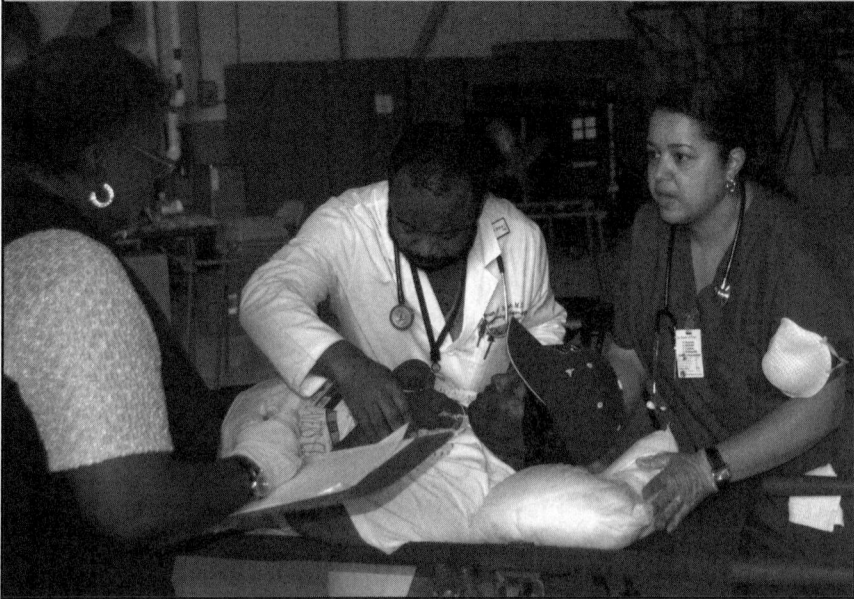

Photo by George Armstrong/FEMA Photo

Some hospitals were short-staffed; those who made it in worked long shifts in adverse conditions. Patient care became exceedingly difficult as hospitals lost power to operate vital equipment such as lab and x-ray equipment, dialysis machines, and elevators. Temperatures rose above 100 degrees in many institutions ... toilets backed up and essential supplies dwindled. Many hospitals reported struggling to care for ventilator-dependent patients after hospitals lost electricity. One hospital told us of emergency surgery being done by flashlight, with little or no anesthesia.[1]

[We learned that] when hospital staff could make use of functional communications equipment, or when they used messengers to relay information, they often did not know whom they should contact to communicate their needs. Was it the New Orleans or Louisiana State Emergency Operations Centers, the health department, a hospital association or the federal government?[2]

You are an emergency manager at one of the nine hospitals in New Orleans that were severely affected by Hurricane Katrina. In review of your hospital's response, it is clear that there were many acts of heroism by both hospital staff and community members in dealing with the crisis. It is also readily apparent that there were multiple levels of failure among emergency response organizations. However, you are troubled by the preceding findings.

You have recently been informed that a Congressional subcommittee is visiting New Orleans, and you have been asked to testify. The subcommittee has graciously shared some of their questions:

What preparations did your facility make before Hurricane Katrina to operate with a limited power supply? Who were your outside partners in this activity? Going forward, who do you need to work with to ensure that you have a plan?

Does your institution have a plan to obtain essential supplies during a crisis? Who do you contact to obtain these supplies?

How does your hospital work with the surrounding community to coordinate in the case of a crisis? Can you accommodate the needs of vulnerable populations likely to use your facility during an emergency?

In retrospect, what kind of coordination would be needed in the future for other disasters? Which government, nongovernment, business, and community contacts do you need to establish?

How should you answer these questions?

gencies will provide examples of how integration should work. Although it may seem counterintuitive to discuss the federal government's capabilities within a chapter on local and community resources, because all response is at the local level, federal response must be understood.

Introduction

Since September 11, 2001, emergency preparedness, once the principle domain of first responders, emergency management organizations, and a few nongovernment organizations, expanded to include hospitals, health departments, businesses, neighborhoods, families, and individuals. This expansion of responsibility presents new challenges to emergency mangers to properly integrate information during all phases of preparing for, responding to, and recovering from disasters. Because most disasters involve injuries, illness, and/or exacerbation of chronic conditions, hospitals play key roles, and need to work with all of these partners in order to maximally respond to the event. The range of coordination potentially needed is vast, and may include the need for obtaining lifesaving medications and equipment, maintaining a safe working environment, arranging transportation for staff and patients, and safely evacuating all patients.

Hospitals have immense financial pressures upon them, and sometimes struggle to provide care on a "normal" day. However, the events of recent years (e.g., September 11th, the Northeast blackout of 2003, Hurricanes Katrina and Rita) dictate that all hospitals need to be prepared for a crisis in their jurisdiction.

Like all emergency planning, coordination does not begin at the time of an event. Good planning involves meeting representatives of all local/regional organizations needed in the response and discussing roles and responsibilities both generally and, if needed, specifically for particular scenarios. Local or state emergency management agencies are a good place to start the process. These agencies are charged with overall emergency coordination and routinely promote partnerships among emergency responders. Finally, state or regional hospital organizations may facilitate planning and promote best practices.

Although all disasters are local, some rise to the level of requiring a broader response, including the involvement of either the state and/or the federal government. Although it may be more difficult to meet in advance with federal planners and responders, hospitals should broadly understand how the healthcare system fits within not only the local and state response, but also within the federal system. This is particularly important in situations where local and state assets are insufficient to meet the needs of the disaster, or when the disaster is a regional, national, or even international one. The following section will review how the federal government weaves together the different levels of response for emergencies that will coalesce at the local level.

National Response Framework

The National Response Framework (NRF), released by the federal government in January 2008[3] (replacing the National Response Plan of 2004), provides the structure for an all-hazards response and functions as the national "playbook" for response. As such, it provides a broad overview of how emergency response integration should occur in the United States. Key principles of the NRF are partnerships, a tiered response, flexible emergency management, unified command, and a readiness to act. Tiered response refers to the concept that all disasters start at the local level and the response can expand to fit the situation. Flexibility stresses the ability to change in response to changing conditions, as well as the ability to go from the response to the recovery stage of the disaster.

Unified command is the process by which different response entities work together during an emergency. Unified command relies on the Incident Command System, which is codified by the federal government under the National Incident Management System (NIMS). Adoption of an incident command system (ICS) is expected of hospitals during disasters, and is critical to an integrated response. Therefore, all hospitals should develop, practice, and use an ICS to internally coordinate their response, as well as to integrate into their jurisdiction's activities. Finally, the doctrine of readiness to act encourages a proactive approach to response.

The NRF has several important appendices. One set, called the Emergency Support Function Annexes (ESF), groups specific functions, such as transportation, communications, public works, and engineering. ESF #8, the Public Health and Medical Services Annex, is directly relevant to all hospitals. It covers incidents involving public health and medical services, including mental health needs. The needs may stem from the incident itself, or from the needs of responders to the event. The lead agency of ESF #8 is the U.S. Department of Health and Human Services (HHS), and its secretary has control of all non-Department of Defense federal assets. The roles of the federal support agency are also detailed. Specific responsibilities in ESF #8 include assessment of public health or medical needs, the need to augment available medical personnel, relevant equipment or supplies, patient evacuation, patient care, oversight of the blood supply, behavioral health care, and mass fatality management. All of these activities may be directly relevant to local hospitals.

Another appendix to the NRF is the support annexes. This details which federal agencies are involved in support of more generic disaster activities, including maintenance of critical infrastructure, international coordination, public affairs, worker safety and health, and volunteer management. Finally, there are a series of incident annexes that provide an overview of specific hazards. These include biological incidents, catastrophic incidents (which include mass casualty incidents), mass evacuation, and nuclear/radiologic incidents. Each annex contains a scope of response, planning assumptions, concept of operations, required actions, delineation of responsibilities, and lists of the cooperating federal agencies.

Federal Assets

Many federal assets relevant to hospitals are housed within HHS,[4] and report to the Assistant Secretary for Preparedness and Response. Disaster Medical Assistance Teams (DMAT) are teams of equipped, trained medical personnel that can be deployed rapidly to provide surge medical care to localities (see Figure 7-2). National Nurse Response Teams (NNRT)

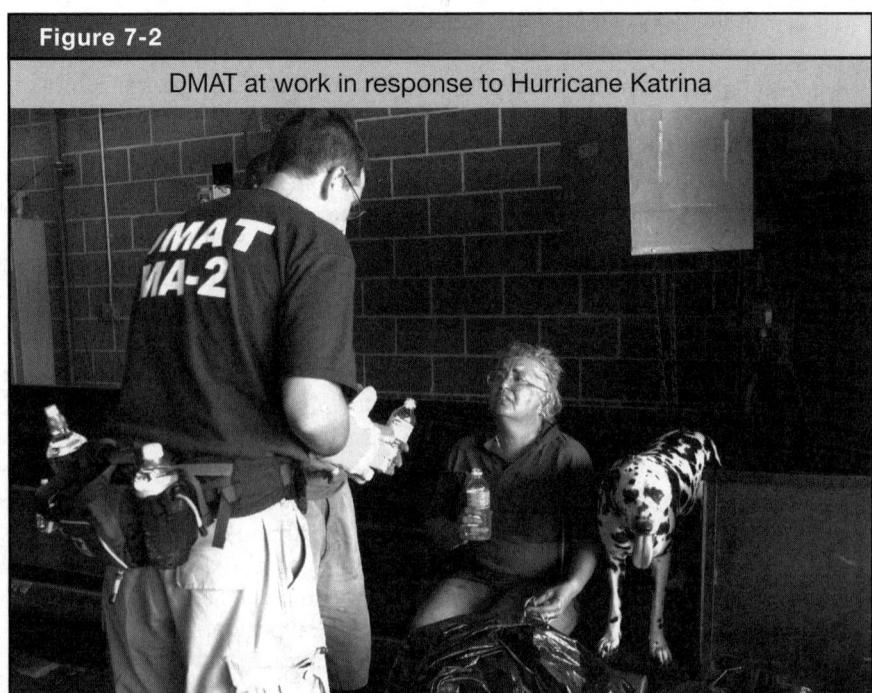

Figure 7-2

DMAT at work in response to Hurricane Katrina

FEMA

Figure 7-3

Loading the Strategic National Stockpile

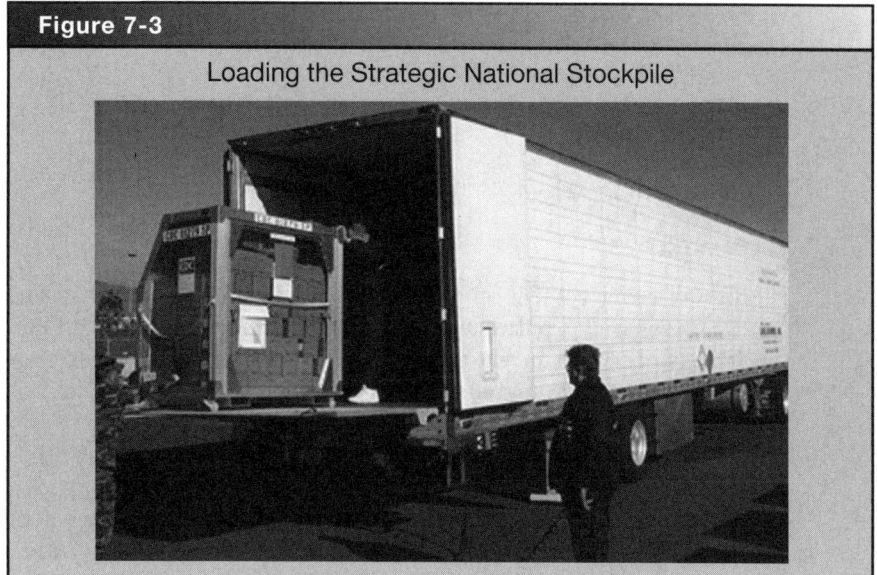

Courtesy of the Strategic National Stockpile/CDC

provide nurses for a wide variety of activities if local nursing capacity is overwhelmed. National Pharmacy Response Teams (NPRT) would respond to situations requiring large numbers of pharmacists, or the need to provide chemoprophylaxis or vaccinations to large numbers of people. The Disaster Mortuary Operational Response Teams (DMORT) provide forensic services for mass casualty events. The National Veterinary Response Team (NVRT) provides veterinary services following a disaster.

Another federal asset directly relevant to healthcare institutions is the Strategic National Stockpile (SNS). The SNS comprises medications, medical equipment, and supplies that may be needed during a disaster (see Figure 7-3). It is overseen by the Centers for Disease Control and Prevention, and maintained at 12 secure locations across the United States. The SNS will provide a "push package" of emergency supplies to any location in the United States within 12 hours of a request by the governor of a state. Push packages contain emergency supplies, and are backed up by a system of vendor-managed inventory that will subsequently supply these materials. Specific kinds of supplies may include ventilators, antibiotics for prophylaxis for agents of bioterrorism, IV fluids, etc.

All states are required to have plans to receive and distribute the SNS to local jurisdictions. There are prearranged delivery warehouses for the assets, and most states will then either directly supply their counties or regional centers, or in some cases, directly supply healthcare institutions. Because hospitals may be recipients of these supplies, they should work with state and local public health or emergency management authorities to determine the logistic and legal issues associated with accepting these critical resources.

State and Local Coordination

COMMUNITIES

Community engagement on emergency preparedness has many advantages.[5] An engaged populace may help spread important messages through social networks[6] and increase social trust between government and constituents. It allows testing of emergency planning assumptions, and provides review and input on difficult decisions. Community groups can encourage resilience to help during the recovery period as well. Unfortunately, many attempts at community outreach have stopped at the brochure distribution and media polling phases, and true engagement has not been attempted in many areas. At times, specific recommendations, such as the need to stockpile food or evacuate, do not recognize the problems that poor communities may have with compliance. A commitment to engagement is needed by government leadership, as well as allocation of resources in order to succeed. Careful attention to process to allow all voices to be heard, as well as discussion of prior experiences during disasters will be needed to achieve this important objective.

EMERGENCY MANAGEMENT ORGANIZATIONS

All states and most local jurisdictions operate emergency management organizations. Those that do not have an emergency management organization will have, at a minimum, an individual who identifies emergency management as either part of their role or their primary role. These agencies typically coordinate emergency response activities in their jurisdiction and run Emergency Operations Centers (EOCs). EOCs function to provide real-time updates and responses to urgent issues during emergencies. EOCs also may host a Joint Information Center (JIC), which is the central point where information is shared with the media about the disaster. In any event, healthcare organizations should either be represented in the EOC, or should know how to contact the EOC for both resource requests and obtaining information. Hospital public relations, marketing, and communications personnel should also attempt to coordinate public messaging with or through the JIC. All hospitals should develop redundant mechanisms to communicate with their emergency management organizations during times of disaster, including special attention for maintenance of communication during power outages or absence of routine telephone connectivity.

Emergency management agencies have other important functions as well. They take the lead in planning for many kinds of events. They also help prepare the public for disasters through community outreach and education. Typically, they are involved in training activities with the public, and may encourage creation of Community Emergency Response Teams. They frequently organize meetings, tabletop exercises, and drills to further emergency preparedness.

STATE AND LOCAL HEALTH DEPARTMENTS

State and local health departments are key contacts for hospitals during an event, but play an important role in preparedness as well. State health departments regulate medical care. As an example, regulatory relief during a disaster may be required to address the need to increase bed capacity. Under this scenario, staffing ratios may need to be relaxed. Healthcare organizations should work in advance with their state to identify regulations that may need to be altered during a disaster.

State health departments conduct mandated surveillance efforts within their state. Typically, infectious diseases are reported through infection control practitioners, but hospital administration and hospital emergency managers should understand all of their reporting requirements. Usually, lists of reportable conditions are located on the health department's Web site. Because disease notification may be the first evidence of disaster, terrorism event, or public health emergency, delays in reporting may increase morbidity and mortality caused by a delayed response. In addition, during prolonged disasters, health departments may need to manage the overall healthcare system and will need information on bed availability, equipment and medication supplies, and staffing capacity. Some states have instituted electronic methods of collecting this information, and hospitals will need to designate personnel to respond to these demands.

The Assistant Secretary for Preparedness and Response of HHS oversees the Hospital Preparedness Program (HPP).[7] This program provides funds to hospitals via state and certain city health departments for preparedness. Specific guidance is given to jurisdictions on preparedness that includes increasing bed and personnel surge capacity, developing decontamination capabilities, and funding drills and exercises. Current priorities for HPP include bed tracking, fatality management, and hospital evacuation.

Health departments have valuable subject matter expertise on a wide range of issues. Frequently, they will provide clinical guidance on infectious and chronic diseases related to the disaster. Just as important is the expertise they possess on issues that are generally not the domain of healthcare institutions. For example, environment cleanup, advice on waste disposal, and suggestions on personal protective equipment may be valuable to healthcare institutions during a disaster. Laboratory support, as shown in the following details, may also be crucial. Finally, health departments may be conduits to further information relevant to the disaster through contacts with federal agencies such as the Centers for Disease Control and Prevention.

The Laboratory Response Network (LRN)[8] is a nationwide network of laboratories that support laboratory emergency preparedness and response. Hospital laboratories are considered "sentinel labs" because of their frontline status with the public. They need to develop advance relationships with reference laboratories, typically state or local facilities, to refer concerning specimens to them. To do so, they must become proficient in proper specimen collection as well as the ability to safely package and ship specimens.

Many communities have a Medical Reserve Corps (MRC),[9] some of which are overseen by local or county health departments. MRCs differ by community, but generally are volunteer health professionals that may provide health services during a disaster. MRC volunteers register in advance, are credentialed, and may receive training on their potential involvement. The kinds of disaster they may participate in include mass prophylaxis, surge capacity in hospitals, and emergency sheltering operations. MRC personnel participated in the response to Hurricane Katrina. Another initiative, the Emergency System for Advance Registration of Volunteer Health Professionals (ESAR-VHP),[10] provides standards for credentialing of volunteer health personnel. Proper credentialing will allow deployment of volunteers within a state, and ultimately facilitate increasing surge capacity.

In studies of the emergency preparedness relationships between healthcare institutions and health departments, several criteria were identified as important in ensuring success.[11,12] Having preexisting relationships was an important factor found in current successful collaborations. Both parties need to believe they can benefit, and strong leadership needs to step forward to promote the collaboration. A process that acknowledges all of the stakeholders and results in more formal written plans or agreements that will outlive changes in personnel were other hallmarks of good collaborations. All successful efforts should result in joint training and drills to maximize effectiveness. After-action reports from all drills or real events should be agreed upon by participants to ensure that corrections are made for the future

FIRST RESPONDERS

Hospitals deal with first responders daily. Disasters will stress this coordination. Rapid sharing of information is important: for example, prehospital providers and agencies will need to get clear information about hospital capacity during a mass casualty incident. Coordination on the need for decontamination should flow from the field to hospitals rapidly to properly address the needs of patients who self-refer to hospitals even before ambulances with casualties arrive. Enhanced security from local police forces may be needed because hospitals have been targets of terror attacks.

BUSINESSES

All healthcare institutions rely on businesses for needed resources. During disasters, it may be difficult or impossible to obtain these resources. For example, during an influenza pandemic, it may be difficult to maintain the supply chain for items that are manufactured overseas. Exacerbating this problem is the practice of just-in-time inventory, which limits the amount of materials that a hospital has "on hand." During these situations, hospital emergency managers will be pressured to look for new suppliers. Obviously, understanding the limitations of key suppliers beforehand is needed, and insisting on reviewing their emergency preparedness plans will help inform when a backup business should be identified. Developing relationships with local hotels may be useful. During the SARS outbreak, hospital personnel were willing to work, but did not want to go home, and they needed to be housed. Alternatively, in other types of disasters, staff may be willing to work, but want to be assured that their families are taken care of. In both of these scenarios, availability of hotel space may be valuable.

NONGOVERNMENT ORGANIZATIONS

There are many not-for-profit organizations that provide valuable services during disasters. One example of a national organization that also provides local activity through its chapters is the American Red Cross (ARC). In addition to providing disaster relief across the United States for situations ranging from home fires to regional or nationwide disasters, the ARC has a vital role in helping maintain the blood supply. The ARC provides shelter, food, and mental health services as appropriate, and will also provide these services to emergency responders and help with clean up and restoration. All healthcare institutions should also identify and maintain relationships with local community and faith-based organizations that can also help during emergency disaster.

MEDICAL EXAMINERS

During a mass casualty incident or infectious disease outbreak, the ability of hospitals to properly manage the deceased may be overwhelmed. In response to this problem, many medical examiners are developing capabilities for storage of decedents until proper identification, examination, and burial can take place. This will require coordination between health-care institutions and medical examiners on proper supplies, protocols, and communication should such an event occur.

Vulnerable Populations

The effects of a disaster on persons at higher vulnerability to the effects of disaster depend on a number of factors, including the kind of event, underlying health and socioeconomic status of the population, geographic location, age of the population, whether the group is institutionalized or not, immigration status, and degree of social or linguistic isolation. In general, groups that are currently disadvantaged in accessing health care will have the same problem during a disaster. In some regions, identifying these populations may be simple, but in complex urban environments, even locating these groups may be extremely difficult. They may be hard to characterize because not all of a particular group may be at increased risk. For example, well-off elderly persons may be at lower risk than the elderly living in poverty for certain kinds of disasters.

There are preparations that all healthcare institutions and government agencies can do in advance of a disaster to address the needs of vulnerable groups. The first step would be to identify potential vulnerable populations in a community and stakeholders. Many local or state health departments or social service agencies have either data or lists of involved groups that can assist in this process. Healthcare institutions should maintain this kind of community profile, and get input from their community advisory groups. Priority should be placed on contacting and working with organizations that meet the needs of these groups on a day-to-day level to gain from their experience.

Specific preparedness activities based on the community profile may be undertaken. Of course, many of these may be a routine part of community service. For example, translation of written materials into languages spoken by the community occurs normally. This daily need to effectively communicate is no less important during a disaster, and methods to rapidly translate materials should be developed. Similarly, meeting the everyday needs of institutionalized populations (nursing homes, prisons, etc.), should lead to developing specific appropriate preparedness plans.

Another generic need may occur when persons are sheltered either outside of their home or have to stay home for prolonged periods and have run out of their prescription medications. It is likely that hospital pharmacies may be expected to provide information on prescriptions and rapidly refilling them. No matter what the disaster, persons who must remain in bed and attended by relatives or home health agencies will need extra support. Coalitions between healthcare institutions and home health agencies may be valuable in dealing with the needs of this special care population.

Published recommendations for addressing the needs of specific populations, such as the disabled[13] or the elderly,[14] are useful tools for emergency planners. For example, it is possible to predict the needs of the hearing impaired or visually impaired populations during disasters. Accommodations may include special signage in Braille, or directions on how to handle service animals in shelters. Shelter supplies should include items for the disabled such as wheelchairs. For the elderly, special attention to transportation issues, management of chronic conditions, and mental health needs, are examples of the kinds of issues that will likely arise in a disaster.

Disaster-specific planning may be advisable. Emergency management organizations, for example, can predict flooding zones associated with coastal storms. Persons who cannot self-evacuate will need assistance from authorities, and hospitals will likely become involved in meeting the health needs of displaced persons. Influenza pandemics, with their associated morbidity and mortality as well as their prolonged course, will also provide unique challenges to vulnerable populations. During the 2009–2010 season, the Association of State and Territorial Health Officials has released a useful review of pandemic influenza and vulnerable populations that will help all emergency planners on this issue.[15]

Integration with Local and Community Resources in Specific Scenarios

This section provides an overview of the kind of local and community resources that need to work together during specific disasters. It is not meant to represent a complete review of these needs, but rather to use as a starting point in thinking about scenario-specific problems. It also doesn't identify the specific scenarios that may be most important in your community, which should be identified through a thorough vulnerability assessment exercise with local emergency planners.

ELECTRICAL OUTAGES

Obvious needs for healthcare institutions will occur during a power outage. Contact with the local emergency management organization should occur to advise on the extent and projected length of the outage, effect on services, and the potential need for evacuation. Emergency management can be the conduit for information to regional utilities to prioritize hospitals for electricity and to deliver fuel for generators if needed. During the outage, some important surveillance reporting to health departments may need to be maintained. If food spoilage has occurred, directions about discarding food and safe food practices may be obtained from the local health department. In some cases, laboratories may need to ask public health laboratories to locate alternative testing facilities. Because hospitals may be one of the few working institutions in a community, they may be flooded with persons, requiring extra security services from local law enforcement. Persons who are forced to relocate because of the power outage may not have their prescribed medicine, and those who suffer effects from extreme heat or cold may be vulnerable populations to consider during a power outage. Coordination with the ARC or Salvation Army may be needed for the displaced populations.

BIOTERRORISM

During a suspected or real bioterrorism event, communication and coordination with the state or local health department is critical to report suspect cases, facilitate safe laboratory specimen submission, and receive up-to-date patient care guidelines. Guidelines to protect staff, including appropriate personal protective equipment, level of isolation, and need for prophylactic antibiotics will also be issued by the health departments. If the SNS is ordered, hospitals should coordinate the drop-off of supplies or antibiotics with the state health department or emergency management organization. Coordination of messaging between the community, emergency management officials, and hospitals is needed to advise the public what to do, and to reduce unnecessary crowding at emergency departments. Cooperation with local law enforcement may be needed if they wish to interview some of the victims, as well as for additional security. Housing for staff may need to be obtained with local hotels. Vulnerable populations may include the immunosuppressed for some agents (such as smallpox) and all those without good access to care if widespread prophylaxis is indicated.

RADIOLOGIC DISPERSAL DEVICE

Coordination with local first responders and emergency management is critical to properly decontaminate and treat transported victims as well as walk-ins. Isotope characterization, as well as screening and treatment guidelines, will be provided by health departments or other first responder agencies. The medical examiner will provide information on proper management of contaminated corpses to hospital morgue personnel. As in the preceding scenarios, coordination of messaging to the public through the JIC will be critical. Federal agencies such as the CDC, the Department of Defense, and the Radiation Emergency Assistance Center/Training Site will respond to this disaster as well. All of the local, state, and federal agencies will be involved in decisions on long-term recovery and re-occupancy issues as well as long-term follow-up of those exposed.

PANDEMIC INFLUENZA

Pandemic "waves" are estimated to be about 8 to 12 weeks in duration, and a pandemic may be comprised of several waves. Therefore, pandemics present unique challenges because of their duration. Guidance from health departments on clinical care, level of respiratory protection, and collection of specimens will be crucial early in the pandemic and may be modified over time by public health authorities as more information from around the world is tracked and understood. Coordination with health departments and emergency management will be needed to track resources, as well as to obtain antiviral medications from government stockpiles. Regulatory relief from state health departments to decrease staffing ratios may be sought. MRC volunteers may be asked to help in hospitals if there are staffing shortages. Hospital morgues will need guidance from medical examiners to deal with the increased mortality during this time period. There may be shortfalls of critical supplies, which will require outreach to alternative suppliers. Vulnerable populations may include those without routine access to care, those who have more barriers in getting antivirals, institutionalized populations (because of the potential for rapid spread of influenza in these environments), and those dependent on medications for their chronic illnesses, if the supply of these medications become compromised.

COASTAL STORMS

Flooding will require the evacuation of low lying areas. If healthcare institutions are in these areas, they will need extensive assistance from first responder agencies and contracted providers to evacuate their patients. These activities will need to be coordinated through the local emergency management organization. Shelters will be set up for the affected community with the assistance of the health departments, emergency management, and nongovernment entities such as the ARC. Although MRC personnel may work in shelters, it is likely that hospitals will need to assist those who fall ill in the shelter system, or who have chronic disease management problems and need medical assessment. Vulnerable populations include those with chronic diseases, those who cannot leave their homes, and persons without the means for self-evacuation.

Conclusions

During a disaster, all organizations need to work together to minimize morbidity and mortality in their community. It is extraordinarily difficult to do this in the absence of a prior process to agree on roles, responsibilities, and expectations of all responding groups. Therefore, identification of all stakeholders (and the ability to communicate with them during an emergency), and development of a routine meeting schedule is the first step. This should be followed by a vulnerability analysis for the community and a frank assessment of capabilities to respond to these vulnerabilities. All agreements should be codified in written protocols, and all written protocols should be tested by tabletop exercises or drills, with the involved agencies present. After-action reports should list suggested improvements in the response, and protocols should be modified if needed. In this way, even in the absence of a crisis, improvements in response can be achieved.

Special emphasis should be made to address the identification and needs of vulnerable populations in a community. Much of the information needed to identify these populations may be requested from the organizations that work with them routinely. The ability to meet the needs of vulnerable populations will likely define the success or failure of the response.

Finally, in the post 9/11 world, the public rightfully expects that institutions created to protect them—the government, hospitals, and voluntary organizations—will rise to the challenge to meet their needs, despite the economic challenges of our time.

References

1.   Gray BH, Hebert K. *After Katrina: Hospitals in Hurricane Katrina. Challenges Facing Custodial Institutions in a Disaster.* Washington, DC: The Urban Institute; July 2006. http://www.urban.org/UploadedPDF/411348_katrinahospitals.pdf. Accessed January 11, 2010.

2.   Franco C, Toner E, Waldhorn R, Maldin B, O'Toole T, Inglesby TV. Systemic collapse: medical care in the aftermath of Hurricane Katrina. *Biosecur Bioterror.* 2006;4(2):135–146.

3.   NRF Resource Center. Federal Emergency Management Agency Web site. http://www.fema.gov/emergency/nrf/. Accessed January 11, 2010.

4.   National Disaster Medical System (NDMS) Response Teams. U.S. Department of Health and Human Services Web site. http://www.hhs.gov/aspr/opeo/ndms/teams/index.html. Accessed January 11, 2010.

5.   Schoch-Spana M, Franco C, Nuzzo JB, Usenza C; for the Working Group on Community Engagement in Health Emergency Planning. Community engagement: leadership tool for catastrophic health events. *Biosecur Bioterror.* 2007;5(1):8–25.

6.   Eisenman, DP, Cordasco, KM, Asch S, Golden JF, Glik D. Disaster planning and risk communication with vulnerable communities: lessons from Hurricane Katrina. *Am J Public Health.* 2007;97(suppl 1):S109–S115.

7.   The Hospital Preparedness Program (HPP). U.S. Department of Health and Human Services Web site. http://www.hhs.gov/aspr/opeo/hpp/index.html. Accessed January 11, 2010.

8. The Laboratory Response Network Partners in Preparedness. Centers for Disease Control and Prevention Web site. http://www.bt.cdc.gov/lrn/. Accessed January 11, 2010.

9. Office of the Civilian Volunteer Medical Reserve Corps Web site. http://www.medicalreservecorps.gov/HomePage. Accessed January 11, 2010.

10. *Integration of the Medical Reserve Corps and the Emergency System for Advance Registration of Volunteer Health Professionals.* The Office of the Civilian Volunteer Medical Reserve Corps. Web site. http://www.medicalreservecorps.gov/File/ESAR_VHP/ESAR-VHPMRCIntegrationFactSheet.pdf. Updated April, 2008. Accessed January 11, 2010.

11. Davis LM, Ringel JS, Cotton SK, et al. *Public Health Preparedness: Integrating Public Health and Preparedness Programs.* Rand Center for Domestic and International Health Security. 2009. http://www.rand.org/pubs/technical_reports/TR317/. Accessed January 11, 2010.

12. Lerner EB, Cronin M, Schwartz RB, et al. Linking public health and the emergency care community: 7 model communities. *Disaster Med Public Health Prep.* 2007;1(2):142–145.

13. Markenson D, Fuller E, Redlener I. *Emergency Preparedness: Addressing the Needs of People with Disabilities.* National Center for Disaster Preparedness. March 2007. http://www.ncdp.mailman.columbia.edu/files/DISABILITIES.pdf. Accessed January 11, 2010.

14. Fernandez LS, Byard D, Lin CC, Benson S, Barbera JA. Frail elderly as disaster victims: emergency management strategies. *Prehosp Disaster Med.* 2002;17(2):67–74.

15. At-Risk Populations. The Association of State and Territorial Health Officials Web site. http://www.astho.org/page.aspx?id=2685&terms=%22at-risk+populations+project%22. Accessed January 11, 2010.

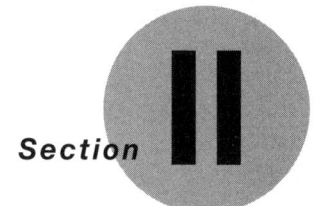

Section **II**

Hospital
Workforce
Issues

Chapter 8

Education and Training

Sean M. Kelly, MA, CCEMT-P and Lindsey P. Anthony, MPA, CEM, CHEC-III

Photo by Marvin Nauman/FEMA photo

Learning Objectives

- Establish effective methods to educate adult learners in topics of emergency management.
- List education and training requirements for various types of healthcare facilities.
- Provide examples of appropriate implementation of classroom, online, or hybrid learning methodologies to specific healthcare personnel and facilities.
- List the best approaches for teaching all styles and levels of adult learners, including visual learners, audio learners, and psychomotor learners.

Introduction

Emergency management and emergency preparedness require the careful coordination of multiple resources in response to various events.

Often, these resources are human resources and their knowledge of disaster preparedness, emergency management, and any other aspects of preparedness is minimal. By default, it becomes the job of the emergency management professional to educate others on the roles and responsibilities of the emergency manager and the responsibilities of the employee during emergencies. It is often required by state and federal law that this education and training take place in order to be compliant with preparedness regulations. The type of learner that must be educated can differ in multiple aspects: students can range in age from teenagers to elderly adults, and education can range from less than high school through post-graduate professionals. The student populations will even range in respect to primary languages spoken and literacy. This creates a huge obstacle for the emergency management professional to overcome. Add to these existing issues the fact that most emergency management professionals have received no formal training in education, and a real dilemma seems to appear. This combination of wide-ranging student populations, lack of formal education or training, training deadlines, and the potential of incurred overtime can make the issue of training healthcare facility personnel a very stressful and time-intensive situation.

The approach to education and training will vary based on numerous factors across all types of healthcare facilities. The emergency management professional should specifically be knowledgeable on how to educate everyone, from physicians and nurses to housekeeping and custodial to staff and volunteers. This will require different approaches in teaching methodologies, and it will also require various approaches in how the content is delivered to the students. Today, these methods mostly consist of traditional classroom training and technology-based approaches such as online learning. All of these approaches and their associated costs will be discussed in detail. Furthermore, today's emergency management professionals, who are responsible for training and education, must operate within strict financial boundaries. Education must be cost-effective, and in an operating environment that is often 24 hours a day, seven days a week, the desire to keep overtime at a minimum is often a priority among senior administrators. Further this responsibility by the fact that consistent documented training in multiple venues is a requirement for preparedness grant funding and continued accreditation, making this a very difficult endeavor to approach.

Traditionally, the approach to the adult student varies. In order to best prepare the educator and trainer, we will first look at what students need to learn based on their work environments. Specific healthcare areas, such as hospitals, emergency medical services, outpatient clinics, and retirement/rehabilitation facilities have different needs and requirements in terms of emergency management/preparedness education and training. The roles and responsibilities of employees in these healthcare facilities differ. Furthermore, as an adult educator, it is the duty of the instructor to provide the knowledge needed to perform required tasks to each student. Though each student presents a different level of experience, desire to learn, maturity level, intelligence, and set of abilities, it is the instructor's job to disseminate the information in a way that allows each student to walk away with the required knowledge. This requires that the trainer have a working knowledge on the different types of learners, as well as an understanding of the diversity among students, different potential instructional strategies, and methods of remediation.

Emergency management professionals need to take a careful look at their methods for training and instructing. They need to understand that training is not just a grant-funding requirement to check off, but that a well-trained workforce is the core of the facility's response in disaster situations. With this in mind, it is very important that students of all levels be taught appropriately so that each individual learns, and no shortcuts are taken to accomplish these requirements. The shortfalls in education will only be illustrated when the students are required demonstrate their knowledge either in a simulated or actual disaster scenario. If training programs are not rigorous, then the entire response could fail at a critical point.

Pay attention to needs and requirements in each healthcare facility. Understand how adult learners differ in many ways. Try to tailor the education approaches to offer equal and consistent training to all learners of every level. Understand that the instructor's method of learning may not apply to each of the students. We will examine various methods of instructing, including the use of computer-based training, online classes, traditional classroom training, and hybrid approaches to learning. The benefits and pitfalls of each approach will be discussed, as will attention to costs and support. The emergency management professional will come to understand that the needed education and training will require more planning and time than most expect. However, the results that will emerge with successful training and the true education of each individual student will make the time, effort, and money well worth it. When a disaster or other event occurs, and all the personnel in the prescribed medical facility have not just taken the training, but have learned their roles and responsibilities, there will be a smoother transition into and out of the disaster response modes.

This chapter will cover various education models that can be used in a variety of education situations. The emergency management environment is fraught with numerous obstacles that would trouble even the most professional educator. This chapter will help you better understand your students, the best approach to technology, and the best methods to help the student actually learn. Discussions will cover financial responsibility and learning style approaches, as well as handling the troublesome students that you may encounter. Furthermore, understanding how to deal with failure on the part of the instructor and the student will be discussed. Remediation must be understood to access the desired results for the students.

Frank discussions regarding issues with current models of education, including the online environment will be developed. Various methods of dealing with disruptive students, cheating, and identity verification will also be touched upon. Overall, this will include much needed information that will help you manage your students and successfully provide quality education in a variety of education environ-

Case Study

Crim Dell Hospital in Anytown, NJ just hired a new hospital emergency preparedness coordinator. Crim Dell Hospital is a 255-bed acute care hospital, with a 35-bed emergency department, which has 24-hour-a-day 7-day-a-week coverage. Typically, 5 physicians, 13 nurses, 6 patient care technicians, and 3 environmental service specialists (housekeepers) run the emergency department, which operates in 12-hour shifts. The hospital has a paramedic service that maintains 24-hour-a-day, 7-day-a-week 911 coverage with 5 fully staffed Advanced Life Support trucks that have 2 paramedics on duty 8 hours a day for 3 shifts. The hospital also runs 10 Basic Life Support ambulances that are staffed with 2 EMT-Basics 8 hours a day for 3 shifts. The hospital also has an attached dialysis center that sees approximately 50 patients a day, and is staffed 7 days a week, 8 hours a day. The hospital has numerous administrative and professional staff members, such as administrative assistants, information technology professionals, coders, and management; clinical staff, such as nurses, doctors, radiology technicians, paramedics, EMT-Basics, and pharmacists; trade staff, such as electricians, plumbers, environmental staff, and food workers; and volunteer staff.

Coming into this position, the new hospital emergency preparedness coordinator must develop training programs for all of the staff in the hospital. Keeping this in mind, the employees range from 16 years through almost 90 years of age. Their education backgrounds range from some high school through post-professional education. The training programs must be developed and implemented quickly because part of the funding eligibility for many upcoming grants depends on the hospital's compliance in terms of education and training. Also, to test the effectiveness of the training, the hospital has been asked to take part in numerous multiagency drills later in the year.

The new hospital emergency coordinator was told in no uncertain terms that overtime must be limited to as little as possible. The hospital emergency preparedness coordinator does have a small budget set aside for education and access to information technology staff. The emergency preparedness coordinator has a small staff of seven people, five of whom have direct emergency preparedness experience, and two administrative personnel.

In all, the hospital has approximately 1200 employees who work various shifts and times. Staffing in many departments is limited, and it can be very difficult to arrange time for these employees to be off of their shifts. Much of the work that is done is clinical patient care, and workloads in several clinic areas cannot be projected with any accuracy.

What are the best methods to train all of the employees of the hospital? Should there be live training, computer-based training, online training, videos, books, or a blended approach? Who will provide the instruction, and how will you provide time for the staff members to take the training without incurring massive overtime or affecting clinical duties? What are the financial impacts of providing the training or failing to provide the training?

ments. Furthermore, the desired success of the student's learning, not just the instructor's teaching, will be established.

Adult Learning

The educator needs to understand the basic principles involved in adult learning in order to successfully teach the vast array of employees they are going to encounter. The majority of the employees in the healthcare environment will be adults. The science of adult teaching is called andragogy, and it is based on basic assumptions about the adult learner.[1] Educators have to be cognizant that adult learners have life experience to draw from, and it is this life experience that allows the students to equate what they are learning with real life examples. It also allows students to be able to share their experiences with others and help in the education of their peers. Adult learners also tend to take an active role in the direction of their education. Adults are used to the freedom of choosing the direction of their lives, and the same goes for education.

Adults do not like to be told what to do. They prefer to have a hand in forming the path that they are going to follow. The educator's role is to facilitate the learning. The education process for the adult is more a path of discovery and self-direction than being handed facts. The educator helps guide adult learners down the right path, but should allow adult learners to maintain their independence. Furthermore, as part of their independence, adult learners will often be critical of activities that waste time, or are deemed incongruent with the education goals. It is often difficult to teach mandated material to adult learners because adult learners must accept that there is a good reason for the education before they are open to learning. Understanding this means that the educator must teach by showing how the required education solves an issue or problem at hand, and how it is relevant to the adult students. This can be difficult to do and the adult learners may not understand that emergency management is relevant to their tasks, until they see how they may face a disaster in their specific position. Simply put, adults that are required to attend classroom or online teaching want to know what is in it for them. Do the end results justify the means of the education? The adult learners want to put into practice what is being taught, and if the adult learners do not equate the material they are learning to their required tasks at hand, they will often be resistant to learning. The adult learners want to see the end goal, and they will work toward that goal if they see the relevance of the material. The adult learners are very different, and it is most important for the instructor to understand that the learning they are engaging in is student-centered. The adult students are the ones who drive the education, and the teacher should be nothing more then a facilitator.

No discussion on adult education can be complete without understanding what motivates adult students to learn. Intrinsic or extrinsic motivators may drive these adult learners toward education. Understanding what the motivator is, and how it affects the adult learner is very important. Intrinsic motivators are internally driven behaviors, a desire to better oneself or the community through their education. This motivator tends to be the more powerful of the two.[2] However, when the education becomes required for the employees to maintain their employment or to avoid facing punitive actions, or it is driven by other external forces, we are facing extrinsic motivators. Regardless of the motivator, the educator must try to have a basic understanding of the underpinnings that drive their students. The simple knowledge of whether a student is intrinsically or extrinsically motivated to attend the class will help the educator better teach that specific individual.

This discussion simplifies the whole of human motivation, which is far more complex overall. There have been decades of research performed and put together that goes in-depth about the things that motivate humans. The most famous of this research was performed by

Maslow. Maslow provides an evolving theory that describes the ascending order of human motivation. The human motivation is first driven by the most basic needs for survival: food, water, oxygen, and thermoregulation. From here, his hierarchy expands and the next level can only be attained after the initial level has been met, with self-transcendence and self-actualization topping off the hierarchy.

We are learning that the adult learner is an entirely complex individual who has numerous reasons, motivators, and tendencies. However, more often than not, we are unaware of the extraordinary aspects of human cognition, and just as easily as we overlook the accumulation of technology that permits use of the Internet on our computers and phones, so too can we forget the sophistication of adult learners and their cognition.[3]

To attend to this sophistication, we must understand that each adult learner may have his or her own key to learning, or learning style. This means that although all of your adult students sit in a lecture, not all of them are learning optimally from that auditory type of teaching. A learning style is a plan or framework that helps to distill raw information that a student is exposed to and form it into knowledge. There are numerous types of learners: auditory, visual, kinesthetic, analytic, global, social, and independent learners.[4] Adult learners may subscribe to more than one of these learning styles. However, many adult learners do not even know that they favor certain learning styles, and whether the adult learners know what works best for them or not, it is up to the educator to cater to all of these learning styles when they teach. Furthermore, it is imperative that as an instructor you find out which learning styles are best equated with success for your individual adult students. In order to do this, the educator must understand each of these learning styles in more detail.

Auditory learners, as the name implies, means adult learners tend to retain information better by hearing it through discussion and presentation. Auditory learners will often favor this type of learning through their actions, as well as oral clues. The auditory learner may prefer having sound or narration playing or explaining their way through a process.

Kinesthetic learners process information best through touching and handling things. The kinesthetic learners are the students who like hands-on activities, and may need to take something apart and put it back together before they can really process their learning. Educators can use supplements like labs, scenarios, and models to provide psychomotor (touch and feel) feedback to these students so they will be able to better process the learning.

Visual learners process information best through sight. Visual representations, such as graphs, slide presentations, handouts, illustrations, DVDs, and computer modeling provide the visual information to these students. They often need to see the words to best process the information and learn.

Analytic learners are the students who do best with step-by step-algorithms and need to have an order to everything. They need to process information in a logical or sequential manner in order to learn. These students will need to systematically identify and analyze the knowledge they are looking at and fit it into some sort of pattern or sequence to best understand it. Teaching in a sequential manner, or providing an outline that sequences the information can be a great aid to these learners.

Global learners like to look at the entire process and work from the outcome back to the beginning or the cause. These learners tend to be more creative and artistic in their endeavors and the idea of following step-by-step protocols may be more difficult. They will want to try to picture the entirety of the process and work from the intended results backward.

Finally, the last set of styles that you may come across is the independent versus social learners. As their names imply, independent learners tend to work better on their own without distractions from other individuals, and social learners draw off of interpersonal interactions. It is important for the educator to understand that he or she will encounter both of these student types. The instructor should encourage students to try to study in groups to foster the social learners, but the instructor should also provide opportunities for the independent learners to learn outside of the group environment.

Whatever the students' learning styles, the educator must try to touch upon and foster all learning styles when he or she teaches. This means using a variety of approaches to the education process. Furthermore, many students may not know "officially" which learning style works best for them. It is important that the educator listens to how students approach education and how they respond to the variety of approaches used. The students need to be key players in their education, and teaching in a method that helps them learn will ultimately benefit you as the educator.

Another issue at hand when dealing with adult students is intelligence. This especially comes into play when working with large organizations, such as healthcare facilities, because you are dealing with such a cornucopia of individuals. The definition of "intelligences" for the purpose of education is varying degrees of ability in eight areas: logical-mathematical, spatial, bodily-kinesthetic, linguistic, musical, naturalist, intrapersonal, and interpersonal.[5] Each individual will have varying abilities in each of these categories, and the sum total of this variety of ability is what defines his or her total intelligence.[5] It is important for an educator to understand these basic compositions of their adult students, and to attempt to vary their material presentation so that each student will have the ability to foster his or her own growth, by using his or her dominant category of intelligence during the learning process.

This touches on the basics of understanding which approaches will help when teaching adult learners. It is obvious that you will have a multitude of adult learning styles and intelligence levels to cope with when instructing adult learners in the emergency management environment. Understand that most educators spend years studying the best approaches to teaching the adult learner, and here it is given to you in a few pages. These are the basics, and understanding just these basics alone will help you better teach the students that you come in contact with, catering to their specific needs and learning styles. You will be able to create more diverse presentations and classes that will appeal to a greater audience than just the emergency management professional. By understanding your students, what motivates them to learn, and how they learn best you will reach your ultimate goal of not just teaching to these individuals, but having them learn. In the long run, the more preparation and consideration you give to these aspects of all of your students, the more likely the important tasks and regulations that you impart to them will be heeded in time of disaster. You and your facility will function in a smoother, more professional manner in time of disaster because you educated your students and they learned.

Behavior Issues

No discussion on educating the adult learner can be complete without discussing the potential for behavior issues among the students. These issues may be destructive or constructive in their appearance in your classroom, and it takes a savvy educator to learn how to deal with good and bad behavior without losing self-control or control of the classroom. The behavior that students portray in class can be linked to the motivation that inspired the student to take the class.

In the healthcare environment, the individual responsible for education will often come in contact with the student who is motivated by extrinsic factors to take mandatory training. The individual who is forced to be in the class will often present in a defiant manner and this is one of the most difficult students to handle. He or she has no desire to be at the training; however, he or she is mandated to be there. The goal for the educator in this instance is to seek a way to have this student accept the training and take an active role in it. After this type of student is identified, it is important that the educator seek out his or her assistance and try to feed off of the student's life experiences to help teach the rest of the students. After the instructor has successfully made this student a value-added part of the class, handling him or her will be much easier. It is also important that the instructor not minimize the situation at hand. The instructor must acknowledge the reasons for this training and communicate to the students that he or she understands that this is not the ideal task for everyone on hand. Setting basic rules for the class, and sticking to those rules for each and every student, will help prevent unnecessary disruptions in the training.

Another student type that may be encountered is the student who demonstrates boredom or no interest in the material being presented. This is identified through the lack of attention the student displays in class, as well as other aspects such as body language. A solution to this issue can only be encountered when the root cause is discovered. There are a variety of reasons why the student may be preoccupied or less attentive in class; these reasons can range from incomprehension of the material at hand through personal issues at home or at work. If the issue at hand is class-related, such as the class moves too slowly for the student or there is not enough hands-on activity to keep his or her interest, then it would benefit the instructor to empower this student with a portion of the presentation or class activity. Have the student prepare a presentation for a future class to help empower him or her, and build the student into the classroom pace and activity.[4] Regardless of the problem, as the instructor, it is important that you privately cousel the individual so as not to create an affront to the student in the class, where irreparable damage can occur in the instructor–student relationship. Above all, remember that this is student-centered learning, and all students must buy in for success. If the problem at hand is of a more personal nature, offer assistance where you can as instructor, and help lead the student toward more professional services that might be able to solve his or her issues.

Another student behavior issue that actually impacts the class as a whole is students who habitually come late to class.[4] These students disrupt the learning process after it has already begun, and divert student attention away from the material at hand because students who arrived in class in a timely manner wonder why the habitual lateness does not affect the offender in any way. This can be difficult to handle, but it must be handled initially through private counseling of the student. The instructor must understand if there are valid reasons for the habitual lateness, such as day care issues. After the problem is identified, the instructor and the student must come up with a plan of action to correct the issue. The student must be made aware that there are repercussions to the habitual lateness.[4] The instructor might want to include more group projects or graded material due at the start of class to pressure the habitually late student into conforming to the schedule or the student will face repercussions that will affect his or her final grade or the ability to pass the mandatory training.

In an emergency management environment, you will have to teach students who work a variety of different shifts. Some of your students may be coming off of busy night shifts and may be sleep deprived. It is important to understand how to deal with the tired student because you want to avoid one of the biggest disruptions in the classroom, which is a sleeping student. The best method for handling this is to approach the class as a whole and offer a number of ways to avoid sleeping. This can be accomplished by offering a variety of activities in class and allowing students to perform hands-on actions that will get them up and moving around. You should avoid the traditional lecture-only format if you believe that wakefulness is a problem in the class. Also, allow breaks to be built in to the class schedule, and allow the students to keep you, as the instructor, honest with these breaks. Have them remind you what time the breaks are supposed to happen and stick to them. Finally, after laying the ground rules in the class and making all the students realize that you understand the wakefulness issues because of the shift schedules they may encounter, but falling asleep in class is not going to be tolerated. Allow students to get up and stand in the back of the classroom if they start feeling as though they may fall asleep; this will keep them awake and paying attention, and it will avoid the potential disruptions that a sleeping student can cause for you, as the instructor, and for the rest of the class.[4]

Finally, one of the last types of students you will encounter is the student who has done it all and knows it all. This student can either be very helpful in class or be a major disruption. Working in the emergency management field, you will come across this type of student. He or she will have a story for everything that you teach, and this can be a major hindrance in the education process. The initial approach to this student, like the many others we have encountered thus far, is a private consultation with the student to explain the effect of the stories or attitude on the class. As an instructor, you can also focus this student's energy into small group projects, as long as the other students in the group receive this student well.[4] Finally, the instructor can also use this student as a resource to help teach or set up the class; however, it is important that this treatment of the problem is not perceived as special treatment by other students, so the instructor must walk a careful line when handling this type of student.[4]

Finally, it is important to understand how to handle the potential for failure, from students, and from you as the instructor. In order to appropriately determine reasons for failure, a true remediation process must exist. Remediation means to correct a deficiency.[6] However, it is important for the instructor to understand the concept that remediation does not just mean taking an exam again; it is a defined and important process that helps to identify the root cause of failure and to find a solution to that cause, so the student or instructor can be successful.

Remediation is often something that has been missing from many education programs. However, according to one study, 30–90% of students enrolled in a community college program are in need of remediation.[7]

This shows the glaring inadequacy that many education programs have when it comes to dealing with students who have problems in assimilating the knowledge required for success. There are several steps that must be followed in order to establish a remediation plan for each student, and the remediation plans for these students must be customized. The first hurdle in the process is to understand exactly what caused the failure. This requires both the instructor and the student to look at the program and at themselves to see where there was a disruption in the learning process. After this gap has been identified, the instructor must decide if the student is open and capable of remediation. The instructor must understand if the cause is something that can be remediated. If the cause is very difficult to overcome, the instructor must consider the possibility of dismissal from the program if that is the only adequate solution. However, this decision cannot be made lightly because program dismissal can have devastating effects on the student, especially if extrinsic factors are motivating attendance and the program. If a cause of the student's failure has been identified and it is a cause that they can remediate, the instructor and the student must form a plan for remediation. The instructor and student must then work together to implement this agreed-upon plan. The final step will be for the student to once again undergo evaluation. With a well thought out program and strong commitment by the instructor and the student, remediation should be a strengthening process for all involved. However, the possibility does exist that a student, even after thorough input into the remediation process, will not be successful. It is the duty of the instructor to understand that, in theory, it would be great for everyone to successfully complete courses, but not everyone is cut out to successfully accomplish everything. It is up to the instructor to weed out those who will not be successful in applying the training to real life. Though this decision is one that should be made only after very careful consideration because of the impact it will have on the student and the program, it is a necessary decision that must be made. Having a student who is not capable or is negligent in applying the training he or she learned in your class to real life situations will be a poor direct reflection on the quality of your training programs, and in the end, on the instructors as well. All things considered, a strong program with a good remediation plan that is already established and individualized to the students will produce better trained and happier students in the long run. This step in the education process is not something that can be overlooked, no matter how many students go through your course or take your training.[8]

Classroom versus Online Learning

In today's world of computers, the Internet, and technology, a decision must be made on how to best apply these tools to the learning environment. There are a number of education technologies that can assist in the presentation of materials, and save time and money. This requires certain considerations to be made regarding the delivery of the instruction to students. The question of delivery mainly revolves around three overarching categories: classroom lecture, online learning, or a hybrid approach.

Classroom lecture follows the format of in-person instruction, in which an instructor leads the learning in a classroom where all students and the instructor must meet at prescribed times. The quality of this instruction often depends on the abilities of the instructor, but it allows the students to be better monitored in terms of their progress, information assimilation, and success. Because students are required to attend in person, time management becomes less of an issue for the students because they have to build classroom time into their own schedule to successfully complete the course. However, this category of instruction also has its pitfalls. If there are a large number of students in the healthcare environment that require the knowledge, this process can become very time-intensive and expensive. Students may have to incur overtime in order to attend classes that are held at prescribed times. Furthermore, numerous classroom options will have to be enabled in order to meet the various shift requirements of the students. This may create an unfair burden on the instructor or instructors because they will have to accommodate these varying schedules, and they will often have to hold multiple sessions for the same material.

The second overarching concept is to use an online or computer-based curriculum. Though many instructors tend to cringe at the idea of online learning, statistics show that this is becoming more and more commonplace in education. In 2001, reports show that close to 80% of colleges and universities in the United States are offering a Web-based component to their curriculum and more than 60% of large corporations offer training that uses the Web.[9] This shows that this concept is no longer novel, because in 2010 these numbers have begun to rise higher. This approach to learning, if correctly implemented, will decrease the need for overtime, decrease the requirement for classroom real estate, and allow students to complete didactic requirements more easily, either during "downtime" or on their own time. Furthermore, this approach to learning will provide better documentation and tracking of student performance, and ultimately can help the instructor better understand a student's learning needs. However, as with any concept, there are important caveats to consider. First, the online approach must be extremely well-planned, the information technology support must be present, and the course must not be put together in haste. Secondly, students must be made extremely aware of the time commitments and requirements that still exist in the online environment. Students can perceive that the lack of their required presence in a physical classroom equates with less time required for the class. This is not true. In fact, student participation in an online course can be more intense than in the classroom, because of the students' requirement to set aside time in their personal schedule to commit to the classroom. This time can be 3 AM if the student so desires, but the time commitment is required. Thirdly, no online course is successful for the student or the instructor unless multiple lines of interactive communication are open between instructors and students, as well as among the students themselves.[9] The students must be able to communicate with their instructor in a manner that is as effortless as possible, and interactive communication is encouraged because it will help retain student participation. Online learning is not a solution that allows the instructor to walk away from his or her responsibilities. Finally, the fear exists that students will cheat when instructors do not directly supervise them during the class or exams. This fear is legitimate. With new technologies, such as randomized tests, timed tests, and extensive question banks, these fears can be somewhat minimized, but never completely refuted. Part of the solution to this process is strong codes of conduct that are made clear to the students early in the class, and are adhered to during the class. For instance, FEMA's online learning initiative makes it very clear that students who cheat on their online tests will not receive credit, and furthermore, their agencies could face disciplinary action.[10] Though FEMA can implement better technology to deter cheating, the rules and guidelines are a good start. The detriment of cheating is the potential life that can be lost when this training must be used in real world situations, and the student who has cheated actually is not proficient in the material. This is a real situation that all emergency management instructors must consider, because it may have been a contributing factor to the loss of lives in past disasters.[11]

When deciding whether to implement an online or computer-based learning system, the instructor must be able to push past the boundaries that are normally comfortable. The instructor must also think carefully about the qualifications of their students and understand that the following obstacles will be encountered: student access to technology, student retention in program, student isolation, student learning style adaptation, student motivation, student time management, and, as we already discussed, student academic integrity.[9] As long as the instructor plans well for these potential obstacles and the instructor maintains strong two-way interactive communication with his or her students, the online or computer-based training is a potential training solution. Multimedia instruction offers powerful learning technology,

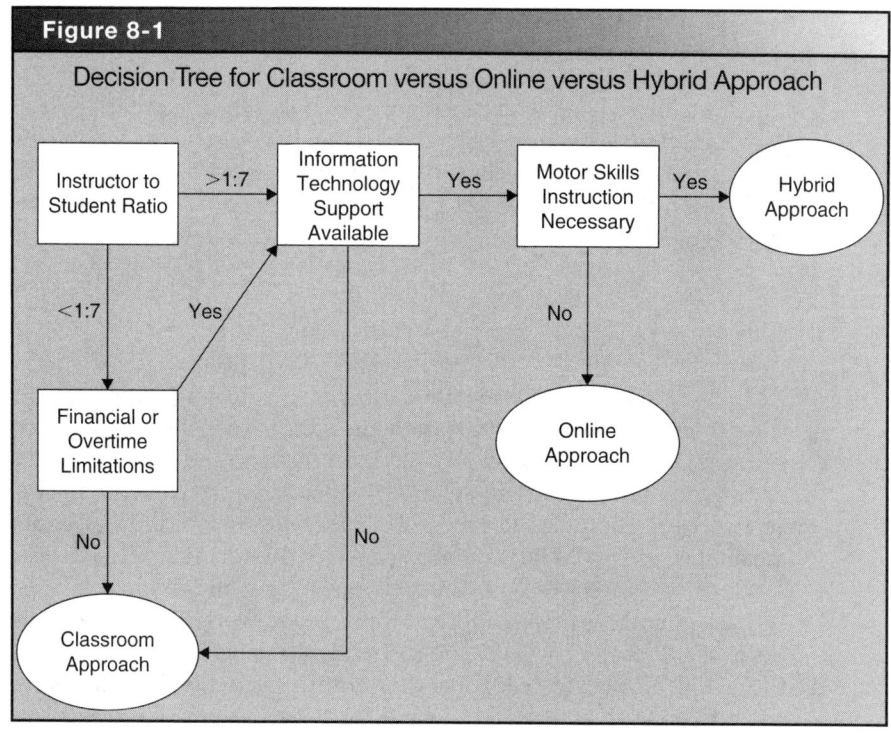

Figure 8-1

Decision Tree for Classroom versus Online versus Hybrid Approach

a system for enhancing human learning.[12] In order to have a successful approach to the online learning environment, the instructor or instructional designer of the content must consider important criteria regarding content. The content must present the information that you intend to convey, the aesthetics of the presentation must be appropriate, and the content delivery must be of satisfactory sophistication, in that it uses the latest technology available and does not depend on outdated technology that will date your program.[12]

Online training may be great for didactic training, but often the curriculum involved in emergency management has the required need for mastery of motor skills. Motor skills are very difficult to teach in a distance environment, so the instructor may opt to combine the online environment with a shorter in-person classroom period of instruction. This approach is called a hybrid approach to learning. Student didactic instruction can still be accomplished through the use of online media. However, special in-person classroom sections, which require instructor oversight, will be used to allow students to attempt mastery of any required motor skills. This allows students to prepare the foundations of learning through online access to the didactic learning, and it should decrease required classroom instruction time because only the motor skills need to be taught in person. This approach to learning has successfully been used in a number of education initiatives, both at the collegiate level and at the technical level of training.

It can be difficult to decide the type of instruction approach to use. However, based on some basic criteria, such as instructor to student ratio, financial limitations, information technology support, and motor skill requirements, the instructor can examine potential paths to follow (see Figure 8-1).

Clinical Healthcare Considerations

Hospitals across America and abroad have been dealing with disasters since their creation; in the past, these disasters have included the yearly influx of influenza patients, smallpox outbreaks, and the occasional community disaster. During the terrorist attacks on the United States on September 11, 2001, healthcare providers saw just how easily a large catastrophic event could impair not just a major metropolitan city, but also the support systems the hospitals rely on, such as the ability to obtain supplies, transfer patients, and staff reporting to work. This proved that hospital personnel needed to be trained and able to handle a mass influx of people needing care, in a shorter time period with limited staff and other resources. After 9/11 came the release of Homeland Security Presidential Directive 5 (HSPD 5) with the explicit purpose: "To enhance the ability of the United States to manage domestic incidents by establishing a single, comprehensive national incident management system."[13] The policy laid out under HSPD 5 states that "The objective of the United States Government is to ensure that all levels of government across the Nation have the capability to work efficiently and effectively together, using a national approach to domestic incident management."[13] From HSPD 5, the National Incident Management System (NIMS) was formed. Doing so created the NIMS Implementation Objectives for Healthcare Organizations, and from HSPD 8 came the requirement that "all hospitals and healthcare systems receiving Federal preparedness and response grants, contracts, or cooperative agreements ... must work to implement the National Incident Management System. Hospitals and healthcare systems are defined as all facilities that receive medical and trauma emergency patients on a daily basis."[14] HSDP 8 "establishes policies to strengthen the preparedness of the United States to prevent and respond to threatened or actual domestic terrorist attacks, major disasters, and other emergencies by requiring a national domestic all-hazards preparedness goal, establishing mechanisms for improved delivery of Federal preparedness assistance to State and local governments, and outlining actions to strengthen preparedness capabilities of Federal, State, and local entities."[15] After the release of HSPD 8, hospitals and healthcare facilities began looking for funding to train their workforces and meet the NIMS requirements now placed on those receiving funding. The Hospital Preparedness Program (HPP) is federally funded under the Department of Health and Human Services Assistant Secretary for Preparedness and Response (ASPR) and it is just one way to secure funds to accomplish the NIMS Implementation Activities.

It was not until 2005 that Hurricane Katrina showed us that hospitals themselves need to be prepared to take action during an emergency involving a hospital or healthcare facility. One such example was Charity Hospital in New Orleans, where more than 200 patients and healthcare providers were trapped for days after withstanding the fury of Hurricane Katrina. On September 17, 2006, a little more than one year after Hurricane Katrina battered the Gulf Coast and wreaked havoc on hospitals and healthcare facilities, the NIMS Integration Center published the NIMS Implementation Plan for Hospitals and Healthcare. They attached a deadline of September 30, 2007 for all hospitals and healthcare facilities to be NIMS compliant. There were 17 objectives deemed necessary for becoming NIMS compliant in the original release, four of which were considered critical enough that without compliance by September 2007, a facility would not be eligible for receiving federal funds. The four include: (1) revising and updating plans to ensure incorporation of NIMS components; (2) completing IS-700 NIMS: An Introduction; (3) completion of IS-800 NRP (National Response Plan—now known as the National Response Framework [NRF]): An Introduction; and (4) completion of ICS 100 and ICS 200 training. The remaining 13 objectives included in the original release were items pertaining to preparedness exercises, resource management, command structure and communications, standard terminology, and preparedness planning.

For FY08–09, the NIMS objectives have been condensed and restructured into 14 objectives for hospitals and healthcare facilities. The objectives were as follows:[16]

Adoption

1. Adopt NIMS throughout the healthcare organization.
2. Ensure federal preparedness awards support NIMS implementations (in accordance with the eligibility and allowable uses of the awards).

Preparedness: Planning

3. Revise and update Emergency Operations Plan (EOP), standard operating procedures, and other plans to include NIMS and NRF principles.
4. Participate in interagency mutual aid and/or assistance agreements, including agreements with public and private sectors as well as nongovernment organizations (NGOs).

Preparedness: Training and Exercises

5. Identify the appropriate personnel to complete ICS-100, ICS-200, and IS-700.
6. Identify the appropriate personnel to complete IS-800.
7. Promote NIMS concepts and principles, and ICS into all organization-related training and exercising.

Communications and Information Management

8. Promote and ensure that all equipment, including communication, and data interoperability, are in the organization's acquisition programs.
9. Apply common and consistent terminology, including plain language standards for communications.
10. Utilize systems, tools, and processes that facilitate the collection and distribution of accurate information during an incident or event.

Command and Management

11. Manage all events (emergencies, disasters, and exercises alike) in accordance with NIMS doctrine.
12. ICS implementation must include use of an Incident Action Plan (IAP).
13. Adopt the principles of public information as facilitated by a Joint Information System (JIS) and Joint Information Center (JIC) during an event or disaster.
14. Ensure that public information policies gather, verify, coordinate, and disseminate information during an event or disaster.

Understanding NIMS is just one of the many integral parts of comprehending emergency management (EM) both outside and within hospitals. Another vital component is understanding EM as it relates directly to hospitals. While many of the standard emergency management principles apply to hospitals, they also face some very unique challenges and considerations.

First, a grasp of the basis of emergency management is required. Emergency management is defined as an integrated, all-hazards approach to the management of any emergency or disaster and to the programs and activities surrounding them. An emergency, as defined by Merriam-Webster, is "an unforeseen combination of circumstances or the resulting state that calls for immediate action."[17] Disaster is a word commonly interchanged with emergency events, but disasters are more correctly situations that overwhelm local resources or capacity, thereby necessitating a call for external assistance. When considering emergencies and disasters, and beginning the process of conducting activities in relation to them, we organize the activities in four groups.

These four groups are known as the Emergency Management Cycle or disaster phases. The four groups are mitigation, preparedness, response, and recovery.

Mitigation is the prevention of disasters through reducing vulnerability to a particular risk or hazard. Steps for mitigating disasters are generally physical or structural in nature, though they can include laws and guidelines. The addition of wind retrofits, such as placing film on glass to prevent breaking or adding functional shutters to a facility, would be considered mitigation efforts. Both structural and nonstructural mitigation efforts should be undertaken in order to remain operational.

Preparedness is the building up of capabilities to manage the impact hazards inflict, as well as a state of being prepared for specific risks. It is often referenced hand-in-hand with mitigation. Preparedness is accomplished through training, education, exercising, planning, and stockpiling. Common preparedness measures include communications plans with easily understandable terminology, chain of command development prior to an incident, practicing multiagency coordination, exercising a facility's Emergency Operations Plan, training on the plan, and educating staff on the plan.

The second two phases in the Emergency Management Cycle are response and recovery. Like mitigation and preparedness, they are often discussed in tandem. Response is decreasing or stopping the ongoing negative effects of disasters, including the mobilization of necessary emergency services for a disaster. Activating a facility's Emergency Operations Plan is an action seen in the response phase. Also included in response is the triage and treatment of patients and management of victims. Response is, in most instances, a short-term operation, unlike recovery that begins simultaneously but continues on until normal operations resume. Recovery is the short- and long-term restoration of the damages caused by a disaster with the aim of restoring the affected area to its previous state, such as reopening a wing of a hospital restored after being damaged by a tornado. These include both operational and business recoveries. It differs from the response phase in its focus; recovery efforts are concerned with issues and decisions that must be made after the immediate needs are addressed. In the United States, the National Response Framework dictates how the resources provided by the Homeland Security Act of 2002 will be used in recovery efforts.

The ability of a healthcare facility to plan for a disaster is determined by many variables. These include funding, a willing and knowledgeable staff, and the ability to determine a facility's risks. Before determining the risk posed by various hazards, a facility must first determine the hazards that are most likely to affect the facility. In following with current doctrine pertaining to types of disasters, an all-hazards approach must be taken. An all-hazards approach is an approach that considers all types of possible hazards to a facility, so that each may be analyzed and assigned both mitigation and preparedness efforts. These hazards are commonly broken down into two categories: natural and man-made hazards. Natural hazards may include thunderstorms, ice storms, hurricanes, tornados, and many more naturally occurring events. Man-made hazards are more complex to analyze and anticipate because they can come in the form of a chemical spill, a power outage, or more sinister and harder to predict occurrences, such as active shooters or terrorist attacks.

Now, with an increased understanding of hazards that may affect healthcare facilities, it is vital to be able to evaluate your hazards in terms of probability of affecting a facility, the impact to said facility, and the level of risk associated with the combination of these two variables. Developing a hazard vulnerability analyses (HVA) is the most analytical process of evaluating a healthcare facility's risk. An HVA should be completed in a formal and organized manner. Knowing the risks likely to impact a facility is the first step to completing an HVA. To begin, search the local weather history, check with the local emergency management agency, and examine other historical data, as well as looking to possible threats within the community. These may take the form of nearby railway yards where train cars holding potentially hazardous materials are located, or it might be that a particular hospital or healthcare facility lies within a 500-year flood plain. All hazards and their associated risks should be based on valid facts and reasonable assumptions. After selecting the hazards most likely to occur, the next step is to determine the probability of each hazard occurring as well as the potential impact from each hazard. When these are analyzed, an outcome of accept, plan, manage, or reduce will occur.

For a hazard with a high probability and a high impact on a hospital, the outcome will be reduced. Regardless of the outcome, it is important to ensure the mitigation efforts surrounding it are proper in relation to the associated risks of the hazard. The outcomes resulting in accept, plan, and manage are results of the following combinations: (1) For a low probability and low impact hazard, a facility should accept the risk. (2) For a hazard that has a combination of high probability and low impact, a facility should manage the risks. (3) For a hazard that has a combination of low probability and high impact, a facility should plan for the risks of the particular hazard.

If a hazard risk is such that mitigation and preparedness efforts are warranted, then some measures a healthcare facility's emergency coordinator should use for the respective facility are an organization's available resources and the ability of the organization to utilize such resources. Furthermore, an organization should evaluate its current preparedness level for each hazard, reevaluate its Emergency Operations Plan as it specifically relates to each hazard, and ensure that the most current mandates, laws, regulations, and standards are being considered.

After a hospital or healthcare facility has an HVA, it is time to move forward in the process and write an Emergency Operations Plan (EOP). An EOP is a written document that outlines individual and department responsibilities when an emergency or disaster exceeds the capability or routine functions. The EOP is not meant to govern routine, day-to-day operations of the hospital or healthcare facility; rather, it may be used during a disaster, when the resources will be quickly overwhelmed. An EOP is a living document that assigns responsibilities to departments and individuals for carrying out specific duties, setting up lines of authority, showing coordination, describing how property and people will be protected, identifying resources, identifying steps to take during all phases of the emergency management cycle, and citing legal basis for its existence.

Following the creation and implementation of the EOP, training and education of the staff must begin. Staff members need to know when and why the plan is used and what roles they will play when the plan is activated. Training and education of staff can be accomplished through many means. One way to train on the EOP is to speak with the hospital's training coordinator, human resources, or the compliance officer. With the aid of these departments, training can be made a simple yearly requirement, much the way many hospitals require staff to do a yearly Health Insurance Portability and Accountability Act (HIPAA) refresher. The ICS and IS courses can be added as base requirements for all new hires, and then specific roles as they relate directly to staff positions/responsibilities during activation of the EOP can be included in yearly training requirements. This ensures the training is taken seriously and time is put aside for such items—items that are generally difficult to get staff to take time out of their daily obligations to complete. It also can gain support and acceptance from the hospital's administration.

Attending a course or courses designed specifically for hospital and healthcare facility emergency coordinators is another option, and one much preferred over simple refresher-style training. In-person, side-by-side training allows productive discussions on how issues facing a facility vary from place to place. The administration's views on emergency management's role in a facility and as part of the bigger picture also vary widely from place to place.

Conclusion

Education is a very involved process that often requires years of experience and training in order to be applied successfully. Most professional educators achieve graduate degrees in their quest for successful application of their craft. However, as we have seen, emergency managers, often without the proper teaching experience, are often handed the responsibilities for educating a diverse workforce, with excessive constraints.

This chapter has illuminated a number of approaches and considerations that emergency management educators can add to their toolbox in order to successfully complete required education for their students. There are many aspects to the education of a diverse student body, and the educators must be prepared to initiate the appropriate implementation of best practices for the teaching of visual learners, audio learners, and psychomotor learners the educators may encounter in their healthcare careers. The considerations that have been highlighted provide a means for allowing the educators to establish effective methods, which allow the education of adult learners in topics of emergency management. Furthermore, the educators can understand how the application of technology can assist in the delivery of education. However, specific criteria must be considered when determining the appropriate implementation of classroom, online, or hybrid learning methodologies to specific healthcare personnel and facilities. The educators now have a better comprehension of specific education and training requirements for the clinical healthcare setting. There are numerous considerations to be made when understanding required policy regarding education in the healthcare and emergency management environments. There are a number of solutions that must come together, including government policy, education approaches, and student comprehension, to allow success in education. Above all, the emergency management educators must understand how their students learn and attempt to successfully train their students, not just teach them. Successful training equates to the proper application of skills in a real world emergency, and the students must learn in order for this to occur. The educators must use all of the tools in their toolbox to allow their students the best opportunity to learn.

References

1. Knowles MS. Andragogy, not pedagogy! *Adult Leadership.* 1968;16(10):350–352.
2. Mendler AN. *Motivating Students Who Don't Care: Successful Techniques for Educators.* Bloomington, IN: Solution Tree Press; 2000.
3. Anderson, JR. *Cognitive Psychology and its Implications,* 5th ed. New York, NY: Worth Publishers; 2000.
4. Cason D. *Foundations of Education: An EMS Approach.* St. Louis, MO: Elsevier; 2006.
5. Gardner H. *Frames of Mind: The Theory of Multiple Intelligences.* New York, NY: Basic Books; 1983.
6. Remediation. *Riverside Webster's II Dictionary,* revised ed. New York: Berkeley Books; 1996.

7. Brenner P. From novice to expert. *Am J Nurs.* 1982;82(3):402–407.

8. Spann MG Jr. *Remediation: A Must for the 21st-Century Learning Society* [policy paper]. Denver, CO: ESC Distribution Center; 2000.

9. Lynch M. *The Online Educator: A Guide to Creating the Virtual Classroom.* New York, NY: RoutledgeFalmer; 2006.

10. Frequently Asked Questions. Emergency Management Institute. http://www.training.fema.gov/EMIWeb/IS/ISFAQ.asp#improperconduct. Updated April 26, 2007. Accessed January 14, 2010.

11. Menchaca R, Smith G. Fire training ripe for cheating. *The Post and Courier.* August 12, 2007. http://www.charleston.net/news/2007/aug/12/fire_training_ripe_cheating12823/?print. Accessed January 14, 2010.

12. Mayer RE. *Multimedia Learning.* New York, NY: Cambridge University Press; 2001.

13. Bush GW. Homeland Security Presidential Directive 5: Management of Domestic Incidents. Homeland Security Web site. http://www.dhs.gov/xabout/laws/gc_1214592333605.shtm. Published February 28, 2003.

14. NIMS Implementation Activities for Hospital and Healthcare Systems Implementation FAQS. FEMA Web site. http://www.fema.gov/pdf/emergency/nims/hospital_faq.pdf. Updated April 20, 2007. Accessed January 14, 2010.

15. Bush GW. Homeland Security Presidential Directive 8: National Preparedness. Homeland Security Web site. http://www.dhs.gov/xabout/laws/gc_1215444247124.shtm. Published December 17, 2003. Accessed January 14, 2010.

16. FY 2008 & 2009 (October 1, 2007—September 30, 2009) NIMS Implementation Objectives for Healthcare Organizations. FEMA Web site. http://www.fema.gov/emergency/nims/ImplementationGuidanceStakeholders.shtm. Posted June 10, 2008. Accessed January 14, 2010.

17. Emergency. *Merriam-Webster's Online Dictionary.* Merriam-Webster Web site. http://www.merriam-webster.com/dictionary/emergency. 2010. Accessed February 24, 2010.

Chapter 9

Functional Roles of Hospital Workers in Disasters and Public Health Emergencies

Tony Garcia, RN CCEMT-P

Learning Objectives

- Identify the roles and responsibilities of key hospital personnel and departments during an emergency event.
- Describe how departments interact with each other and community facilities during an emergency.
- Explain how typical functional roles may change during a disaster, act of terrorism, or public health emergency.

Introduction

Disasters come in all shapes and sizes and they are likely to occur when the community is least prepared. Sometimes, the healthcare facility can be the epicenter of the disaster when there is some type of catastrophic loss to the facility. Other times, resulting from ineffective preparation, an external disaster is "relocated" to the hospital, serving only to incapacitate the response. Regardless of the situation, it has become painfully clear that all healthcare facilities, large and small, are a crucial spoke in the larger wheel of community disaster preparedness and response. Healthcare facilities and workers have acquired a larger role in the face of all types of disasters. As such, all employees of a healthcare facility must be trained and capable of functioning in various capacities during a critical event.

Key Personnel

HOSPITAL CHIEF EXECUTIVE OFFICER

The hospital's senior administrator is the chief executive officer (CEO), who will have the ultimate authority for the overall operation of the hospital during the disaster or emergency. The CEO must possess a fundamental knowledge of the traditional four phases of emergency management in order to be able to commit and allocate resources for mitigation, preparation, response, and recovery from an emergency. The CEO will work closely with the hospital emergency management program manager prior to an event to ensure that the hazard vulnerability analysis (HVA) is current and that the Emergency Operations Plan is also up-to-date and corresponds to the current HVA. The CEO will ensure that hospital emergency plans and personnel are prepared to interface with the local emergency response community as required by The Joint Commission on the Accreditation of Healthcare Organizations (JCAHO). The CEO will be responsible for implementing and establishing a hospital emergency incident command system for all hazards or emergencies consistent with the National Incident Management System (NIMS) and determine suitability of personnel to fill the key positions for Hospital Incident Command System (HICS) implementation, a form of institutional responder credentialing in line with the national responder credentialing system that is currently under development. During a disaster situation, the CEO could serve as the incident commander or could designate another qualified person to fill that role.

HOSPITAL CHIEF FINANCIAL OFFICER

The costs associated with a disaster or other emergency must be captured as accurately as possible for various reasons. For starters, and most important of all, the level of federal disaster reimbursement will be directly linked to the completeness of required paperwork. In today's financial times when hospitals are forced to cut costs, a significant disaster with or without a large influx of casualties can bankrupt an institution without federal aid. This has been shown with Charity Hospital in New Orleans after Hurricane Katrina and UTMB Medical Center in Galveston after Hurricane Ike. It will be the responsibility of the chief financial officer (CFO) to develop a plan for cost distribution tracking during the event (overall event vs. department). A large-scale disaster will require a significant amount of resource cost tracking to include personnel time, durable equipment usage, disposable supplies, etc. The CFO will work with the hospital emergency manager to determine budgetary requirements in order to maintain compliance with all applicable rules and statutes while taking into consideration the impact of emergency management on the budget of other hospital operations. During an event, the CFO is the most qualified candidate to fulfill the role of "Finance/Administration Section Chief" within the Hospital Incident Command System structure. The CFO can explore innovative ways to fund or underwrite the hospital emergency management program through grants, foundations, or alternative sources of philanthropy.

CHIEF MEDICAL OFFICER

The chief medical officer (CMO) will serve as the primary medical advisor to the incident commander in all aspects related to the appropriate medical care of victims. The CMO will determine when the hospital will begin diverting all noncritical admissions and cancellation of elective surgeries. The CMO will have final approval authority in the designation of alternative treatment locations within the hospital facilities. The CMO will identify the staff medical experts in infectious disease, toxicology, and radiation illness. The CMO can be the hospital liaison with other members of the local medical community, including other hospitals, emergency medical services, and the public health authority. The CMO will work with the human resources department in planning for medical staff surge during emergencies and oversee the development of a policy for emergency authorization of outside or retired healthcare personnel (physicians, nurses, pharmacists, EMTs) to assist in the event of a large-scale disaster. The CMO is responsible for developing a plan to educate the medical staff about their roles and responsibilities during different kinds of emergencies.

CHIEF NURSING OFFICER

The chief nursing officer (CNO) will maintain overall authority of all nursing personnel as they deliver patient care within their respective care areas. In planning for an event, the CNO will work closely with the hospital emergency manager to accomplish several goals including, but not limited to, the following:

- Identify primary and alternate treatment locations for disaster patients.
- Determine the number and locations of surge isolation rooms for contagious patients.
- Develop a plan for housing and feeding the staff.
- Develop a plan for a surge in hospital bed capacity during emergencies.
- Develop a protocol for the disposition of patients from a discharge area.
- Coordinate with Social Services to assign locations for a "Family Support Center" during the emergencies.
- Work with the pharmacy section chief to develop a plan for the administration and distribution of prophylactic medications and/or immunizations to staff.

The CNO will also need to work closely with the human resources department in planning for a surge in the nursing staff capacity and other support staff (unlicensed assistive personnel) capacity during emergencies. The plan should include notification and "callback" procedures in the event of a disaster. The CNO will consult with other senior administrators (CEO/CMO) to develop a protocol for transferring patients during an emergency caused by capability, capacity, or contamination issues. The CNO is also responsible for developing a plan to educate the nursing staff about their roles and responsibilities during different kinds of emergencies.

HOSPITAL EMERGENCY MANAGER

The hospital emergency manager will be the focal point for the development and implementation of the overall program. The program should be comprehensive, utilizing an "all-hazards" approach in accordance with accepted "best practices" and compliant with JCAHO standards. The emergency manager will perform a hazard vulnerability analysis for the healthcare institution. The HVA will serve as the foundation for the written Emergency Operations Plan (EOP), which is reviewed and updated annually. The EOP will address mitigation, preparedness, response, and recovery for all anticipated events based on the results of the HVA and will incorporate the Hospital Incident Command System. The emergency manager will ensure that the hospital EOP integrates with the local emergency management plan of the community agencies and resources. The emergency manager will serve as a liaison with other local emergency managers and coordinate planning with them as well. The emergency management program should also address training of facility personnel and the emergency manager should ensure that all individuals are trained to the appropriate level for the work they will be expected to perform. This will include compliance with Occupational Safety and Health Administration (OSHA), Environmental Protection Agency (EPA), and JCAHO mandates, as well as any other local requirements from an authority having jurisdiction. During a disaster, the hospital emergency manager will interface with other local hospitals and the local Emergency Operations Center (EOC) to obtain or share resources. This position has become an integral function within a hospital as JCAHO standards related to emergency management have evolved.

PUBLIC INFORMATION OFFICER

In today's world of 24-hour news, the duties of a public information officer (PIO) during a disaster could be like trying to play with alligators. The PIO will have a difficult job trying to provide essential public information while maintaining patient privacy and confidentiality. The PIO should establish good working relationships with local media personnel well ahead of any event. The PIO will be the "public face" of the hospital during a disaster and will be the point of coordination to grant or deny media access to the hospital. The media and the public will develop their impression of the competency of the institution based upon the composure of the PIO. The media can also assist the PIO in delivering risk communications to the public throughout the life cycle of the event. During a significant event, the PIO should coordinate the delivery of information within a Joint Information System (JIS) as designated by local protocol. The PIO should establish and maintain constant two-way communications with the Joint Information Center (JIC) while keeping a close eye on alternative information sources. The PIO should refrain from providing any information that is not specific to the institution he or she represents. At the same time, the PIO should work diligently to squash rumors and dispel myths that will only serve to excite the public and possibly incite panic and fear.

Medical/Technical Specialists

During an incident, these positions will be staffed to support the incident commander providing subject matter expertise. These positions are staffed as dictated by the incident.

HEALTH PHYSICIST

A health physicist (HP) will be of crucial importance in the event of radiological disaster involving exposed and/or contaminated victims. The HP will be the definitive subject-matter expert in the management of these specialized patients, especially with respect to biodosimetry. The HP will be responsible for developing a Radiation Safety Plan, as a component of the whole emergency management (EM) plan, for suspected or established radiation emergencies in coordination with the hospital emergency manager. The HP will acquire dosimeters and radiation monitoring equipment for the staff doing assessment and monitoring. The HP will also develop the radiological decontamination plan, in consultation with the CMO/CNO, and designate a location within the institution where the affected patients will be decontaminated and housed. The HP will need to work with other radiation health and safety professionals within the community to establish area-wide plans to handle one of these unique situations. Because radiation emergencies tend to invoke considerable fear (usually related to a lack of knowledge), the HP will need to develop and deliver education/training programs to the hospital staff to enhance their abilities to care for these patients. Because of the potential long-term consequence of radiation exposure, the HP will need to establish and maintain procedures to prevent exposure to hospital staff and track/follow up those employees who do receive an occupational exposure.

PEDIATRIC SERVICES

Because the needs of children will vary from those of adult patients, a technical specialist specific to the needs of children (pediatrician, child psychologist, etc.) will likely be needed during all disasters. Specialized medical knowledge specific to pediatric exposure to chemical, biological, or radiological materials will be beneficial to the incident commander (IC) or the CMO advising the IC. Additional guidance that can be provided relates to the social service issues of reconnecting children who have been separated from their parents because of the disaster. In dealing with neonatal issues, staff with expertise in this area will need to be recruited to manage this very specific subpopulation of patients. The care of pediatric patients will need to be in a designated area that has equipment and supplies that are specific to pediatric patients.

RISK MANAGEMENT

The risk manager will work closely with the hospital emergency manager in development/revision of the EOP to ensure compliance with the Health Insurance Portability and Accountability Act (HIPPA), Emergency Medical Treatment and Active Labor Act (EMTALA), OSHA, EPA, and other local/state/federal regulations affecting the emergency management of the facility. In doing so, the risk manager will review the institution's liability exposure during all phases of the EOP and establish a plan to minimize impact. With respect to the utilization of volunteers, the risk manager will need to identify any liability that could arise from the use of outside physicians and nurses who assist during a disaster. Issues related to employment law and practices will need to be coordinated with the hospital emergency manager, the human resources department, CNO, CMO, and the employee health Department to ensure compliance with all applicable contracts, laws, and regulations. During the crisis, the risk manager will work in conjunction with the safety officer, as well as all the aforementioned personnel, to minimize risks and liability to the institution.

LEGAL SERVICES

Advice from legal services (corporate counsel) during an event will be necessary when the presenting issue is not clearly defined or addressed in the EOP and the matter could present a liability issue to the hospital. This specialist has the requisite knowledge and experience to research those issues and provide advice to help work out EMTALA, HIPPA, OSHA, EPA, and other regulatory issues related to patient care during a disaster.

Clinical Care Areas

EMERGENCY DEPARTMENT

The emergency department (ED) is likely to be the first area of care that will be impacted immediately following a disaster. Personnel working is this department will need to be intimately familiar with all facets of HICS and be capable of implementing it at a moment's notice. ED personnel must acquire the specialized knowledge to manage casualties from all types of disasters, including weapons of mass destruction (WMD) events. As such, they should possess the competency level to provide care to patients while wearing personal protective equipment (PPE). ED personnel must plan for and be prepared to establish an alternate site in case the main ED becomes contaminated, damaged, or destroyed by a secondary terrorist attack. In preparation for a mass casualty incident (MCI) or disaster, the ED should perform the following actions:

- Institute protocols to evaluate, stabilize, and, if needed, transfer victims of the disaster to other facilities.
- Establish procedures to procure equipment and supplies needed for the decontamination of patients, staff, and bystanders.
- Coordinate with the CNO and hospital emergency manager to plan for ED surge capacity.

- Plan for continuity of services to the existing ED patients unaffected by the disaster and implement ED diversion to avoid saturation.
- Work with security to develop a plan to control access to the ED.

In addition, because of the specialized knowledge and experience found within the ED, its personnel are likely to be assigned to augment other areas of the hospital.

CRITICAL CARE UNITS

Like the ED, the medical intensive care unit (MICU), surgical intensive care unit (SICU), critical care unit (CCU), etc., will need to adequately prepare for the rapid influx of acutely ill or injured patients from the disaster event. The staff in these units will need to be trained to provide care to patients who are suffering from exposure to WMD agents. The units will have to be equipped to isolate patients who pose a hazard to other patients or staff either from contagion or contamination. Existing Intensive Care Unit (ICU) patients will still need continuous care, despite the influx of disaster patients, and the institution must have a plan developed to quickly increase critical care beds through alternative care sites (ACS) within the institution for conversion into ICU beds if the need arises. Prior identification of the equipment/supplies needed to convert an area into an ICU will need to be readily available for rapid mobilization.

SURGICAL SERVICES

During a disaster, routine surgeries will have to be postponed. When there is no advance warning and the surgery suites are occupied at the onset of the event, the hospital will need to establish protocols and procedures to address these events in accordance with standard medical and ethical practices. Part of that plan can be identifying alternative sites where emergency surgeries can be performed when the operating rooms (ORs) are full or become unusable because of contamination. This plan should also include increasing OR and anesthesia department capacity in the event of a patient surge to meet the needs of the disaster victims. Department managers should work with engineering personnel to ensure that the hospital ventilation system is capable of isolating the surgery suites to prevent contamination.

BEHAVIORAL HEALTH/CASE MANAGEMENT/PASTORAL CARE

Large-scale disasters will be very taxing on the most important resource, the hospital staff. Besides the stress imposed by the magnitude of the event, the entire healthcare team will be worried about loved ones, pets, homes, and any other personal belongings. As such, the hospital should provide support for staff to communicate with family members during a disaster. The patients will also be concerned about the long-term impact the event will have on them and how they will be able to recover. Prior to any event, the hospital should provide behavior health training for all hospital professionals, emphasizing disaster stress, normal reactions, and support resources. A professional crisis counseling team should be available throughout the event to serve the needs of the staff and, possibly, their families.

The staff must be prepared to handle the surge of patients who will all be seeking care. In a biological, chemical, or radiological terrorism event, many of those seeking care will be psychological casualties or "worried well." In other words, they show no signs of exposure or illness, but they seek reassurance. This can present a real problem for facilities because clinical symptoms may not be immediately apparent in some cases. The staff will need guidance regarding procedures for dealing with a possible surge of fearful patients and family members during disasters, as well as triage protocols to attempt to distinguish actual casualties from psychological ones. The hospital will need to work with other community mental health agencies and social services to provide mental health counseling and treatment to victims and their family members, pastoral or spiritual counseling to victims and their family members in emergencies, and plan to assist families in identifying and locating victims, including communicating with the Red Cross and the medical examiner. An area should be establish as a family assistance center (FAC) to provide these services.

These services will be assigned to different functional areas within the Hospital Incident Command System (HICS). The provision of mental healthcare to victims falls under the direction of the mental health unit within the medical care branch of the operations section. Additional duties for patient mental health or social work could also be assigned to the clinical support services unit, which is also in the medical care branch. Tending to the needs of the hospital staff occurs through the employee health and well-being unit within the support branch of the logistics section, and the needs of employees' families is assigned to the family care unit, which is also within the support branch of the logistics section.

Clinical Support Functions

CLINICAL LABORATORY

Laboratory services can quickly become overwhelmed during a disaster. Therefore, procedures should be implemented in the planning phase to determine how much toxicologic and microbiologic testing will be performed at the hospital and how much will need to be outsourced. In consultation with all clinical departments, establish minimum, absolutely necessary blood/lab work required for different types of disaster casualties without compromising care. In the event of an influx of contaminated casualties, protocols will need to be in place for obtaining samples from contaminated patients and for the safe transportation of contaminated samples to the point where they will be tested. Personnel will need to be familiar with Centers for Disease Control and Prevention (CDC) and Federal Bureau of Investigation (FBI) procedures for collecting specimens that could also be criminal evidence.

Laboratory services will need to work closely with hospital infection control professionals. Public health officials may provide presumptive, early recognition of unusual health events. Labs must be familiar with the CDC Laboratory Response Network (LRN) and the procedures for sending samples and obtaining confirmation from an LRN lab.

In the planning phase, alternative labs for use will need to be identified in the event the hospital lab becomes saturated with samples to test or the hospital lab inadvertently becomes contaminated. Also, in advance of the event, ensure that laboratory personnel who will be handling potentially contaminated specimens are properly educated, trained, and equipped.

HOSPITAL EPIDEMIOLOGY/INFECTION CONTROL

Infection control personnel within the hospital will serve a dual role during a disaster. They will assist public health officials in early recognition of bioterrorism agent syndromes and they will serve as safety advocates for the healthcare staff. This will be accomplished through various preparatory efforts such as the following actions:

- Identify personal protective equipment for biological agents on the CDC category A, B, and C agent lists and provide training and respiratory protection fit testing for the hospital personnel who use respirators.
- Establish protocols/procedures for isolation and movement of any exposed or potentially contagious patients.
- Educate hospital staff in precautions for infection control.
- Coordinate syndromic surveillance with public health officials.
- Establish a HIPPA-compliant protocol, in consultation with risk management, for information exchange with other healthcare facilities and the health department.
- Work with facilities and engineering to identify areas where air flow can be restricted or isolated in order to establish isolation areas for contagious victims.

PHARMACY

In preparation for a possible disaster involving the use of WMD agents, pharmacy services will need to stockpile an inventory of antidotes, antibiotics, and vaccines needed for the treatment or prophylaxis of patients or staff exposed to various chemical, biological, radiological, nuclear, and explosive (CBRNE) agents. Plans for distribution will be coordinated through the use of HICS to ensure timely allocation within the institution. The institution can establish contracts with outside vendors, pharmacies, and/or other institutions for augmenting the hospital's inventory by obtaining additional supplies. The pharmacy should be the primary department to oversee the receipt and distribution of the Strategic National Stockpile (SNS) in coordination with the local and state SNS plans. Procedures must be well-established to provide for the department's acquisition, accountability, and billing for the stock during a disaster. Accurate documentation and records retention will be the responsibility of various units within HICS.

RADIOLOGY

Similar to laboratory services, establish minimum, absolutely necessary radiologic studies to be performed for different types of disaster casualties without compromising care. This should be done in consultation with all clinical departments. Plans should also be established to identify possible alternative locations with X-ray capability in case the primary department becomes contaminated. This could include the use of portable equipment in the areas without contamination. In consultation with manufacturers, develop a plan for the decontamination of all radiologic equipment in the event of contamination by patients.

MORTUARY SERVICE

Most hospitals don't have the storage capacity to handle a large number of fatalities. It will be essential to include a contingency plan for storage of contaminated bodies or to identify sites within the facility that will be suitable alternatives. The EOP will also need to indicate procedures for security and access to the morgue in order to ensure that potential evidence is not disturbed. In developing the EOP, the hospital emergency manager must coordinate the hospital's plan for mass fatalities with the local medical examiner's plan and the state mass fatality annex. The plan should enlist the assistance of local funeral homes and directors to assist with surge capacity. Protocols should also be established and coordinated with social services/pastoral care to address appropriate religious rites or cultural practices for the deceased.

Hospital Infrastructure

FACILITIES AND ENGINEERING

Within the context of the HICS framework, the facilities and engineering functions will be managed by various units within the infrastructure branch of the operations section and will be the lifeline of the facility. It is in this area that failure to identify vulnerabilities and mitigate their effects will become painfully obvious during a disaster. A prime example of this is the Texas Medical Center (TMC) during Tropical Storm Allison. The primary and secondary sources of electrical power for many of the TMC hospitals were located underground. The sump pump system proved woefully inadequate for the torrential rains and flooding that occurred in such a short span of time. Consequently, all power was lost within the TMC, forcing the evacuation of entire hospitals.

If not already performed, the facility will need to be evaluated for vulnerabilities identified in the National Institute for Occupational Safety and Health (NIOSH) May, 2002 document *Guidance for Protecting Building Environments from Airborne Chemical, Biological or Radiological Attacks* and fortified accordingly. In addition, the following items need to be considered:

- Develop plans to isolate the ventilation system/air handlers in selected areas of the building, if needed, due to contamination.
- Determine the need for high-efficiency particulate air (HEPA) filters on the heating, ventilation, and air-conditioning (HVAC) system.
- Determine the number and location of the negative pressure isolation rooms.
- Implement a plan to control the elevators during an emergency.
- Plan for the redistribution or installation of medical gases, vacuum, and water for newly created patient care spaces in an emergency.
- Develop an alternate plan for providing electricity, water, air-conditioning, medical gases, and suction in case these are lost during an emergency.
- Identify a location and/or establish a chemical/radiological "decontamination area" for the facility. Provide warm water and the ability to contain water at the decontamination sites within the institution. In the event that the contaminated water holding tank becomes full, provisions will need to be made to pump out the tank or re-route the contaminated water to the municipal sewer system.
- Plan for continuity of critical functions during an extended power outage.

- Identify the capacity of the central sterile supply area for cleaning and sterilizing the instruments and/or equipment during emergencies (consider disposable instruments/supplies).
- Identify possible alternative sites for sterilization in case the primary central sterile supply site becomes inoperable.
- Designate individuals and locations for decontaminating durable equipment under the auspices of the facility/equipment decontamination unit within the hazmat branch of the HICS organizational structure.

ENVIRONMENTAL SERVICES

Personnel within this department are ideally suited to perform duties associated with the hazmat branch of HICS. It is a mistake to plan on exclusively utilizing clinical personnel (physicians, nurses, or technicians) to function in this capacity because their expertise will be stretched too thin and their turnover rate is greater (constantly have to train new staff); the labor pool within this department is more stable and consistent. In order to perform these duties, personnel will need to be trained to the operations level. They can then be assigned to perform not only decontamination, but detection and monitoring throughout the facility. The EOP will need to address a protocol to institute callback of personnel in order to support increased surge capacity.

BIOMEDICAL ENGINEERING

The biomedical engineering department in most hospitals is responsible for the inventory of durable medical equipment. Durable medical equipment can include such devices as IV pumps, portable suction devices, portable ventilators, cardiac monitor/defibrillators, or pulse oximeters. The industry has become dependent on the space-age technology these devices provide, making them invaluable in the care of patients. These devices are also very expensive and, therefore, in limited supply within any facility. The disposable supplies required for the operation of these devices can also be limited. The devices and supplies will really become scarce during a disaster surge of patients. If one of these devices becomes nonfunctioning, having a staff member who can inspect and repair the equipment will be ideal. Procedures for contamination avoidance should be established. In the event that contamination does occur, plans consistent with manufacturer's recommendations for decontamination must be researched and developed. A plan for emergency resupply of equipment should be prearranged with vendors, other hospitals, or manufacturers. During an event, these devices will be coordinated through the medical devices unit within the infrastructure branch of the operations section.

FOOD AND NUTRITION SERVICES

Food and nutrition services will have a daunting task during disaster operations. They will have to feed an increased number of patients, increased staff who have also become residents of the facility in disaster mode, and possibly the families of staff members who have become displaced because of the incident. Plans to obtain additional food and water in a timely manner will have to be included within the EOP. This might involve food and water supply/resupply agreements with local commercial food suppliers or other hospitals. If local water treatment facilities become inoperable, the plan must provide for the stockpiling of potable water and sources to maintain an uninterrupted resupply.

SECURITY

In order to maintain the integrity and usability of the hospital, security measures will have to be instituted at the first sign or notification of an incident. The facility must be protected from contamination, civil unrest, and secondary attacks. The EOP should address the protocols and procedures to restrict or deny access to the facility in order to protect staff and existing patients. Several items need to be considered and addressed:

- controlling access to the facility and decontamination site
- augmentation of the security force
- media control
- patient screening for contamination at all possible entrances to the healthcare facility
- performing security duties while wearing full PPE
- positive identification of authorized personnel (100% ID checks)
- communications with local law enforcement agencies
- control of vehicle access to vulnerable and/or sensitive structures
- restricted parking areas close to buildings (stand-off restrictions) and plans for towing unattended vehicles
- barriers to protect entrances
- security screening of all visitors
- plans for inspection/searches of all bags, suitcases, briefcases, and packages at each access point
- strict enforcement of visitor policy

The hospital security force should have a close working relationship with community law enforcement agencies; the security portion of the EOP should be developed and coordinated with the assistance of local law enforcement.

Logistic Support

HUMAN RESOURCES

The human resources (HR) department will need to continuously maintain accurate contact information for all full-time and part-time staff to ensure that callback rosters are current. Prior to an event, the HR department can develop plans to utilize a "phone tree" callback procedure. HR personnel will need to be available throughout the incident in case access to personnel records becomes necessary, questions about employment regulations arise, or worker's compensation expertise is required. The HR department will also need to assist with the credentialing and authorization of volunteers.

EMPLOYEE HEALTH/OCCUPATIONAL HEALTH

The primary function of this department before and during a disaster will be to prevent work-related injuries and promote workplace safety. This could be accomplished through several mechanisms such as the following:

- pre-event immunizations, when appropriate
- maintaining employee immunization statuses to all appropriate vaccines
- compliance with all regulatory agency requirements for healthcare worker safety
- monitoring employee well-being during and following the event
- post-exposure immunizations and/or prophylaxis
- post-event employee evaluation and follow-up

MATERIAL MANAGEMENT/PURCHASING

The capability of a facility to continue to provide care will be impacted by the amount of supplies that are available. The EOP should identify the amount of supplies to be stored for use in an emergency. A system for purchasing, handling, inventorying, inspecting, and delivering materials on short notice should be included within the EOP. This department should work in conjunction with the pharmacy to obtain additional support from any local supply/equipment stockpiles or the Strategic National Stockpile program. Joint purchasing plans through mutual aid agreements with other hospitals could be explored prior to an event as a remedy to possible situations.

PATIENT TRANSPORT

Plans will need to be established for the orderly movement of patients through the various areas where patients will receive care. This must be performed safely despite the ensuing chaos. Alternate routes to move patients, staff, and equipment need to be identified if contamination of an area of the hospital prohibits normal pathways. Additionally, plans must be identified to move patients vertically within the institution when power failure prevents the use of elevators.

VOLUNTEERS

The assistance of volunteers will be essential in the event of a disaster. Prior to the event, volunteer assistance can be solicited from the community and those individuals can then be credentialed. However, the plan will need to address the assistance of spontaneous volunteers and procedures to credential them during the event. The Medical Reserve Corps (MRC) is an ideal source for healthcare volunteers. The EOP should also designate a location where existing volunteers can check in and spontaneous volunteers can be credentialed.

Tracking (Planning) with Medical Records

Medical records will be an integral part of any event. A mechanism to generate the medical record for patients who present at all potential points of care in the facility will have to be implemented. Because many institutions have converted to electronic record systems (ERS), a backup system of paper records is necessary in case the EMS system is not functioning. Patients, beds, supplies, and personnel will all have to be continuously tracked in order to advise the IC of capability status of the facility. Other items should also be considered:

- security of medical records and HIPPA compliance
- handling and transcribing records from contaminated patients
- proper identification of patients to avoid mixing records
- appropriate documentation of incident activities on HICS forms

Conclusion

The roles and responsibilities of healthcare workers are diverse. All departments within a facility will have a function in the smooth operation and success of the facility during a crisis. Disasters can present with notice (hurricane) or without notice (bombing) and the planning and preparedness of the staff will directly impact their performance during the event.

References

Bowers PJ, Maguire ML, Silva PA, Kitchen R. Everybody out. *Nurs Manage.* 2004;35(4):50–54.

Braun BI, Wineman NV, Fin NL, Barbera JA, Schmaltz SP, Loeb JM. Integrating hospitals into community emergency preparedness planning. *Ann Intern Med.* 2006; 144(11):799–811.

California Emergency Medical Services Authority. Disaster Medical Services Division—Hospital Incident Command System (HICS) Web site. http://www.emsa.ca.gov/HICS/default.asp. August 2006. Accessed January 16, 2010.

Cocanour CS, Allen SJ, Mazabob J, et al. Lessons learned from the evacuation of an urban teaching hospital. *Arch Surg.* 2002;137(10):1141–1145.

Department of Homeland Security. Federal Emergency Management Agency. National Emergency Responder Credentialing System—Job Titles. http://www.fema.gov/emergency/nims/ResourceMngmnt.shtm#item3. Published March 2008. Accessed January 16, 2010.

Hatton MA. Tropical Storm Allison recovery: a facilities and operations perspective. *Internet J Emerg Intensive Care Med.* 2002;6(1). http://www.ispub.com/journal/the_internet_journal_of_emergency_and_intensive_care_medicine/volume_6_number_1_9/article/tropical_storm_allison_recovery_a_facilities_and_operations_perspective.html. Accessed January 04, 2009.

Hospital Emergency Standards Enhanced: A Good Model Gets Better. Suburban Emergency Management Project Web site. http://www.semp.us/publications/biot_reader.php?BiotID=525. Published June 05, 2008. Accessed January 04, 2009.

The Joint Commission. Emergency management (EM). In: The Joint Commission. *2009 Hospital Accreditation Standards.* Oakbrook Terrace, Illinois: Joint Commission Resources; 2009:47–68.

Lessons Learned from a Hospital Evacuation during Tropical Storm Allison. Suburban Emergency Management Project Web site. http://www.semp.us/publications/biot_reader.php?BiotID=216. Published May 21, 2005. Accessed January 04, 2009.

Mackler N, Wilkerson W, Cinti S. Will first-responders show up for work during a pandemic? Lessons from a smallpox vaccination survey of paramedics. *Disaster Manag Response.* 2007;5(2):45–48.

Masterson L, Steffen C, Brin M, Kordick MF, Christos S. Willingness to respond of emergency department personnel and their predicted participation in mass casualty terrorist events. *J Emerg Med.* 2009;36(1):43–49.

Meade C. Planning the safety of healthcare structures. http://www.rand.org/pubs/working_papers/WR309/. RAND Health working paper series. WR-309. Published October, 2005. Accessed January 16, 2010.

Risk Management Solutions. Tropical Storm Allison, June 2001. http://www.rms.com/publications/ts_allison.pdf. RMS Event Report. Risk Management Solutions Web site. Updated September 10, 2004. Accessed January 16, 2010.

Romans JF. Tropical Storm Allison: the Houston Flood of June 9th, 2001. Internet J Emerg Intensive Care Med. 2002;6(1). http://www.ispub.com/journal/the_internet_journal_of_emergency_and_intensive_care_medicine/

volume_6_number_1_9/article/tropical_storm_allison_the_houston_flood_of_june_9th_2001.html. Accessed January 04, 2009.

Thorne CD, Curbow B, Oliver M, Al-Ibrahim M, McDiarmid M. Terrorism preparedness training for nonclinical hospital workers: empowering them to take action. *J Occup Environ Med.* 2003;45(3):333–337.

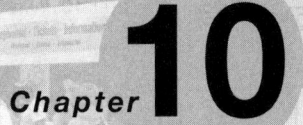

Chapter **10**

Credentialing and Management of Volunteer Health Professionals

Deborah Viola, PhD, MBA and Peter Arno, PhD

Learning Objectives

- Identify the importance of a fully integrated emergency preparation plan that includes all stakeholders within the local public health system.
- Define the linkages between the hospital and the local public health system in all-hazards planning.
- Discuss the Emergency Systems for Advanced Registration of Volunteer Health Professionals (ESAR-VHP).
- Propose strategies for managing volunteers during all phases of an emergency or public health threat.

Overview

One of the biggest challenges facing hospitals today is ensuring that adequate resources and appropriate personnel are in place for emergency preparedness, planning, and response. As hospitals are integrated into community-level, all-hazards emergency planning, it is incumbent upon hospital management to develop policies and initiatives for credentialing and managing volunteers. The extent of volunteerism of course can vary. During major disasters like the 1989 Loma Prieta Earthquake in California, thousands of residents from surrounding areas appeared as willing volunteers; in New York City approximately 40,000 volunteers from the city and around the country arrived in the aftermath of 9/11.[1,2] Conversely, even though models and strategies exist to increase patient care surge capacity in hospitals by 20–30%, the problem of staffing remains largely unresolved.[3]

A proactive approach to identifying and credentialing volunteers also ensures the adequate supply of "recruited" volunteers, i.e., volunteers with known capabilities given specific assignments, as opposed to an over-reliance on unsolicited or spontaneous volunteers who show up when an emergency occurs. Obviously, hospital leadership must be prepared to effectively manage volunteers because their manpower will undoubtedly be needed.

Introduction

Since our nation was founded, Americans have volunteered to help each other. In 1736, Benjamin Franklin began the first volunteer firefighting company; today, almost two-thirds of all fire departments utilize volunteer firefighters. In 1881 the American Red Cross began its mission to "provide relief to victims of disaster and help people prevent, prepare for, and respond to emergencies."[4] People volunteer for many reasons, but during a tragedy or crisis the primary motivators are to help out friends and families, whether we know them personally or not, simply because "they could be us."

Managing volunteers is important because unsolicited or spontaneous volunteers do not show up knowing what they need to do. During an emergency, volunteers may very well end up requiring assistance (food, shelter) and care (medical, psychosocial) as well as the victims they are trying to help. For volunteers to be an effective part of all-hazards emergency planning, hospitals would be better served by integrating their preparedness plans with those of the local public health system and by taking a proactive approach to identifying and credentialing volunteers to ensure an adequate supply of recruited volunteers (i.e., volunteers with known capabilities given specific assignments). Integrating hospitals into community emergency planning will also facilitate the registration of volunteer health professionals and first responders with training and experience responding to actual disasters.

It is critical that hospital management consider the local public health system. This involves a more systematic, ecological approach to all-hazards planning. Hospital management must identify all sectors involved in the local public health system (e.g., public health agencies, healthcare providers, public safety agencies) and their organization and resource capabilities to respond to a crisis with public health consequences. This facilitates the identification of essential measures of public health system preparedness for the community, including: resilience (availability of resources), effectiveness (capacity, capability, and competency), and strength of public health partnerships. To ensure an adequate supply of trained volunteers, hospitals must take the initiative in developing systems to register and utilize all levels of volunteers, including medical and healthcare professionals. To ensure that volunteers are deployed efficiently, registries should be able to classify volunteers according to emergency credentialing standards. Finally, hospitals must consider human resource management in dealing with volunteers, including training, liability insurance, and worker's compensation if these individuals become victims themselves.

Involving All Stakeholders

The need for a systems approach to public health preparedness is emphasized in the reports by the Institute of Medicine (IOM), *The Future of the Public's Health in the 21st Century,*[5] and *Research Priorities in Emergency Preparedness and Response for Public Health Systems: A Letter Report.*[6] Public health emergency preparedness has been defined by Nelson et al and adopted by the IOM as

> "the capability of the public health and health care systems, communities, and individuals, to prevent, protect against, quickly respond to, and recover from health emergencies, particularly those whose scale, tim-ing, or unpredictability threatens to overwhelm routine capabilities. Preparedness involves a coordinated and continuous process of planning and implementation that relies on measuring performance and taking corrective action."[7]

Despite many improvements in emergency preparedness, planning, and coordination among public health entities, communities, and the private sector—particularly since 9/11 and Hurricane Katrina—the existing linkages are far from robust, the optimal organization structures to meet critical preparedness goals are still unknown, and the evidence base for assessing progress reaching these goals remains elusive.[4–7,8,9,10] The local public health system (LPHS) plays a critical role in communities' emergency preparedness activities. The CDC has defined an LPHS as the "constellation of individuals and organizations in the public and private sectors that provide information and assets to promote population health, provide health care delivery, and prevent disease and injury (including health care providers, insurers, purchasers, public health agencies,

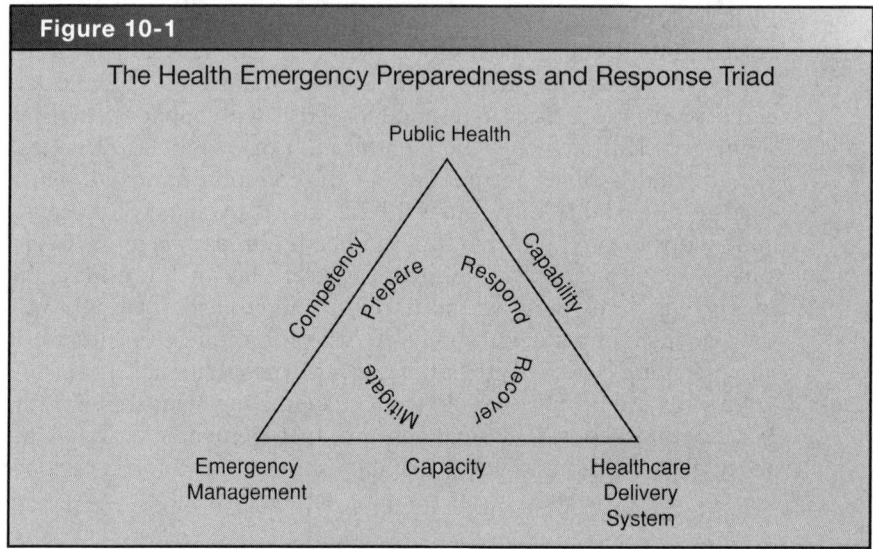

Source: Agency for Healthcare Research and Quality

community-based organizations, and entities that operate outside the traditional sphere of health care)."[11] In addition, integration of preparedness with other public health functions involves the regionalization of public health resources. According to Koh et al, "regionalization of local public health preparedness seeks to advance functions of networking, coordinating, standardizing, centralizing, and generating new local capacity."[8]

In efforts to enhance regionalization and further integration of public health preparedness, the National Incident Management System (NIMS) was developed by the Federal Emergency Management Agency (FEMA). Its objectives are to facilitate responders from different jurisdictions and disciplines working together to respond to disasters and major emergencies, and includes a unified approach to incident management; standard command and management structures; and an emphasis on preparedness, mutual aid, and resource management.[12] For the most part, these regionalization and integration initiatives are evolving and systematic efforts to quantify and assess their impact on public health preparedness.

The development and nurturing of formal and informal networks within the LPHS is central to effective coordination and public health preparedness. We know that health partnerships are important, and that the pattern of partnerships in a community is likely to affect communication and collaboration throughout the system.[13] Because these community-based networks sometimes develop over long periods of time, they tend to embed extensive knowledge of members' capabilities and preferences. This knowledge streamlines cooperative efforts, particularly under time pressure. Furthermore, these relationships sustain themselves with little outside intervention needed to support them. To maximize their contribution, government and healthcare organizations should develop more effective mechanisms for informing community networks of public needs and for integrating their competencies into emergency planning. (See Figure 10-1.)

Hospitals as Partners

The local public health system (LPHS) is composed of organizations or facilities that contribute to the delivery of public health services within a community. We will use the National Public Health Performance Standards Program (NPHPSP) definitions for the sectors that are identified and described in this chapter.[14] These include: public health agencies, healthcare providers, public safety agencies, environmental agencies or organizations, human service and charity organizations, education and youth development organizations, recreation and arts-related organizations, and economic and philanthropic organizations. (See Figure 10-2.)

Regional and local coordination is an integral part of response to major public health emergencies. As defined in the *Medical Surge Capacity and Capability (MSCC) Handbook*, healthcare coalitions are "composed of healthcare organizations . . . and other healthcare assets that form a single functional entity to maximize MSCC in a defined geographic area coordinating the mitigation, preparedness, response, and recovery actions . . ."[15]

Critical to all-hazards preparedness is an understanding of existing capacity and infrastructure within the LPHS and the notion that "incidents are generally handled at the lowest jurisdiction level possible."[16] This requires the following information:

1. A physical inventory of assets and resources

2. A qualitative description of public health partnerships within the local public health system with particular emphasis on intra- and inter-sector organization networking

3. A quantification of public health preparedness, including resilience, effectiveness, and strength of public health partnerships

Local stakeholders and facilities must be identified by sector. A directory should be compiled that includes the facility name, address, and ownership status (i.e., public, private, non-profit). In the case of larger geographic jurisdictions, a sample should be drawn from the directory based on preexisting partnerships (e.g., cooperative agreements, medical

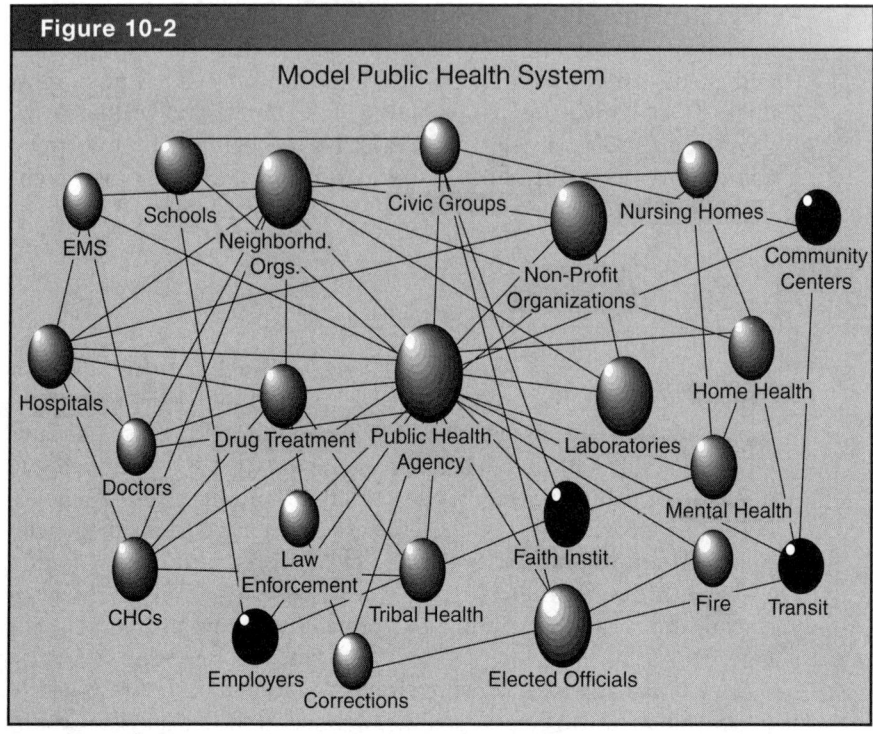

Figure 10-2

Model Public Health System

Source: Centers for Disease Control and Prevention, National Public Health Performance Standards Program (NPHPSP)

mutual aid agreements), common risks and vulnerabilities, proximity, and willingness to participate. Interviews with senior-level managers and staff responsible for emergency planning, as well as focus groups of organization leadership across sectors, will secure the following types of information: existing written emergency response and recovery plans (including resource and capabilities assessment); training and/or exercise procedures; and evaluative and corrective action processes. Resource inventories would include medical/surgical supplies, staffing, registry of volunteer health professionals, number and types of beds ("bed tracking"), evacuation plans, NIMS compliance, etc., as relevant to a particular facility.

Emphasis within communities should be on the interoperability of the volunteer fire, ambulance, and rescue squad, and paid police force. Model community initiatives, using criteria developed by the TIIDE Project (Terrorism Injuries: Information, Dissemination and Exchange) established by the CDC, can facilitate integration on local levels that can be tapped into by hospitals "to integrate public health and the emergency care community."[17] Intrinsic to improving partnerships between the LPHS and the emergency care community are seven

Table 10-1

Seven Elements of Successful Partnership

1.	Strong working relationships between community leaders of emergency care and public health
2.	Regularly scheduled meetings with personnel from both constituency groups as well as other nontraditional partners
3.	Cross-education and training on expertise and roles during disaster or crisis
4.	Shared response plans that reflect unique local circumstances
5.	Maintain ongoing collaboration on disaster and nondisaster activities
6.	Identified leader who has prioritized collaborative efforts between groups
7.	Resource sharing and leveraged funding to accomplish mutual goals

Source: Lerner EB, Cronin M, Schwartz RB, et al. Linking public health and the emergency care community: 7 model communities. *Disaster Med Public Health Prep.* 2007;1(2):142–145.

elements that also ensure sustainability of local and regional emergency planning when factored into partnership building by stakeholders. (See Table 10-1.)

Specific services are also assessed, including *Investigation and Response to Public Health Threats and Emergencies*.[18] Assessment of local and state public health systems are based on responses to questions such as:

Question 2.2.3: "Has the LPHS designated an individual to serve as an Emergency Response Coordinator within the jurisdiction?"

Does the individual:

2.2.3.1 Coordinate with the local health department's emergency response personnel?

2.2.3.2 Coordinate with local community leaders?

Hospital leadership should be aware of the model standards to optimize their own performance and to ensure a broader view of the public health system. They should network with their local public agencies, specifically departments of health, to participate in the survey and assessment process. Information can be used to determine the capabilities of the local public health workforce, the resilience and strength of local partnerships, and overall areas of concern, even in the absence of emergencies, such as education and research needs.

Register Volunteer Medical and Healthcare Professionals

The Emergency Systems for Advance Registration of Volunteer Health Professionals (ESAR-VHP) program is an advance registration and credentialing system of health volunteers developed by the Department of Health and Human Services and the Health Resources and Services Administration to support "a health care workforce emergency surge capacity" as an essential component of emergency healthcare preparedness. The health volunteer is defined as the "medical or healthcare professional that renders aid or performs health services, voluntarily, without pay or remuneration."[19] The volunteers consist of clinicians as well as behavioral health professionals. The ESAR-VHP program is a state-based approach to ensuring a national system. It primarily allows identification and preplanning for qualified, licensed providers to care for victims. It is predicated on the tradition of mutual aid and cooperation that has served communities across the United States for more than two centuries. The guidelines provide standards and protocols to create a national network of compatible systems that can be fully integrated to respond to national disasters. Table 10-2 identifies the key topics that states must address to ensure effective development of the ESAR-VHP system.

The hospital community is a critical part of state-level planning and is encouraged to participate in the state's program advisory group. As discussed in the previous section, hospitals are an integral part of the local public health system with knowledge of various emergency management agencies and providers, local health departments, state licensing boards, and volunteer organizations such at the American Red Cross and Medical Reserve Corps. The hospital, therefore, has a critical role in all key areas of establishing the ESAR-VHP system within its state.

System design involves the registration, emergency credentialing, and verification of health volunteers and may incorporate other registration processes used by organizations such as the American Red

Table 10-2	
Ten Key Topics	
1.	System design
2.	Emergency credentialing standards
3.	Training and situational orientation
4.	Recruitment and health volunteer advocacy
5.	Funding and cost
6.	Security and privacy
7.	Authorities and emergency operations
8.	Regionalizing and nationalizing the ESAR-VHP program
9.	Data definitions and naming conventions
10.	Operations and maintenance

Source: U.S. Department of Health and Human Services, Health Resources Services Administration. *ESAR-VHP Interim Technical and Policy Guidelines, Standards, and Definitions.* Version 2. Washington, DC: U.S. Department of Health and Human Services; June 2005.

Cross. States are required to have a central database of all volunteers and their records before credentialing and verification can take place. For the hospital, these volunteers are important if effective surge capacity is to ensure optimal patient care during an emergency. However, despite the emergency credentialing level given a volunteer, "the assignment of clinical privileges is the responsibility of the hospital authority."[19] It is also imperative that hospitals have access to the system to electronically verify information about volunteers that should be available on ID cards.

Emergency credentialing standards involve implementing emergency credentialing standards for clinicians and mental health professionals. Essentially, they represent the volunteer's qualifications and are the basis for determining the type of deployment and privileging granted by a hospital for a volunteer to provide patient care. The ESAR-VHP program emergency credentialing standards include whether a volunteer has disaster preparedness training or direct experience. The credentialing protocol uses a systematic methodology to classify personnel as summarized in Table 10-3. Suffice it to say, ensuring proper credentialing has legal implications for volunteers and the hospital.

Training and situational orientation focuses on defining formal activities and courses necessary for volunteers to optimize their ability to perform their jobs during a crisis. Volunteers may be trained for specific situations or emergencies, but should have a core set of competencies that allow them to provide health services in a disaster. Training is available through organizations like the American Red Cross. Competency-based training is a critical benchmark of the National Bioterrorism Hospital Preparedness Program for adult and pediatric hospital and outpatient care. Training is provided for all hazards.[20]

Health volunteer recruitment and advocacy involves activities geared toward attracting, recruiting, retaining, and providing protective measures for volunteers. Mutual aid programs within communities and volunteer programs, such as the Medical Reserve Corps and American Red Cross, provide hospitals the opportunity to build upon and integrate existing

Table 10-3	
Summary of Emergency Credentialing Standards	
Metric	Verified credentials based upon occupation
Occupation	Health profession definitions based on Standard Occupational Classification codes
Emergency and Credentialing Level	Based on metric for each volunteer; highest level is 1 (of 4 possible levels), which indicates volunteer has all required, verifiable credentials.

Source: U.S. Department of Health and Human Services, Health Resources Services Administration. *ESAR-VHP Interim Technical and Policy Guidelines, Standards, and Definitions.* Version 2. Washington, DC: U.S. Department of Health and Human Services; June 2005.

volunteer databases. Hospital management should encourage all volunteers to seek relevant training, participate in local drills, and periodically communicate to ensure that volunteers are updating their records. It is imperative that hospital management is aware of state-level initiatives, not only for training, but also in the area of precautions and protections offered for volunteers if they become injured while responding to an emergency, e.g., workers' compensation. Similarly, hospital management must be conversant in liability protection related to allegations of malpractice or other medical negligence. Information should be provided to volunteers prior to registration and credentialing. If nothing else, this nation's 9/11 experience taught us the need to consider not only the care of victims, but of the responders who so selflessly heeded the call. Tens of thousands of Americans affected by the toxic exposure of 9/11 still suffer chronic bronchial disease, cancers, and post-traumatic stress, and have difficulty receiving and paying for appropriate medical treatment. Registering volunteers is one way of helping them secure state-level workers' compensation benefits by classifying volunteers as "emergency workers."

Funding and cost, security and privacy, authorities and emergency operations, operations and maintenance are key topic areas that reside with the state-based ESAR-VHP system. However, critical points are worth mentioning because of their applicability to the participating hospital or hospital system. Security and privacy of volunteer records should be obvious; local registration should be accompanied by informed consent on behalf of the volunteer. Hospitals should issue unique identifiers for each registered volunteer because the use of social security numbers is restricted in many states. Access to volunteer information should be limited to authorized individuals and system security must ensure the integrity of data transfer via the Internet to other systems, such as hospital databases updating the state-level ESAR-VHP system. Most states have legal structures in place for declaring emergencies or disasters; however, hospital management must be clear as to who will be responsible for deploying volunteers. These procedures must be established in advance through mutual aid agreements, coordination with other agencies such as the American Red Cross, and in particular, planning with state-level representatives of the ESAR-VHP system. After formal state authority has been clarified, it is anticipated that, in local, contained emergencies, the state may delegate power to local authorities to administer assignment of emergency resources, including volunteers.

Whether a hospital is part of larger state programs depends in part on the availability of these programs. Nevertheless, many key topic areas have traditionally been addressed as part of a hospital's accreditation process or standard, non-emergency participation in the local communities they serve (e.g., credentialing, mutual aid agreements,

Table 10-4

Competencies for Successful Partnerships

Manage and implement the hospital's emergency response plan during drills or actual emergencies within your assigned functional role and chain of command.

Describe the collaborative relationship of your hospital to other facilities or agencies in the local emergency response system and follow the planned system during drills and emergencies.

Describe the key elements of your hospital's emergency preparedness and response roles and policies to other agencies and community partners.

Initiate and maintain communication with other emergency response agencies as appropriate to your management responsibilities.

Source: Emergency Preparedness for Hospital Workers. Available at: www.ncdp.mailman.columbia.edu/files/hospcomps.pdf. Accessed October 24, 2008.

training). Other areas, like emergency preparedness competencies for hospital personnel and healthcare volunteers, are newer and need to be evaluated and considered as part of hospital administration.

Recently, the Center for Public Health Preparedness, Mailman School of Public Health, Columbia University in collaboration with the Greater New York Hospital Association produced a set of competencies based on focus groups with leadership from New York hospitals.[21] The competencies distinguish between two core groups: hospital workers and hospital leaders. The four competencies for a hospital (Table 10-4) support the critical components of establishing hospitals not only as partners in the LPHS, but ensuring their interoperability with all volunteer and responder organizations to facilitate the recruiting, registering, credentialing, and training of the existing hospital workforce as well as volunteers.

These same competencies take on even more significance for hospital leadership as they consider effective volunteer management pre-emergency, when leadership has the luxury of dealing with recruited volunteers; during an actual crisis, when additional spontaneous volunteers may converge on a scene; and postevent, when volunteers have the potential to become victims themselves.

Managing Volunteers

The management of volunteers is particularly important to ensure the timely and appropriate deployment of medical personnel to disasters. Much of the chapter has discussed pre-event activities, with particular emphasis on ensuring an adequate supply of recruited volunteers or personnel. As noted, discouraging the arrival of hundreds or thousands of spontaneous volunteers during an actual emergency is just as significant. The concept of "convergent volunteerism," i.e., "the arrival of unexpected or uninvited personnel wishing to render aid at the scene of a large-scale emergency incident"[22] has been studied with respect to the unintended detrimental impact spontaneous volunteers can have. Further, as the 9/11 response revealed, even physicians were compromised when involved in situations where they lacked training. Several other problems presented themselves as a result, including, but not limited to, violation of dispatch and response protocols, liability, and safety.[23]

Ideally, the use of registries such as the ESAR-VHP should ensure an adequate supply of recruited volunteers. Furthermore, integrating hospitals with the LPHS can ensure timely and coordinated communications with the incident commander or medical operations officer responsible for crisis management. This should allow incident commanders and hospital leaders to focus on effective volunteer management during and immediately following a crisis.

First and foremost, volunteers must be deployed commensurate with appropriate credentialing and training. Equipment and supplies should be provided to allow volunteers to perform the service or provide the care that is part of their mission and charge. Volunteers should be informed as realistically as possible of the potential hazards they face and their time commitment. The better prepared the volunteers are for the situation they will be responding to, the less the likelihood of suffering later as a result of stress reactions. During the response phase, stress is mitigated and performance optimized when there is clearly defined leadership, and it has been shown that "credible experts keep fearful and anxious reactions" on the part of volunteers (as well as the greater population) from spiraling out of control.[24] The recovery phase is an extended period to monitor volunteers to ensure time for physical and psychological recovery and to identify when vulnerable volunteers may become victims of the crisis themselves.[25]

However, nothing will prevent spontaneous volunteers from arriving at disaster scenes. Incident commanders or medical operations officers should have plans in place to mitigate the potential strain these volunteers may cause. In the short term, volunteers should be encouraged to participate in helpful ways when personnel shortages are legitimate. In the long term, they can be registered in the volunteer management system for follow-up after a crisis so they can be credentialed appropriately for deployment in future disasters.

This is no small task. During the preparedness phase, there must be accommodation in the local volunteer registration system, or at a minimum, the local system used by hospital leadership, to directly include spontaneous volunteers. This is not a specific component in the ESAR-VHP, but that doesn't mean that regional and state-level system designs cannot accommodate this modification, similar to other organizations that have done so, such as the American Red Cross.

Table 10-5	
Additional Competencies for Successful Partnerships	
Describe your responsibilities for communicating with other employees, patients and families, media, the general public, or your own family. Demonstrate them during drills or actual emergencies.	
Source: Emergency Preparedness for Hospital Workers. www.ncdp.mailman.columbia.edu/files/hospcomps.pdf. Accessed October 24, 2008.	

The Centers for Law and the Public's Health, a collaboration between Johns Hopkins and Georgetown Universities, has published a Universal Checklist for identifying "legal and regulatory issues related to the implementation and organization of a volunteer registration system."[26] View the following five sections of the checklist that should be used during the preparedness planning phase (see Appendix). It is also helpful to refer to this list during and after an actual emergency event. Deficiencies in the checklist can be used by hospital leadership to advocate with state-level partners to ensure that all requirements are satisfied and accommodated in emergency plans.

It is worth noting the impact the media has on encouraging volunteerism during disasters. It is absolutely critical to ensure that the incident commander or local leadership accurately communicates the need for volunteers and defines the skills required of those volunteers who may report. The request for spontaneous volunteers should be specific, e.g., where volunteers should report, what identification they should bring to the scene, even how they should dress. It was difficult to accommodate spontaneous physician volunteers during the 9/11 disaster when many of them showed up wearing clogs and scrubs.

Additional competencies for hospital leaders who support successful partnership with the media are noted in Table 10-5.

Conclusion

Emergency response evaluation and assessment require a comprehensive look at the entire public health system's level of preparedness, as well as a coordinated and integrated review of "response linkages." It requires a continual and sustainable plan for maintaining community linkages, employing the use of planning groups, drills, communication with state-level stakeholders, and clearly defined roles in the incident command system.[10] Significantly challenging to hospitals is ensuring that adequate personnel, including volunteers, are in place for emergency preparedness planning and response. This includes identifying, training, credentialing, and tracking volunteers to ensure a sufficient supply of *recruited* volunteers are available during a public health emergency. Without this, there can be no assurance of successfully integrating and managing volunteers, the most critical component of the overall effectiveness of even the best emergency plans.

References

1. O'Brien PW, Mileti DS. Citizen participation in emergency response following the Loma Prieta Earthquake. *Int J Mass Emergencies Disasters.* 1992;10(1):71–89.
2. Illinois Terrorism Task Force Committee on Volunteers and Donations, Community Guidelines for Developing a Spontaneous Volunteer Plan (February 2005). http://www.ready.illinois.gov/. Accessed September 28, 2008.
3. Hick JL, Hanfling D, Burstein JL, et al. Health care facility and community strategies for patient care surge capacity. *Ann Emerg Med.* 2004;44(3):253–261.
4. American Red Cross. Mission statement. http://www.redcross.org/portal/site/en/menuitem.d229a5f06620c6052b1ecfbf43181aa0/?vgnextoid=f5195032f9 53e110VgnVCM10000089f0870aRCRD&vgnextchannel=d18859f392ce8110 VgnVCM10000030f3870aRCRD. Accessed October 13, 2008.
5. Institute of Medicine. *The Future of the Public's Health in the 21st Century.* Washington, DC: National Academies Press; 2002.
6. Altevogt BM, Pope AM, Hill MN, Shine KI, eds. *Research Priorities in Emergency Preparedness and Response for Public Health Systems: A Letter Report.* Washington, DC: National Academies Press; 2008. http://www.nap.edu/catalog.php?record_id=12136. Accessed, April 1, 2008.
7. Nelson C, Lurie N, Wasserman J, Zakowski S. Conceptualizing and defining public health emergency preparedness. *Am J Public Health.* 2007;97(S1): S9–S11.
8. Koh HK, Elqura LJ, Judge CM, Stoto MA. Regionalization of local public health systems in the era of preparedness. *Annu Rev Public Health.* 2008;29:205–218.
9. Lurie N, Wasserman J, Nelson C. Public health preparedness: evolution or revolution? *Health Aff.* 2006;25(4):935–945.
10. Braun BI, Wineman NV, Finn NL, et al. Integrating hospitals into community emergency preparedness planning. *Ann Intern Med.* 2006;144(11):799–811.
11. Emergency Preparedness and Response. Centers for Disease Control and Prevention Web site. http://emergency.cdc.gov/planning/faq2008foa.asp. Updated May 5, 2008. Accessed, April 15, 2008.
12. National Integration Center (NIC) Incident Management Systems Integration Division Web site. http://www.fema.gov/emergency/nims/index.shtm. Accessed, April 20, 2008.
13. Gibbons DE. Interorganizational network structures and diffusion of information through a health system, *Am J Public Health.* 2007;97(9):1684–1692.
14. Centers for Disease Control and Prevention. *NPHPSP: National Public Health Performance Standards Program: User Guide Fall 2007.* http://www.cdc.gov/od/ocphp/nphpsp/Documents/NPHPSPuserguide.pdf. Accessed, May 1, 2008.
15. Institute for Public Research. *Medical Surge Capacity and Capability: A Management System for Integrating Medical and Health Resources During Large-Scale Emergencies.* Alexandria: The CNA Corporation; 2004.

16. U.S. Department of Homeland Security. National Response Framework. January 2010. http://www.fema.gov/emergency/nrf/. Accessed February 18, 2010.

17. Lerner EB, Cronin M, Schwartz RB, et al. Linking public health and the emergency care community: 7 model communities. *Disaster Med Public Health Prep.* 2007;1(2):142–145.

18. Centers for Disease Control and Prevention, Public Health Practice Program Office, National Public Health Practice Program Office, National Public Health Performance Standards Program. http://www.cdc.gov/od/ocphp/nphpsp/. Accessed November 1, 2008.

19. U.S. Department of Health and Human Services, Health Resources Services Administration. *ESAR-VHP Interim Technical and Policy Guidelines, Standards, and Definitions.* Version 2. Washington, DC: U.S. Department of Health and Human Services; June 2005.

20. Bioterrorism Training and Curriculum Development Program. U.S. Department of Health and Human Services Web site. http://www.hhs.gov/aspr/opeo/nhpp/btcdp/btcdp.html. Accessed October 19, 2008.

21. Greater New York Hospital Association. *Emergency Preparedness and Response Competencies for Hospital Workers.* http://www.gnyha.org/31/Default.aspx. Accessed October 19, 2008.

22. Cone DC, Weir SC, Bogucki S. Convergent volunteerism. *Ann Emerg Med.* 2003;41(4):457–462.

23. Cook L. The World Trade Center attack: the paramedic response: an insider's view. *Crit Care.* 2001;5(6):301–303.

24. Fernandez LS, Barbera JA, van Dorp JR. Strategies for managing volunteers during incident response: a systems approach. *Homeland Secur Aff.* 2006;Vol II(3).

25. Laurendeau M, Labarre L, Senecal, G. The psychological dimension of health and social service interventions in emergency situations. *Open Med.* 2007;1(2).

26. The Centers for Law & the Public's Health: A Collaborative at Johns Hopkins and Georgetown Universities. Legal and Regulatory Issues Concerning Volunteer Health Professionals in Emergencies. Universal Checklist. http://www.publichealthlaw.net/Research/PDF/ESAR%20VHP%20Universal%20Checklist.pdf. Accessed November 1, 2008.

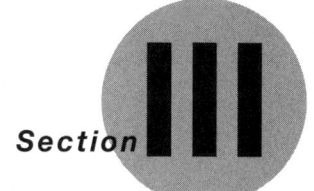

Hospital Operations During Disasters and Emergencies

Quantitative Planning for Epidemic and Disaster Response: Logistics and Supply Chain Considerations

Nathaniel Hupert, MD, MPH; John A. Muckstadt, PhD; and Wei Xiong, PhD, MS

Photo by Barry Bahler/FEMA

Learning Objectives

- Explain why emergency response logistics systems need improvement.
- Identify the principles for improved disaster supply chain management for healthcare facilities.
- Define the research agenda for emergency response logistics.

Overview

The focus of this chapter is the challenge of building logistics systems to support emergency response for public health and healthcare delivery. We present and illustrate general principles addressing the role of information systems in sustaining medical care during disasters.

Case Study

It was New Orleans in September, 2005. Working in 100°F+ weather, often without electricity, adequate water pressure, or communications capabilities, multiple teams of dedicated healthcare providers at hospitals throughout New Orleans and surrounding areas succeeded in maintaining care for and eventually evacuating more than 120 neonatal intensive care unit patients to safety within one week of Hurricane Katrina's landfall. Nearly every report to emerge from this Herculean effort describes an information-poor environment in which the healthcare infrastructure's continued function depended on individual improvisation and luck.[1] But the successful rescue of these sick newborns came with numerous costs, including the separation of children from their parents in the chaotic airlift that occurred days after the hurricane struck. Disasters thrust unexpected and, as in this example, occasionally dramatic demands on existing hospital patient and resource management systems. How these systems are designed in "peacetime" will largely determine their capability to sustain surges in demand for services during crises. This chapter discusses general principles for the creation of these resilient and flexible hospital logistics and supply systems.

The Need for Improved Health System Emergency Response Logistics Systems

Many have argued that the health emergency response infrastructure in the United States is in a state of preventable crisis.[2,3] Emergency planners, service providers, and hospital managers contend on a daily basis with massive patient and data flows in an environment that does not effectively employ technology to manage resources. For example, emergency surge capacity, even in the largest hospitals of our major cities, typically is managed with manual bed counts (sometimes augmented by data from the nightly automated census from the emergency department's registry log) and phone calls.

While this level of situation awareness may suffice as standard procedure for the occasional local emergency, it clearly risks catastrophic failure when situations escalate in scope and severity shown, for example, in the U.S. Gulf region after Hurricane Katrina. Despite heroic medical care, hospitalized patients in New Orleans died for lack of adequate means of interstate transportation and clearly defined regional transfer protocols.[4] In the aftermath of the storm, a consensus arose in this country and abroad that such loss of life was unaccept-

Table 11-1
The science of logistics combined with medicine and public health, where logistics is defined as:
■ the set of physical and human infrastructures;
■ materials and supplies;
■ transport resources;
■ information and communication systems;
■ business processes;
■ decision support systems;
■ and command and control systems
. . . required to respond quickly and appropriately to a public health emergency.

able in twenty-first–century America and should have been avoided.[5] This unprecedented natural disaster revealed a cascade of public health and hospital system failures that may have been foreseen, planned for, and overcome, in part, if local officials had access to and were trained to use adequate tools needed to manage such a complex task.

Given the current threat of intentional mass casualty events in addition to natural catastrophes, clearly more needs to be done. A first step is to clearly demarcate what is meant by health system emergency response logistics. (See Table 11-1.)

Armed with such a definition, a reasonable next step is to define those components of hospital and public health practice that enable successful response processes and that may be addressed through targeted research and training. (See Table 11-2.) As we will discuss, perhaps the most critical concept underlying these processes, from a supply chain perspective, is the probabilistic nature of demands, which determine the necessary quantity and placement of assets to deliver services under uncertain conditions. Hospital and public health authorities must have the means to comprehend this changing operation environment and the interaction of that environment with response

Table 11-2	
Elements of Response Logistics Systems for Hospitals and Public Health	
Hospital Systems	**Public Health**
Surge treatment capacity	Capacity planning
Supply chain management	Supply logistics
Staff management	Scale-up of permanent and temporary clinics
Interface with public health	Interface with hospital systems
Inventory control	Mass prophylaxis
Financial resiliency	Quarantine and containment
	Ambulance routing

mechanisms employed in order to engage in effective tactical decision making during disasters. In the remainder of this chapter, we describe several ways in which this state of affairs will impact healthcare logistics during disasters, and several principles, called the Laws of Supply Chain Physics, which may guide effective healthcare supply chain modeling and management to support disaster response.

Principles for Improved Disaster Supply Chain Management for Healthcare Facilities

Since World War II, modern supply chain management practices have revolutionized manufacturing and service industries by reducing the uncertainty of demand and improving the quality (including timeliness) of work products to fulfill that demand. Today, these methods are applied to manage activities ranging from jet engine maintenance to Internet-based retailing; in all cases, improving operational capabilities results in "lean" production and warehousing characterized by minimal on-site inventory and rapid demand fulfillment. In these settings, smaller inventories generally translate into improved profitability. As a consequence, hospitals and healthcare delivery organizations have often attempted to alter their supply chain and logistics systems to just-in-time materials management systems. These systems typically provide immediate benefits—reduced internal workforce requirements for hospitals and occasionally cost savings—at the expense of flexibility and control over logistics and resupply stocks.[6] The danger of implementing these systems in the unpredictable environment of healthcare management is that any deviation from the assumptions of predictability and consistency of demand— such as that encountered in public health emergencies and disasters—has the potential to destabilize the entire system, making it unable to provide needed services or able to meet those needs only at extraordinary costs.

Mounting an effective hospital response to public health emergencies and disasters requires appropriate strategic and tactical planning as well as operational flexibility. The only sure thing in disasters is that they are unpredictable; unknowns during disasters range from knowing what resources may be required to determining where and when those resources will be needed in the course of emergency response.[7] This is captured in the first Law of Supply Chain Physics: "To forecast is to err." (See Table 11-3.)

Consequently, the only sure thing about resource requirement models based on predicting the future in this setting is that they will be wrong. And, because some form of demand forecast is the basis for virtually all just-in-time supply arrangements, modern hospital supply chain systems turn out to be exquisitely fragile in the face of the

Table 11-3	
Laws of Supply Chain Physics for Hospital Emergency Response	
Statement of Law	**Practical Application**
1. To forecast is to err.	Hospital emergency response logistics systems should address uncertainty at all phases of operation planning and execution.
2. Local optimization results in global disharmony.	Hospital logisticians should strive to integrate their emergency supply chain plans into regional strategies that involve extensive linkages between public health and healthcare delivery systems.
3. Collaborative information sharing is critical for supply chain sustainability; its value diminishes only when capacity utilization is either extremely low or extremely high.	Hospital emergency response plans should include clear, capacity-based thresholds for activation of and participation in regional assistance compacts.
4. Keep assets in their most flexible form for as long as operationally and economically possible.	Hospital emergency response planners should strive to maintain the capability for redirection of materials as far down the supply chain as possible.

types of unpredictable demands that arise during health crises. Such situations require the use of probabilistic demand models. Such models may operationalize the hazard vulnerability analysis (HVA) that accrediting organizations and the federal government require hospitals to undertake for emergency preparedness activities. HVAs consider the likelihood that a particular disaster scenario will occur, and overlay that on the risk that such an event would pose to continued operations of the institution. Probabilistic resource and supply chain models consider both the probability of a particular event occurring and the probability that particular resources will be needed in particular quantities at particular times during a crisis response. Undertaking these types of calculations is the only reproducible method for anticipating the range of healthcare needs that may occur over a range of events.

In such an unpredictable environment, it is only natural that each healthcare institution will attempt to optimize its ability to care for patients and increase surge capacity by maximizing its stores of critical resources using preexisting or rapidly determined estimates of the amount of emergency stores that will be needed to meet current or expected demands. Unfortunately, efforts to estimate these quantities in the absence of models that take into consideration the variance inherent in complex hospital system performance will likely underestimate true resource requirements. Paradoxically, recent changes to accreditation requirements have the potential to reinforce this impulse, requiring, for example, that each hospital preparedness plan describe how the facility might sustain operation for up to 96 hours in the absence of resupply (i.e., Joint Commission Standard EC.4.12, Element of Performance 6).[8] One problem with such an individual facility-based approach is that it eliminates possible benefits from collaborative risk-sharing and material stockpiling among geographically proximate facilities. A more fundamental problem is that efforts to improve local response capabilities (potentially at the expense of neighboring facilities) are likely to jeopardize regional or multi-jurisdiction plans, a state of affairs captured in the Second Law of Supply Chain Physics: "Local optimization results in global disharmony." The expectation that an "every hospital for itself" approach will lead to poor outcomes is especially relevant given recent consolidation in the healthcare supply industry, in which a handful of large corporations have multiple, often overlapping obligations for emergency supplies during emergencies. Without a systematic command and control environment and centralized authority for making critical resource allocation and reallocation decisions, one can expect that every hospital will work for itself, hoarding supplies for example, and this will lead to poor outcomes overall.

On the other hand, regional planning alone is not a panacea for emergency response supply chain problems. First, just engaging in planning, even complemented by scripted discussion-based exercises such as "tabletop exercises," is not sufficient to ensure that response mechanisms are flexible enough to be of value in the most extreme of demand scenarios, such as those envisioned during the peak of a global influenza pandemic. In such settings, resource deficits will almost certainly have a negative impact on hospital-based patient care, but the situation awareness afforded by effective supply chain communications channels (i.e., collaborative efforts to ensure communication regarding current and anticipated demand and supply from the manufacturer down to the hospital) may spell the difference between a shuttered and a functioning hospital. Regionalization of planning alone, therefore, will not eliminate the need for hospitals to invest to some degree in risk management schemes and supplies to guard against such unlikely events. Disaster preparedness dollars often are seen as wasted capital when the demand for purchased matériel or emergency response systems fails to materialize. Information systems for supply chain management may be lumped into this category of unnecessary expenditures, but only in periods when hospital resupply is not the bottleneck in surge capability, which can occur momentarily in major disasters such as mass casualty incidents when, for example, supply of trained surgeons or available operating rooms may be the limiting factor. The Third Law of Supply Chain Physics addresses this point directly: "Collaborative information sharing is critical for supply chain sustainability; its value diminishes only when capacity utilization is either extremely low or [as would be expected at certain moments in a major emergency] extremely high."

During disasters, hospital and health system logisticians are likely to be faced with sudden and irregular demands for services and supplies. The complexity of meeting these demands will likely be exacerbated by poor situation awareness and limited collaborative forecasting of future demand by public health and hospital planners. In such circumstances, resource allocation decisions within a healthcare facility or system will be fraught with potential for error, and because the propensity to focus locally will be greater, so the potential for global dysfunction will increase. Given that there will be limited critical supplies, optimal allocation of resources to meet regional demands requires balancing current needs with anticipated future ones. And this requires that systems be created that are capable of redirecting critical resources after they are "pushed" out to regional hospitals. Such systems are aided by management plans that adhere to the Fourth Law of Supply Chain Physics: "Keep your assets in their most flexible form for as long as it is operationally and economically possible." Implementing such a strategy, though, requires a sophisticated system for hospital and health system inventory control, including mechanisms to determine temporal and geographic demand imbalances, track shipments well into end-user environments (such as distributed nursing stations), as well as address issues of fairness and efficiency. Designing such a system requires a thorough understanding of supply chain structure (how material flows to and among locations), communication (e.g., timing and content of reports among locations), resupply capabilities (quantity, location, interval), and demand quantification and forecasting. Even if all these aspects of the supply chain are known, maintaining tactical control over materials is often a challenge. For example, in some large U.S. cities, regional blood centers have only limited ability to recall and redirect allocated blood products because "ownership" (and therefore traceability) changes at the hospital loading dock. This leads to a near-total lack of visibility after the products are within the hospital stock system. In the absence of infrastructure investment to improve information systems, business policies, and operational procedures covering such items, breakdowns in the supply and distribution of critical resources will continue to occur during emergencies, with serious potential consequences.

In considering the principles and recommendations embodied in the Laws of Supply Chain Physics, it is important to remember several key underlying facts about the environment in which hospital material management will occur during disasters. Most important, although the effects of uncertainty can be mitigated to some extent through collaboration and communication, fundamental uncertainty will always exist. For that reason, tactical response systems need to be designed so that they are robust in the presence of this uncertainty. The first step in creating

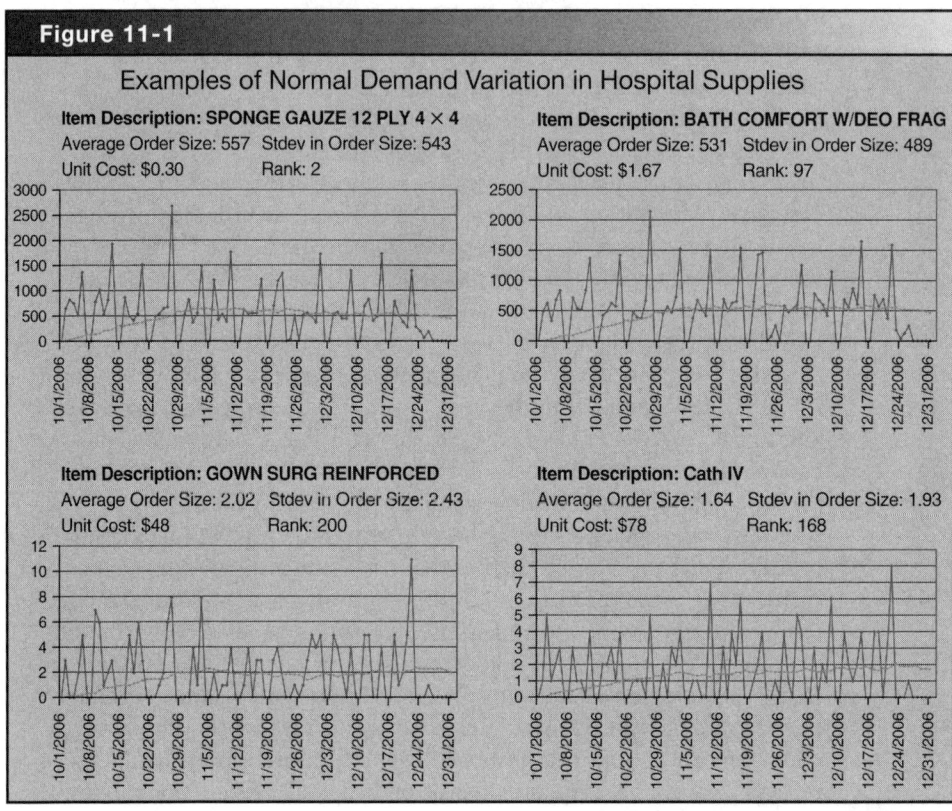

Figure 11-1

Examples of Normal Demand Variation in Hospital Supplies

robust supply systems is establishing methods to understand resupply requirements probabilistically, both for normal daily operations and for emergencies. Figure 11-1 provides an example of analyses of four frequently ordered items in a major U.S. teaching hospital. Note the considerable order-to-order variation, such that the standard deviation is larger than the mean order quantity for two of the four items. Models (both conceptual and quantitative) intended to assist in planning and real-time disaster response should capture and represent the implications of this uncertainty on potential outcomes of specific logistic decisions at single institutions and across affected regional healthcare systems. Such probabilistic models are a common feature of other high-reliability, high-consequence industries requiring real-time allocation decisions, such as finance and revenue management. Because in the United States these systems are typically made up of disparate independently operated entities, effective response strategies will require command and control systems that can coordinate the management of additional resources to ensure adequate response.

Defining the Research Agenda for Emergency Response Logistics

Research in public health response logistics focuses on the design, construction, testing, and deployment of logistics response and decision support systems. Ideally, development of such systems would proceed through three stages. First, creation of integrated data management environments will permit collection, analysis, and structuring of the required information on patient type and location (demand), quantities and disposition of various medical resources (supply), as well as rules for allocating their use in time of need. These resources should include: physical resources such as hospitals, beds, ICUs, emergency departments, and operating rooms; personnel such as doctors, nurses, and other health professionals; other equipment and supplies necessary for emergency and ongoing medical response such as pharmaceuticals; transportation assets such as ambulances and other EMS units; command and control mechanisms that ensure the maximum effective use of these physical assets; and an identification and information system including data required to support the system.

The second stage comprises efforts to use these data structures to construct real-time operations support systems intended to maximize effectiveness of response logistics resources after an emergency occurs. A real-time execution system includes acquisition of state-of-the-system data in real time; evaluation of alternative actions that could be undertaken by personnel in different parts of the response system (hospital administrators, political leaders, police, emergency management personnel, regional government and health system managers, etc.) in real time; dissemination of system status and projected consequences of alternative courses of action to appropriate personnel in real time; and a command and control infrastructure that ensures system performance is maximized.

Given the rarity of actual catastrophic disasters that would stress such decision support systems, the third stage would involve development of simulation environments for constructing and assessing the effectiveness of alternative logistic response system designs (physical elements, information systems, command and control architectures, management rules, etc.) and ultimately, for training personnel to ensure that all management levels of emergency response logistics systems understand and can execute their tasks in a maximally effective manner. These systems may be amenable to validation against data from real-life emergency response scenarios, although data collection during emergencies is often haphazard.

Conclusions

The four Laws of Supply Chain Physics described here derive from extensive work by two of the authors and many others over the past three decades in optimizing service performance in the manufacturing and retail environments, which are by nature more competitive, though arguably less consequential, than hospital emergency response activities. In our work with hospitals in both urban and rural settings, we have found only intermittent awareness of, attention to, and adherence with the principles embodied in these laws. It is our opinion that hospital emergency response logistics is in its infancy, both theoretically and operationally; the overwhelming lesson of Hurricane Katrina is that individual heroics is no substitute for a well-designed, workable regional management plan. A concerted national effort to develop a cross-trained health logistics workforce (in public health and operations research or systems engineering) will help to achieve this goal.

References

1. Bernard M, Mathews PR. Evacuation of a maternal-newborn area during Hurricane Katrina. MCN Am J Matern Child Nurs. 2008;33(4):213–223.

2. Committee on the Future of Emergency Care in the United States Health System, Board on Health Care Services, Institute of Medicine of the National Academies. Hospital-Based Emergency Care: At the Breaking Point. Washington, DC: The National Academies Press; 2006.

3. Woerth G. IOM and ACS warn of the impending crisis in emergency care: emergency departments overwhelmed, underfunded, and dangerously fragmented. Bull Am Coll Surg. 2007;92(3):20–26.

4. Centers for Disease Control and Prevention. Public health response to Hurricanes Katrina and Rita—Louisiana, 2005. MMWR. 2006;55(2):29–30.

5. Brunkard J, Namulanda G, Ratard R. Hurricane Katrina deaths, Louisiana, 2005. Disaster Med Public Health Prep. 2008;2(4):215–223.

6. Molina SL, Figge HL. Protecting the pharmaceutical supply chain. Ensuring an unbroken supply of pharmaceuticals can save lives during times of disaster. Health Manag Technol. 2008;29(8):20–22.

7. Auf der Heide E. The importance of evidence-based disaster planning. Ann Emerg Med. 2006;47(1):34–49.

8. DeJohn P. Hospital supply chain vital part of disaster plan. Hosp Mater Manage. 2002;27(9):14–15.

Chapter 12

Risk Communication and Media Relations

Linda C. Degutis, DrPH, MSN and Lauren Babcock-Dunning, MPH

Learning Objectives

- Describe risk communication theories.
- Identify appropriate media relations techniques and communication channels.
- Understand media activities during the phases of a disaster.
- Implement appropriate disaster responses.

Introduction

Effective risk and media communications are essential to disaster preparedness, mitigation, response, and recovery. Thoughtful communication enhances an organization's ability to act effectively in the face of disaster, while poorly managed communication impedes response or undermines public opinion about an otherwise successful operation. Every organization involved in healthcare emergency management needs a communication plan as part of its emergency management strategy. By providing the public with essential information, effective communication can mitigate the impact of public health crises on healthcare facilities, for instance, by preventing the flood of "worried well" that has been so disruptive during past disasters. Media, such as local television and radio, are paramount to your communication strategy. In fact, in the event of a potential bioterrorist event, people identified these channels as their primary source of information.[1] Consequently, organizations need to develop effective strategies for communicating their messages through the media. This chapter will address risk communication theories, media relations, and materials development, and finally, the phases of a public health emergency, with the goal of enabling you to communicate effectively with the public and the media if disaster strikes.

PRELUDE: WHEN COMMUNICATION FAILS

Hurricane Katrina demonstrated the impact of ineffective communication on disaster preparedness, response, and recovery. While many of the communication shortcomings in Katrina were due to tactical communications failures (downed communications towers, lack of satellite phones, etc.),[2] there are several risk communication and media relations lessons that may be drawn from this disaster.

■ **Addressing the needs of vulnerable populations:** Prior to the hurricane, communicators failed to reach several important target audiences with emergency messaging: the elderly, individuals living in low-income areas, and people with disabilities.[3,4] Authorities did not adequately inform these vulnerable residents or their families how to ensure their safety if they did not have access to a car, financial resources, someplace to stay outside the city.[3]

■ **Unclear lines of authority:** As discussed later in this chapter, the public becomes anxious when it is apparent that those responsible for ensuring their safety do not have a situation under calm control. When Mayor Nagin issued his "desperate SOS," it was evident that the situation had exceeded his office's capabilities to address it competently, and this undermined the public's trust and heightened anxiety.

■ **Inadequate media strategy:** Reports following Katrina indicate that there was no media strategy in place to get ahead of the media coverage to enable authorities to convey effective messages and refute rumors.[2]

■ **Failure to refute rumors:** Authorities' inability to refute inaccurate information reported by the media, and their public repetition of these rumors irrepealably damaged the response and recovery efforts during Katrina.[2] Reports of widespread violence delayed the arrival of needed supplies (e.g., fuel that could have powered communications equipment) and personnel and heightened New Orleans residents' anxiety.[5]

Part 1: Risk Communication Theories

Since 9/11, the field of risk communication has gained increasing prominence.[6] What was once a field focused on environment hazards now has a rich literature dealing with a variety of public health and other risks. As the field has grown and been tested during past emergencies, so has our knowledge of the social and cognitive processes that underlie how people perceive risk and what can be done to influence these perceptions to engender the responses most adaptive to health. However, risk communication is a still-evolving science, with lessons yet to be learned.[6–8] Despite this, four prevailing theories have emerged that form the basis of risk communication: risk perception theory, the mental noise model, trust determination theory, and the theory of negative dominance. These theories, along with knowledge of several other cognitive processes that underlie risk-related behavior, will help to understand how people react during a crisis, and therefore, how to communicate effectively with them.

Risk communicators engage in activities that are dependent on the hazards associated with a risk and the public's emotional response to it. Four categories exist: precaution advocacy, outrage management, stakeholder relations, and crisis communication.[5] If risks generate little public outrage but present serious hazards to public health, then the task of the risk communicator is precaution advocacy. This is largely the domain of health education—convincing the public to protect their health when they have little motivation; for instance, encouraging people to lose weight to prevent diabetes and heart disease. Outrage management occurs when the public has an emotional response out of proportion to the risk, for example, addressing fears of pandemic flu due to avian influenza when there has not been a report of human-to-human transmission. The task of the risk communicator in this instance is to try to align public perceptions with the actual threat posed by a risk. Stakeholder relations occur when both risk level and outrage are moderate. This is the ideal situation because your audience is engaged and the risk is urgent, but not immediate. The final category, crisis communication, occurs when the public is justifiably concerned by a risk that poses a high hazard. The risk communicator's task is to communicate effectively to mitigate the hazard presented by a serious risk.

ASIDE: AVOIDING PANIC

During past risk communication efforts, avoiding panic has been listed as a primary goal;[9] however, studies have shown that, in the face of serious emergencies such as those presented by natural disasters or acts of terror, panic is rare. One danger of thinking of panic avoidance as a communication goal is that it can encourage leaders to behave in ways that are perceived as secretive and dishonest, and this, not emergencies in and of themselves, has been found to generate panic.[10]

THEORY 1: RISK PERCEPTION

There are 16 factors important to understanding the public's perception of risk. Collectively, they are called the "outrage factors."[11,12] The risk communicator needs to understand these factors because they are at odds with the "scientific" conceptualization of risk. While scientists view risk in terms of absolute hazard (morbidity and mortality), this is not how the public perceives it. Instead, risk is viewed through the lens of the outrage factors. These factors shape public opinion regarding a hazard, and they can lead to strong emotional reactions to risks that scientists might otherwise ignore.

1. **Involuntary:** Risks imposed by others or perceived as involuntary are less acceptable than risks that are considered as voluntary.

2. **Uncontrollable:** Risks viewed as outside of individuals' control or for which they cannot take precautionary measures are harder to accept than those perceived as controllable.

3. **Unfamiliar:** Unfamiliar risks are viewed as more hazardous than familiar ones.

4. **Inequitable:** Risks that affect one part of the population more than another are less readily accepted than equitably distributed risks.

5. **Unbeneficial:** Risks that have no or unclear benefits are viewed less favorably than ones that have appreciable benefits.

6. **Difficult to understand:** Risks that are poorly understood are less acceptable than those that arise from activities that are well understood or self-explanatory.

7. **Uncertainty:** Relatively unknown risks or those with greater dimensions of uncertainty are more worrying.

8. **Dreaded:** Risks that cause a dreaded illness or evoke terror or anxiety are more threatening than risks that do not evoke such emotions.

9. **Originate from untrustworthy sources:** Risks associated with untrustworthy institutions or figures are less acceptable than those associated with entities that are perceived as credible and trustworthy.

10. **Cause irreversible and hidden damage:** Risks that result in irreversible or hidden damage (e.g., cause illness years after exposure) are less acceptable that those whose effects are temporary or immediate.

11. **Personal:** Risks that pose a personal threat are less acceptable than those that are not viewed as directly threatening individuals.

12. **Ethical/moral nature:** Risks perceived as ethically or morally objectionable are more likely to cause outrage than those without a moral component.

13. **Human origin:** Risks that originate from human causes are more threatening than those that are naturally derived.

14. **Create identifiable victims:** Risks that create identifiable victims are less acceptable than those that generate anonymous ones.

15. **Affect small children and pregnant women:** Risk that affect small children, pregnant women, or future generations are less readily accepted than those that affect other populations.

16. **Catastrophic potential:** Risks with the potential for creating a catastrophe (those grouped spatially and temporally that produce illness, injury, or death) induce greater fear than those that are viewed as having a random or scattered impact.[12]

While communicating about risk, the temptation is to try to put risks into perspective. For example, one might want to compare the risk of driving a car to some new environmental exposure that is less hazardous to try to illustrate that people encounter more dangerous risks every day. However, risk comparisons such as these are perilous and should be avoided.[8] They are dangerous because they may seem patronizing; they often fail to consider personal values and the outrage factors; and they tell people they should not be scared when they already are, which seems uncaring. Take our car example. Getting into a car is voluntary, controllable, familiar, and the risks that arise from car travel are readily understood. However, if the environmental exposure being compared to car travel is exotic, human-caused, poorly understood by science, and has the potential to cause hidden damage in pregnant women and young children, then these risks may not be comparable at all because they may elicit completely different emotional responses. While it is possible to compare risks that are well matched by outrage factors, given the potential missteps risk comparisons can create, they are best avoided.

THEORY 2: MENTAL NOISE

When people's values are threatened, their emotions and thought processes are affected. This effect is known as the mental noise model.[11] It addresses how people process information during a crisis. When people are alarmed, their ability to assimilate and use information is severely impaired. In fact, mental noise has been found to reduce people's ability to process information by 80%.[13] Greater levels of impairment occur when the risk encountered is associated with one or more of the outrage factors. People become outraged, anxious, and upset and this results in mental noise, which limits their functional abilities.

THEORY 3: TRUST DETERMINATION

Trust is an overarching goal for the risk communicator. To communicate effectively during times of calm, but especially during crises, messengers must establish themselves as trusted sources of information and avoid any action that could undermine the public's trust. Much research has been devoted to understanding the factors that determine trust. Four factors have been shown empirically to determine the public's trust for organizations: perceptions of caring and empathy, openness and honesty, competence and expertise, and dedication and commitment.[14] For government organizations, the most important factor in determining public trust is dedication and commitment; for industry, it is care and empathy. However, all factors are important in establishing the public's trust when communicating about environmental and other risks.[11]

THEORY 4: NEGATIVE DOMINANCE

When people are upset, they develop a negative bias, or a tendency to remember negative things. This is another reason why it so important to avoid violating the public's trust. After they form a negative opinion regarding an organization, negative dominance renders it even more difficult to change their opinion. When risk communicators need to release a negative message—e.g., when the response to a reporter's question must be that the organization is unable to answer a question—at least three positives are needed to counteract this negativity.[9] For example, while the spokesperson may be unable to confirm that a particular pathogen is responsible for an outbreak, the spokesperson could say that

1. contact tracing is taking place;

2. lab results are expected and give a predicted timeframe;

3. he or she has confidence that the investigation will reveal the source of the outbreak.

SOCIAL AMPLIFICATION OF RISK[12] AND VICARIOUS REHEARSAL[15]

Risk is no longer local. What happens in rural Kansas may reach someone as far away as Singapore through today's lightening speed communication networks. This social amplification tends to occur when risks portend future problems, such as severe acute respiratory syndrome (SARS) signaling our susceptibility to global disease outbreaks. Because we live a 24-hour-a-day news cycle and news from around the globe is readily accessible, individuals are increasingly exposed to coverage (and images) of disasters that, while not physically threatening, create emotional turmoil. Given this media exposure, those distant from the emergency's epicenter experience anxiety. One mechanism people engage in to deal with this anxiety is to mentally rehearse the courses of action recommended for disaster victims (aka vicarious rehearsal). Past events have shown that those furthest away—emotionally (from proximity to victims) and geographically—are most likely to engage in vicarious rehearsal. This process is problematic because it leads people to adopt inappropriate behaviors for their personal levels of risk. These behaviors may tax an already burdened healthcare system in the midst of responding to a disaster. For example, the "worried well" may flood emergency rooms demanding treatment when they are not actually at risk. In the sarin attack on the Tokyo subway system, the worried well outnumbered those who were actually ill 4:1[16] and ran into the thousands.[17] One way to address vicarious rehearsal is to give people things to do, and structure these activities based on their proximity to the incident.[15] For instance, for those directly affected, seek medical attention; for those trying to locate loved ones, visit the Red Cross Web site for a list of survivors; for those who wish to honor victims, donate blood or aid, or attend a public vigil. Actions such as gathering aid for victims or attending a vigil help to limit vicarious rehearsal.[15]

PSYCHOLOGICAL PRINCIPLES

There are several psychological principles that underlie how people interpret risk. Several of these are cognitive shortcuts or heuristics. Because the world is filled with more information than we could ever hope to process, we engage in these cognitive shortcuts to help us filter it. While these shortcuts are helpful in our day-to-day activities, they can present challenges to risk communicators because they can lead to errors of interpretation. By understanding these shortcuts, risk communicators can construct messages that account for these, and are thus more effective.

- **Availability heuristic:** People have inherent problems making decisions about statistical probability.[18] Instead of making a decision about what is likely to happen statistically, people interpret what is memorable (i.e., what they have seen and remember) as being the same as what is likely. This is amplified by the media's tendency to focus on events that are rare (e.g., plane crashes, bovine spongiform encephalitis, necrotizing fasciitis) but garner ratings due to a sensational or "newsworthy factor," which will be discussed later in this chapter.
- **Confirmatory Bias:**[19] When people have formed opinions, they are resistant to contradictory information. They do not

seek out information that might disprove their prevailing view, and they have a tendency to find flaws when such information is presented. When presented with ambiguous information, they interpret it as confirmatory. Information that agrees with one's views is readily assimilated and subjected to less scrutiny than contradictory information.

- **The serial position effect:** The serial position effect[20] (or the primacy/recency effect) posits that people have a tendency to recall what comes first (primacy) and what came last (recency) and to gloss over what is in the middle. This is especially true during times of heightened anxiety.[9] (This bias can be used to the risk communicator's advantage: position your most important messages at the beginning of your communications and restate them at the end.)

- **Mental models:** People build cognitive frameworks called mental models to help them understand their world. These frameworks help to interpret and categorize new information. People find it easier to assimilate new ideas when they fit into an existing cognitive framework.[6] For example, if they have a framework for infectious disease and a new threat can be characterized in the same way, they are better able to understand it. Risk communicators have used mental models to help them map out people's existing frameworks, which helps them understand the factors that contribute to the people's perceptions of risk and to help explain novel or complex risks.[21]

Part 2: Materials Development and Media Relations

Effective media relations is more than just responding to media coverage as it happens—it's developing a proactive strategy that ensures messages are reported accurately and an organization communicates effectively.[9]

GENERAL CONSIDERATIONS

When presenting people with information on a risk, communicators must maintain a careful balance. They must avoid providing over-reassurance (which has been shown to erode trust) and creating inaction by inciting fear, because too much information has been shown to lead to cognitive overload that can stop people from taking protective actions.[22]

- **Health literacy**[23,24] **and numeracy:** The public health and medical communities have been aware for some time that a disconnect exists between lay and professional understandings of scientific information;[21] however, following the anthrax attacks of 2001, health literacy emerged as an important theme in public health preparedness.[23,25,26] Healthy People 2010 defines health literacy as: "The degree to which individuals have the capacity to obtain, process, and understand basic health information and services needed to make appropriate health decisions." Health literacy involves a number of skills, including the ability to: read text, use and understand numbers (also called numeracy), and use forms. According to the 2003 National Assessment of Adult Literacy (NAAL), more than 93 million Americans have limited literacy.[24] The NAAL also measured health literacy and found that 36% of adults had basic or below-basic health literacy skills. This means that they were unable to complete tasks such as determining what time a person could take a prescription medication based on information on the prescription drug label related to the timing of medication to eating, or determining a healthy weight from a BMI chart.[24]

- **Plain language:** Whether your organization is developing a Web site, a fact sheet, or holding a press conference, plain language considerations are paramount when developing risk communication messages. As discussed in the previous section on health literacy, the average American has difficulty with complex reading and numeracy tasks, both as they relate to everyday activities (like reading a bus schedule) and health-related tasks (such as understanding nutrition labels). Therefore, it is important when presenting health-related information that your organization does so as clearly as possible. For most audiences, aim to write at the fourth to eighth grade level.[27] To assess your text's reading level, you can use your word processor's spelling and grammar function, or an online assessment such as the SMOG[28] readability assessment. (SMOG is the simple measure of gobbledygook.) When first introduced to the concept of plain language, many people think that it involves dumbing down information and that it results in oversimplified and boring text of the "See Jane run. See Spot play." variety, but this is not the case. Plain language need not be boring language and both advanced and average readers prefer plainly written text.[23] Suggestions for writing in plain language include the following concepts:

  - **Organize material logically.**[27] Organize material in order of importance to the reader. Put the most important information first and use meaningful headings to help the reader find information quickly.

- **Keep sentences short.**[29] Keep sentences between 15 and 20 words each. This does not mean that you cannot vary their length for interest.
- **Use common words.**[27] Choose common words. Pick "more" instead of "supplementary" or "additional." Also, avoid using words commonly understood by medical personnel but not lay people, e.g., people feel sick, they do not "present with symptoms."[17] If a technical term is needed, clearly define it.
- **Use personal pronouns such as "we" and "you."**[27,29] "The West Wind Medical Center advises all patients that they will be contacted in the event of abnormal results" becomes much simpler and friendlier if changed to "We will call you if your results are not normal."
- **Employ terms consistently.**[17] Pick one term and employ it consistently throughout your communication. For example, in a patient handout on MRSA, do not switch among the terms infection, illness, disease, etc. These may mean different things to different readers and switching between terms is confusing.
- **Write in active voice.**[27,29] (This topic is discussed later in this chapter.)
- **Use bullets and tables.**[27,29] To break information into digestible chunks, use bulleted lists. To present complex information clearly, use tables.
- **Use the imperative.**[29] The imperative form of a verb is the form used in giving instructions and is often the most short and direct form. Observe: "Patients are advised to wait in this area until called" versus "Please wait here."
- **Avoid nominalizations.**[29] Nominalization turns verbs into nouns: "discuss" into "discussion," "complete" into "completion." They are harder for the average reader to understand and they take the action out of a sentence, much like passive verbs.

■ **Cultural competence:** In one study, many minority groups expressed mixed trust in national government organizations, noting instead that hospital staff, local civil servants, and emergency personal were trustworthy sources of information.[30] Therefore, these organizations have an important role in communicating with ethnic and cultural minorities prior to and during public health crises. With that in mind, cultural competence is an important consideration when developing messages as part of your organization's communication strategy. Symbols, words, and behaviors can carry different meanings across cultures; consequently, it is important to get to know the community that your organization serves so that your messages, at best, resonate with the many groups you serve, and at minimum, do not unintentionally offend. Some questions to answer regarding cultural sensitivity when developing your materials include the following topics:[9,31]

- Do any words or images convey negative cultural or ethnic stereotypes?
- Are symbols, signs, or words appropriate to the cultural groups your communication is targeting?
- Does your communication conform to differences in norms of interpersonal communication? These include: interpersonal distance (space between speakers), eye contact (maintaining versus avoiding), speech volume, and what is taboo.
- Are recommended courses of action compatible with cultural norms surrounding health, gender, and religion?

■ **Key messages:** One strategy that is often recommended when developing key messages for public and media communications is message mapping. Message mapping is a communication strategy designed to overcome a main barrier to comprehension during a crisis—mental noise.[9] Message mapping helps to overcome mental noise by packaging information in a way that is easier to remember and understand. It also allows an organization or multiple partners to communicate with one voice when they employ the message maps as part of their broader risk communication strategy. Message mapping is a strategy widely endorsed as part of successful emergency communications[9,15] and has been used by many effective communicators, including Mayor Rudolph Giuliani during his communications regarding the World Trade Center attacks.[13]

So, what exactly are message maps and how are they employed? Message maps are risk communication tools that help organize complex information and convey messages succinctly. They are organized in sound bites that conform to the 27/9/3 template:

- 27 words each that can be spoken in 9 seconds[13]
- 3 key messages
- 3 supporting statements for each key message (maximum)

This structure ensures that messages can be quoted accurately and completely in media interviews (because the media will edit longer

244 | Chapter 12 Risk Communication and Media Relations

Exhibit 12-1

Message Map Template

Stakeholder: [e.g., public, long-term care administrators]

Concern: [insert question to address]?

Key Message 1	Key Message 2	Key Message 3
Supporting Fact 1-1	Supporting Fact 2-1	Supporting Fact 3-1
Supporting Fact 1-2	Supporting Fact 2-2	Supporting Fact 3-2 `
Supporting Fact 1-3	Supporting Fact 2-3	Supporting Fact 3-3

Source: EPA

quotes). To develop a message map, address a likely question or concern related to a health risk by filling in key messages that your organization would like to convey to the public along with facts to support your key messages. The following template (Exhibit 12-1) provides a model for developing a message map.

Message maps have been developed to address a number of public health emergency topics, ranging from water safety to pandemic influenza and West Nile virus, and many are freely available for use by public health and other agencies. A more in-depth discussion of message mapping is available elsewhere.[13] Use the message maps that your organization develops to guide all of your communication efforts, be they media interviews, posters, pamphlets, or online fact sheets.

MEDIA RELATIONS

The media landscape is currently changing.[9,32,33,34] This offers the advantage of new and numerous means for communicating with the public, but some of these changes can exert negative pressures on the media that make it more difficult to interact with them. Reporters now have to deal with greater business pressures than ever before and with shrinking traditional media markets. For risk communicators, this has many implications. People have their choice of thousands of media outlets available online; therefore competition is fierce. This can create greater and greater demands for news that must be filled, and if credible experts are not available, then less scrupulous sources will be tapped.[17] Additionally, newspapers, once a daily presence in American households, are dwindling in popularity. To increase profitability, owners are reformatting newspapers, increasing the amount of space devoted to advertising[35] and reducing the number of writers on staff.[36] For those trying to communicate complex health messages, this means two things. First, a smaller news hole means there is less space available for stories. As a consequence, it is more important to convey your organization's messages succinctly. Second, as more newsrooms move away from larger staffs with more salaried employees, fewer seasoned writers are available to cover stories. This means that novice reporters may be deployed with greater frequency[36] and specialized reporters, such as those covering health or science, may be required to take on other topics.

Deadlines

Reporters have tight deadlines. While these vary by medium, one general constraint among reporters is that they have strict timelines that must be met. When the media contact your organization, determine their deadlines and respect them. As a deadline approaches, a reporter will go ahead with a story—regardless of whether your organization has issued a statement. A failure to respond to a media request is a negative development for the following reasons. First, presumably your organization would like its perspective included in any story that relates to its area of practice. Second, it is a missed opportunity to cultivate a good relationship with a reporter. Reporters remember communicators they can rely on for expertise when they are on deadline and communicators who left them in a bind. By responding promptly and providing credible information, you become a trusted source for the reporter.

Conflict in Public Health and Media Perspectives

Media is, first and foremost, a business.[34] While members of the media think of themselves as watchdogs[9] and view themselves as engaging in public service,[37] they are accountable to corporate masters. Public health and healthcare workers focus explicitly on serving the public's needs, and are often frustrated when science is glossed over or risks are sensationalized in the interest of entertainment or marketing. The media also deal in definitives, while science deals in degrees. There is a great deal of debate and uncertainty inherent in many scientific findings, but what the media want is to be able to report on definites, such as causation, cures, and safe levels of exposure.[33] With the exception of highly specialized science and health writers, most reporters do not have a strong science background.[38] The fact that most media are not "sciency"[33,38] means that you cannot make assumptions about background knowledge related to the health risk information you are conveying. Many novice risk communicators assume a background level of health literacy among reporters, do not convey information clearly, and are later annoyed when a reporter uses a quote out of context or misinterprets data. In order to avoid this, it is critical to think about the message that you want to convey, to convey it clearly, and to eliminate as much ambiguity as possible in your responses to a reporter's questions.

Elements of Newsworthiness

The elements of newsworthiness determine the media's interest in a story. If your organization is engaged in precaution advocacy, understanding these elements will help you effectively pitch stories to advance your education campaigns. If you are in the midst of a crisis, they will help you gauge the media's interest and the angles they are likely to focus on. There are 11 elements of newsworthiness to keep in mind:[32,33]

1. **Timely:** Has the story been covered recently and extensively by the media, or is it breaking news? The most compelling stories are those reported as they happen. If a story has been covered extensively, unless it can be presented with a new spin, it will not generate much interest.

2. **Relevance to audience:** Does the story affect a broad audience or is it only relevant to a small group of people? A story may be interesting, but unless it appeals to a wide audience, it is unlikely to garner media interest.

3. **Controversy/conflict:** Are there identifiable villains or controversies? A program that stays on budget, is widely accepted, and saves lives is unlikely to be reported on because there is no controversy. However, one that is grossly over budget, unproven, and contested makes for a great story.

4. **Injustice:** Are there inequities or unfair circumstances? Injustice stories play to the audience's sense of right and wrong, and are a favorite of journalists because they lend themselves to questions of "Who is responsible for the injustice?" and "How will it be rectified?"

5. **Irony:** Is there something ironic or unusual? For example, did the evaluation of a program intended to increase disaster preparedness reveal that the organization is *less* prepared than it was prior to its implementation?

6. **Local:** The more proximate the story is to the media outlet's audience, the greater their interest in it.

7. **Breakthrough or important consequences:** Does the story represent a breakthrough or first-of-its-kind event? Does this event portend a change in the way we view the world from now on as 9/11 or SARS did?

8. **Human interest or personal angle:** Is there a person to interview who can share their story and embody the issue? Stories with personal angles give the audience someone with whom they can empathize, and this makes them more interesting.

9. **Celebrity:** Does the story affect a celebrity or notable figure? In our fame-obsessed culture, any link to a celebrity spells news.

10. **Seasonal peg or anniversary:** Does the story tie into a seasonal peg (for example, fire safety and holiday lights) or important anniversary? Reporters have predictable cycles of seasonal news stories and if you can present an issue in a novel way, then your story is more likely to gain coverage.

11. **Visuals:** Are there compelling images for journalists to shoot?

Developing Media Contacts

Before you are in the midst of dealing with a crisis, get to know the media that serves your area and develop relationships with them. Just as forming partnerships with other organizations who will be involved in emergency response will facilitate future interactions, getting to know the media before a crisis strikes will ensure that you will understand each other better when interacting during times of greater stress.

Identify and Train a Public Information Officer and Spokesperson

There is often some confusion regarding the roles and responsibilities of the public information officer (PIO) and the spokesperson. The PIO is a role assigned as part of the Incident Command System (ICS). The PIO is responsible for coordinating internal and external communications, including coordinating with the Joint Information Center (JIC) and the media. The PIO is the person under the incident command structure to whom media calls are referred. He or she then designates who within the organization is best suited to respond to the media's needs based on the situation, for instance, a subject matter expert (e.g., the hospital's infection control specialist) or the organization's spokesperson. Sometimes, the PIO and the spokesperson are one and the same; however, a spokesperson is always someone high within an organization's hierarchy who the media view as having sufficient authority and expertise to represent the organization's interests. Because the spokesperson may have other organizational duties, he or she may not also be able to fulfill the role of PIO.

Correcting Media Errors[9,17]

During routine communication with the media and during a crisis, you may find that the media have reported errors that you would like to correct. When addressing errors, there are several things to keep in mind. First, remain polite and calm when correcting a media error. Do not assume malice on the part of the media. The media are under incredible time constraints, and errors do occur. Next, decide on the corrective action you would like the media to take so that you have a goal for your conversation. Do you want to correct misinformation so that it is not repeated in subsequent broadcasts? To change the online editions of the newspaper to correct a factual error? To print a retraction or read it on-air? If the error is minor, try to address it with the reporter directly rather than going to his or her editor. Do not make a habit of complaining about trivial omissions or errors. After all, you want to maintain a good working relationship, and this involves being viewed as an asset, not a pest.

If an issue is not adequately resolved by talking directly to the reporter (if for example, he or she refuses to take the corrective action you request or if the error is egregious), then you may want to address it with his or her editor. You want to avoid doing this as a first step because it may damage your relationship with the reporter. (Imagine your response if someone went directly to your boss with an error you committed rather than affording you the professional courtesy of bringing it to your attention first.) Going to the reporter's editor may still damage your working relationship, but factual errors need to be corrected because they will live on in electronic databases and may be repeated in subsequent reports. If the error is reported by several media outlets, correct it during your next news release or press conference, but do not name the media outlet that committed the initial error by name because this will embarrass them and the reporter.

Finally, it is important to recognize the difference between what the media characterize as an error of fact, and what you or your organization may characterize as an error of emphasis or of opinion. If a reporter takes a particular perspective in a story that you do not agree with, or uses a quote out of context, this generally is not grounds for a retraction or other correction. Your recourse in this instance (and the option you will most likely be given if you bring this to the reporter's attention) is to write a letter to the editor. If this is important to you, it is worth the effort, because your letter will likely be retrieved during electronic searches for the original material and will provide context for future stories.[17]

Media Advisories
Media advisories differ from news releases in that they alert the press to a potential story without delving into great detail. They serve to advise the media of your organization's newsworthy event and entice them to show up to cover it. Advisories usually cover the basic information about an event, including

- the location;
- the date;
- the start and finish times;
- a brief description of what will be covered during the event; and
- the names and titles of speakers.

Take a look at the advisory template in Exhibit 12-2 to learn more about format and style.

Writing News Releases
Ideally, your organization will develop news release templates for a number of scenarios before a disaster strikes, so that only the details need to

---

Exhibit 12-2

Media Advisory Template

FOR IMMEDIATE RELEASE

(Today's date)

Contact: Name
(After-hours phone number)

Headline here, initial cap

WHAT:_____ [Two to three sentences describing the event; include information on any photo opportunities]

WHEN:_____ [Date and time of event]

WHERE:_____ [Address]

WHO:_____ [Identify individuals or organizations involved]

WHY:_____ [Two to three sentences emphasizing the newsworthiness of the event]

End or # # #

End your advisory with important organizational information, for example:

Organization name ● Telephone number ● Fax number ● Email address ● Web site

Source: EPA

---

be filled in during a crisis. Crises are inherently chaotic; therefore, the more you can do now, the more likely accurate information will be released quickly during a crisis. A news release is your organization's opportunity to write the ideal news story on an issue that it is involved in. Because reporters often use portions of news releases verbatim in their stories, the more your release is written like news, the more likely they are to use it "as is."[9] When your release is used "as is," it increases the chances that your key messages will be delivered accurately to the public and that your communication goals will be achieved.

- **Write using the inverted pyramid:** Most writing provides supporting arguments before coming to a conclusion, but this is not the case with a news release. Instead, news releases are written in the inverted pyramid style. (See Figure 12-1.) This style places the most important information up front, followed by the supporting facts. Releases are written like this because reporters and the public are busy and inundated with news items. Because of these constraints, reporters may not have the time to read the entire release, and they need to be able to gather the vital information for their stories quickly. If they need further details, they can get those later by reading more of your release.
- **Prefer active voice:** In active voice, the subject does the action. For example: "The hurricane destroyed the neighborhood." Contrast this with passive voice, where the subject of the sentence has something done to it, "The neighborhood was destroyed by the hurricane." Not only is the first sentence more engaging, but it is also more succinct. When writing a news release, use active voice throughout. Be certain to use it in the first paragraph (the lead) because the lead is what grabs the reporter's attention and conveys the story's most important information.
- **Use plain language:** Plain language is not boring language.[29] It is language that conveys your point simply and clearly. When mental noise is present, people's ability to absorb information is already limited. Your message should not am-

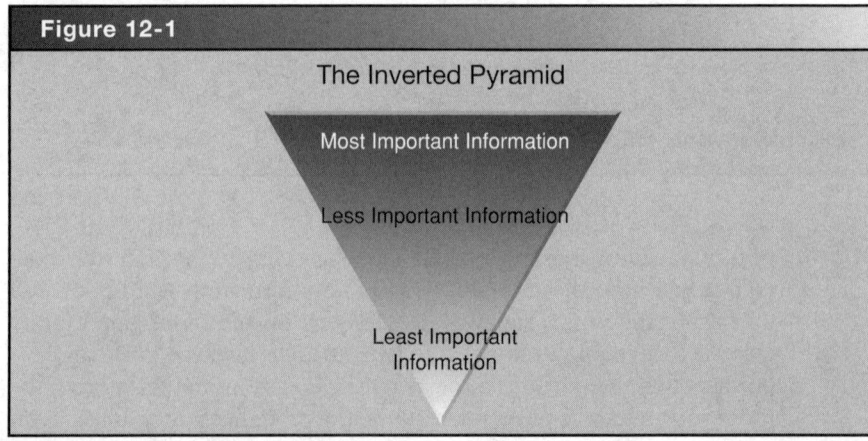

Figure 12-1

The Inverted Pyramid

Most Important Information

Less Important Information

Least Important Information

plify their confusion; it should alleviate it. Use common words. For example, choose "more" rather than "additional," and "use" instead of "utilize."

- **Limit numbers and statistics:** Because the public and journalists have difficulty interpreting statistics,[18] it is best to avoid them unless they are absolutely necessary. Interpreting absolute versus relative risk is particularly difficult. For example, if the absolute risk of contracting an illness over one's lifetime is 1 in 1,000,000, and a study reveals that those exposed to factor X are 3 times more likely to contract this illness, journalists and the public most often focus on the 3-fold increase in risk. However, what is important to note is that the absolute risk from factor X is still minute, now 3 in 1,000,000. This is why, if numbers or statistics must be included in your release, it is best to present them as simply as possible in ways that fit into frameworks people already have. Some examples in Table 12-1 are illustrative.

- **Avoid jargon:** Another component of writing simply is avoiding jargon. Jargon will only limit the impact of your message by confusing your audience. Additionally, it may convey to your audience that you do not care enough to try to communicate understandably.[17] Obviously, during a disaster, some unfamiliar terminology may be necessary. If a new or complex term is needed, define it first. If your release refers to multiple organizations by acronym, spell these out the first time they appear to avoid "alphabet soup."

- **Be precise and concise:** Use precise language that avoids editorializing and is not flowery, because nothing raises reporters' ire faster than a news release that refers to structures that were "completely destroyed" (either a structure is destroyed—there are no degrees here—or it is damaged, severally, moderately, etc.). Do not send a two-page release when you could send a one-page release instead. Cut out unnecessary and repetitious words. Only include what is "need to know," not "nice to know." When you are an expert, you are tempted to try to

Table 12-1

How to Present Statistics

Instead of . . .	Try . . .
10% chance of contracting an illness	One in 10 people will get sick
1/100,000	About 1 person sitting in the Michigan stadium (seats 106,000)
1 part per million	One drop of gasoline in a full-size car's tank full of gas[39]

Source: The Oak Ridge Institute for Science and Education (ORISE)

convey as much information as possible; however, this is not the goal of the news release. You need to spell out what is most important by focusing on your key messages. You can always direct people who would like to know more to your Web site or other information sources. However, if you fail to be concise, someone else will simplify your message.[40] You may not want leave this to the reporters because they may not emphasize the same message you would.

■ **Make sure every pronoun has only one possible antecedent:**[39] The antecedent is the word that the pronoun (it, his, that) stands for, and when it is not clear what the pronoun is standing in for, your writing and the impact of your communication suffers. Consider the following sentence: "The police officer wrestled the suspect for control of his gun."[41] Whose gun were they fighting over? It is not clear because the pronoun "his" could refer to the officer or the suspect because both are possible antecedents of "his." A rewrite that eliminates the pronoun or elucidates who it refers to helps clear up the confusion: "The officer wrestled the suspect for control of the suspect's gun."[41] You do not want your audience struggling to understand what you mean, so make your intent as clear as possible.

■ **Stick to one idea per sentence:** Writers jeopardize clarity and brevity when they try to cram too many ideas into a sentence. Because the goal of a news release is to be both informative and engaging, be sure that each sentence conveys one, and only one, clear idea.

■ **Create a punchy headline:** A headline should give the reader an immediate idea of what the story is about and hook their attention so they want to read more. Headlines are written omitting articles (a, an, the), for example: "Groundbreaking study shows most Americans unprepared for disaster."

■ **Write a strong lead:**[42]

 • **Keep it short:** A good lead is a one-sentence introductory paragraph. It should be 30 words at most and summarize, at minimum, the most newsworthy elements of a story, the: "what," "where," and "when." Example: "A hurricane made landfall in Galveston early Tuesday evening."

 • **Tell them what is what:** Express the main "what" of the story with the lead's first verb and place it among the lead's first seven words. Be sure this verb is in active voice.

 • **Emphasize the "who:"** If the story has a "who," the lead should indicate who this is. Example: "Mayor Giuliani visited ground zero today."

- **Address "why" and "how:"** The lead should summarize the "why" and "how" of the story, but only if there is room.
- **Attribute if necessary:** If the lead must contain an attribution, place it at the end. The newsworthy element of a lead is not that someone stated, disclosed, or announced. It is the content of their statement, disclosure, or announcement, so lead with that. Use "5 million in funding to improve emergency preparedness was awarded to the Connecticut Department of Health, Governor Doe announced Tuesday" rather than "Governor Doe announced Tuesday that 5 million in funding was awarded to the Connecticut Department of Health to improve emergency preparedness."

Be sure to include a release date, contact information, organization boilerplate, and further details of your story. For comprehensive information on formatting a news release, see the template (Exhibit 12-3) that follows.

Disseminate your Release

After you have written, formatted, and proofread your release, you are reading to disseminate it.

- **Obtain approval for your release:** The communication plan in section three outlines the written set of procedures for approving communications that every organization needs before dissemination to the public and the media. At this point, it is important to note that all news releases need your organization's approval before being released.
- **Send your release electronically:** For speed, disseminate news releases electronically rather than by fax, unless a reporter requests otherwise. Sending a release electronically has several benefits:
  - It allows the reporter to quickly use your organization's copy in a story without having to retype it.
  - It provides a record that the information was sent.
  - It allows your organization to target many news agencies at once, saving time.
- Also, be sure to create a press corner on your organization's Web site where you post media releases and other information of interest to the press (e.g., leadership bios, organization facts, etc.).

Media Briefings and Press Conferences

Media events such as briefings and press conferences require organization and forethought to ensure that they go smoothly and meet your

---

Exhibit 12-3

News Release Template

FOR IMMEDIATE RELEASE*   Contact:

(Today's date)   Organization name

Telephone number

After-hours telephone number

Fax number

Email address

Web site

Headline here, initial cap

Sub headline (if using)

City, State – Date [Text follows. Double-space and indent paragraphs.]

[The Lead: Keep it brief—30 words maximum. Put the most important information here. Focus on the "what" of your story. If space allows, include the "why" and "how."]

[Second paragraph: Try to include a quote from the organization's leadership in this paragraph.]

[Body of story: contains further details of the story. During a disaster, include actions the public can take to protect themselves and how your organization will update them on the situation.[9]]

If the news release is more than one page long, use: —more— Center at the bottom of the page, then continue to the next page with a shortened headline and page number. Do not break paragraphs across pages.

* Releases may also be held until a later date. If this is the case, put **EMBARGOED UNTIL (release date/time).**

—more—

[Shortened headline] — Page 2

[Final paragraph: This paragraph is usually organization "boilerplate," which is a brief description of your organization and any other information you would like to share with your readers.[9] For example, in a news release on an immunization program, you might include dates, times, and locations of upcoming immunization clinics, as well as the program's Web site address and contact information.]

At the end of the release put: End or ###

Source: The Oak Ridge Institute for Science and Education (ORISE)

communication goals. Whether you have days, hours, or minutes to plan, taking the time to prepare will ensure that you stay on message and convey what is needed to the public.

Press conferences usually involve the announcement of information by one or more speakers, followed by questions from the media. Therefore, they are typically held to announce newsworthy items that will generate many questions among the media, beyond the information that could be addressed by a news release. They are also held to respond to events when there is a need to address a number of media requests for information at one time. Some events that might necessitate a press conference include a mass casualty event, a disease outbreak, the release of an important report, or a new innovative collaboration among several organizations.

Media briefings are just that, brief. They typically serve to update the media on an ongoing situation. For instance, during the anthrax investigation, the CDC held national daily conference calls to brief the media on the state of the investigation.[43] Organizations can combine press conferences and briefings as part of a successful communication strategy, scheduling daily briefings during a crisis and supplementing these with press conferences when important developments occur.

Preparing for a Press Conference[9,32]

- **Reach out to reporters early:** Identify the journalists you want to invite several days prior to your event and make sure your contact information for them is up to date. Three days before your conference, email or fax a media advisory. Follow up with a second advisory (if possible) at 6:00 AM on the day of your press conference. Media outlets receive hundreds of advisories each day, so you may also want to follow up with a brief phone call.
- **Facilities:** If using a location other than your organization's headquarters, select a venue that is central and well known with adequate parking. Pick a venue that is large enough to accommodate the number of guests you expect will attend (and their camera equipment), but not one so large that there will be many unfilled seats, because this give the impression your event was poorly attended. Cameras are usually placed at the back of the room with speakers up front, so consider this when arranging seating. Be sure the venue you select has adequate lighting for visuals the media will want to film and that there are enough electrical outlets for their technical needs.
- **Press kits:** Put together press kits prior to your conference. The kits should contain organization fact sheets, a press release, background information, and contact information. Have these available at the sign-in table.
- **Timing:** Work around other events that might present conflicts, for instance, major elections. The best days for making news are Tuesdays through Thursdays, and the best time to hold press conferences is generally 10:00 AM. News conferences held after 4:00 PM may be poorly attended because reporters are usually busy finalizing stories.

- **Assign roles:** Determine who will greet the press, moderate, and speak at the conference. Be sure to train these people appropriately for their roles. If possible, prepare speakers in advance with anticipated questions and key messages.
- **Anticipate questions:** During a crisis event, research has shown that the media commonly ask 77 questions that address the facts of the situation (What happened? Who was harmed? How can we protect ourselves?) as well as responsibility and blame (How could this have been prevented? Who is to blame?). A complete list of these questions is available in Hyer and Covello's book, *Effective Media Communication During Public Health Emergencies.*[9]

During the Press Conference[9,32]

- **Sign-in:** Have a sign-in area for media attending the press conference. Assign a staff person to hand out press kits and request that media sign in as they arrive. Having a sign-in requirement allows you to track attendance (so you can monitor for subsequent media coverage) and gather important information for your media contact list.
- **Moderate the conference:** Have the moderator introduce each speaker. The moderator should set the ground rules for the conference, and explain the procedures and timing that will be used for asking questions. The moderator should also act as timekeeper, ensuring speakers do not exceed their allotted time.
- **Keep it brief and on time:** Start the conference on time, respecting the media's time constraints. Limit speakers' prepared comments to 5 minutes at most. Leave time for reporters' questions at the end (generally 10 to 15 minutes).

After a Press Conference[9,32]

- **Have staff on hand:** Be sure that someone is available to answer media calls and direct them to the appropriate person because reporters may have follow-up questions as they are writing their stories.
- **Follow up with the media:** Thank the media for attending. If you were unable to answer questions, explain how and when they will be answered. (Is there another conference scheduled? Can they visit the Web site? Are speakers available for follow-up interviews?) Provide photo opportunities for the print media. Offer to email press kit information to media who did not attend.
- **Evaluate performance:** Use the sign-in sheet to assess the success of your recruitment efforts and to determine which

media were in attendance. Monitor the media coverage following the conference and take note of any errors. Evaluate spokesperson performance and incorporate feedback into future events.

Preparing for Interviews

Interviews are critical media appearances for your organization. They require careful preparation to be successful. This list discusses important questions to ask prior to giving an interview as well as dos and don'ts that will enhance your performance.

■ **Important questions to ask:**
- **What is the subject or topic of the interview?** You have the right to ask this and to receive a reasonable response. Finding out the topic allows you to figure out what the reporter wants, who the appropriate person is to meet their needs (if not you), and allows you to begin putting together key messages.[9]
- **What is the reporter's deadline?** You want to determine this (and if there is any flexibility) so that you can respond in time.
- **Who will be conducting the interview?** If you take the time to do a little research, knowing whom you are dealing with will give you valuable insights into the reporter's perspective. For example, does this reporter only do watchdog stories? Does he or she specialize in health or cover another beat?
- **What is the interview format?** Will the interview be used for print, radio, or television? Will it be live or taped? These important considerations affect how your messages are prepared.

■ **Do:**
- **Practice:** Successful interviews do not happen by accident, they are the result of practice. Enlist the help of colleagues to practice your interviewing skills and obtain feedback on your performance. Practice based on the interview format. For instance, if it is a TV interview, try taping your performance. Anticipate likely questions based on the interview topic and the reporter's past stories and practice answering these using key messages. Be sure to prepare for the hard questions too, because these are bound to come up.
- **Express empathy:** During emergencies and controversies, an expression of empathy within the first 30 seconds engenders public trust.[9]

- **Use bridging statements:** Bridging statements are a communication technique that can help you ensure the interview stays focused on what is relevant and important. Bridging can help you redirect the interview toward your key messages when a reporter asks a question that is inappropriate or off-topic; for example, if it is one you have already answered satisfactorily that asks you to speculate. Examples: "And what's most important to know is . . ." "If we look at the big picture . . ." "What I would like to convey to your viewers is . . ."
- **Admit when you do not know the answer:** A reporter will not fault you for not knowing an answer. Where you will lose credibility is if you try to bluff knowledge that you do not have. If you do not know the answer to a question, say so. If your organization is engaged in a process to obtain an answer, express confidence in the process and give the reporter a timeframe for getting back to him or her with a response.
- **Remember body language:** For an on-camera interview, ask where to look. Also keep in mind that certain postures convey meaning. (Crossing your arms over your body looks hostile. Fidgeting with your hands or wiping your brow appears nervous.) Aim to keep neutral body language by leaning slightly forward and keeping hands and body quiet.[44] Be mindful that you may still be on-camera while someone else is speaking. Do not yawn, roll your eyes, or do anything else that might be interpreted as disrespectful while someone else is speaking.

■ **Don't:**

- **Be put on the spot:** Just because a reporter is calling does not mean you have to give an interview right away. Take the time (even if it is just minutes) to compose yourself and prepare your key messages. If a reporter shows up unannounced at your office or while you are on the way to your car, employ the same tactic. While you prepare briefly in your office, invite the reporter to wait elsewhere (preferably while supervised by another staff member). Always aim to conduct the interview on your terms.
- **Fill the silences:** A favorite technique of reporters is to use silence to prompt their subjects to say more. If you have delivered your key messages in response to a question, wait for the next question rather than feeling compelled to fill the silence and risk saying something off-message.

- **Go off the record:** There is no such thing. From the time you first greet a reporter until you leave each other's company, anything you say is fair game. What this means is that you should not say anything in a reporter's presence that you would not want broadcast or printed. (Also, be certain not to have private conversations when off-air but still wearing a microphone.)
- **Speculate:** When asked to speculate or answer a hypothetical question, bridge back to a key message instead. Examples: "What I think you're really asking is ..." "While I can't speculate, what I can tell you is ..."
- **Use humor:** In the context of an emergency, humor will be viewed as inappropriate and taken as a sign that you do not care. This will jeopardize the public's trust for your organization and thwart further communication efforts.
- **Forget about appearance:** For on-camera interviews, your appearance counts. Wear bright solid colors and avoid busy prints, white, and cream. Men should be sure to shave, wear dark suits and colored ties. Women should wear everyday makeup and avoid heavy jewelry. (It is distracting, and if it catches your eye in the mirror, it will catch the viewers' eyes and may create glare, so take it off.)[44]

MATERIALS DEVELOPMENT

As part of your greater communications strategy, in addition to communicating through broadcast media and newspapers, your organization may want to develop other materials to communicate with the public or your employees. Examples of materials to consider include: fact sheets, posters, newsletters, mailings, training videos, and Web sites.[9] Table 12-2 and the following sections discuss some principles for designing print and Web materials are discussed.

Print Materials
A variety of printed materials may be developed to increase emergency preparedness and to aid in response and recovery. Fact sheets are a particularly versatile tool for communicating with the public, employees, and the media. The types of facts sheets your organization may want to develop may include:[9]

- topical fact sheets (for example: pandemic flu, social distancing measures, treatment, etc.) with resources on where to find additional information;
- organization fact sheets that outline roles, responsibilities, and resources (these are useful for press kits);

Table 12-2

Media Channels: Pros and Cons[33,45]

Medium	Means[33]	Pros	Cons
Television	▪ News broadcasts and programs ▪ Health programs ▪ Talk shows ▪ Editorials ▪ Dramatic programming (edutainment) ▪ Advertising (paid or public service)	▪ Reaches the widest and most diverse audience quickly ▪ Not dependent on audience's ability to read	▪ TV broadcasts are short; therefore, cannot cover complex health issues in depths as easily as print ▪ Reliant on visuals; therefore, may not cover stories that don't have "good visuals"
Radio	▪ News broadcasts and programs ▪ Health programs ▪ Public affairs/talk shows ▪ Dramatic programming (edutainment) ▪ Advertising (paid or public service)	▪ Can reach a wide audience quickly ▪ Paid radio ads are relatively inexpensive ▪ Not dependent on audience's ability to read ▪ Reaches many minority audiences	▪ Reaches smaller audiences than TV ▪ Radio broadcasts are short; therefore, cannot cover complex health issues in depth as easily as print ▪ Public service ads may be broadcast at times that reach few members of your target audience
Newspaper	▪ News ▪ Feature stories ▪ Op-ed pieces ▪ Letters to the editor ▪ Advertising	▪ Can reach a wide audience quickly ▪ Better able to thoroughly convey health messages than television or radio	▪ Coverage depends on newsworthiness of your story ▪ Large circulation papers may only take paid ads ▪ Reliance on audience's ability to read ▪ Less popular among younger readers
Magazines	▪ Feature stories (cover story) ▪ Health or lifestyle stories ▪ Editorials ▪ Letters to the editor ▪ Advertising	▪ Extremely targeted to audience's interests ▪ Provides greater depth of coverage than TV or radio	▪ Reliant on audience's ability to read ▪ Paid advertising is expensive ▪ Reaches a narrower audience than other media ▪ For breaking information, develops slower than newspapers

Internet/electronic	▪ News Web sites:
	  ● Feature stories
	  ● Health or lifestyle stories
	  ● Editorials
	  ● Letters to the editor
	  ● Advertising
	▪ Own Web site:
	  ● Fact sheets, FAQs, etc.
	  ● Email alert sign-up
	  ● Chat rooms
	▪ Text messaging
	▪ Video Web sites (e.g., YouTube)
		▪ Can inform many people quickly
		▪ Can be updated instantaneously
		▪ Can be tailored for multiple audiences
		▪ Makes use of multiple media formats (audio visual interest of radio or TV with self-pacing of print[45])
		▪ Can serve as a portal for more detailed information as part of your broader communication strategy.
			▪ Reliant on audience's ability to read
			▪ Reliant on users' access to technology
			▪ May not reach elderly audiences as readily
			▪ For internal Web sites, your organization must maintain and update them
			▪ Reliant on audience to be proactive and search for information

▪ lists of frequently asked questions (FAQs) for various emergency scenarios (these can be used to help prepare hotline operators to answer questions from the public);
▪ fact sheets offering advice to employees and other relevant groups on handling post-traumatic stress and media enquiries; and
▪ holding statements (messages prepared in advance) for various emergency scenarios.

Keep organization key messages in mind as well as the principles of plain language when you develop print materials. If time and resources allow, test your materials to be sure they are clear and resonate with your target audience before disseminating them.

Web Materials

What so often happens with Web sites is that organizations take what works in a print publication and simply post this directly onto a Web page. However, this is problematic for two reasons. First, it does not take advantage of the interactivity of the Web format. Secondly, it does not work. People view information on the Web differently than printed text; therefore, what works as a printed fact sheet in a hospital waiting area probably will not translate well when posted on a hospital's Web site. When viewing materials on the Web, people tend to skim rather than thoroughly read text,[33] so Web materials need to be presented in a format that can be scanned. The following list presents some tips on presenting materials on the Web.

▪ Use the Web's interactivity to your advantage. If you envision multiple audiences, tailor your home page to meet their needs, for instance, design pages for patients, health professionals, and the media.
▪ Put the vital information at the top, where it is immediately visible without having to scroll down. Put the "nice to know" information (that which is beyond what the typical user would require) on secondary pages.
▪ Present information using the inverted pyramid (putting the most important information first).[33]
▪ Use the principles of plain language.
▪ Use half as much text as you would for print material[33] and make liberal use of headers and bullets to make materials easy to skim.
▪ Create a glossary with hyperlinks to unfamiliar terms used throughout the site that allows users to learn while they surf.
▪ Follow the principles of good Web design: have a consistent look for pages, text, headers and footers; employ uniform navigation; identify your organization on each page; and clearly label links.

Part 3: Phases of a Public Health Emergency[9,15]

A public health emergency can be divided into four distinct phases:[15] pre-crisis, initial, crisis maintenance, and recovery. The phases of a crisis necessitate different communication responses. This section discusses the phases of a crisis, the likely media response, and the activities that organizations need to undertake during each phase.

PHASE 1: PRE-CRISIS PHASE

During the pre-crisis phase, lay the groundwork for a successful communication response to disasters that are likely to affect your area. This phase is where most of the work should happen. The last thing an organization needs in a crisis is to be scrambling to figure out how to clear information before it can be released to the media, or realize that is does not actually have the capacity to staff a hotline. These and other considerations are the things to address now, during times of relative calm.

Create Partnerships

In the pre-crisis phase, it is vital to develop partnership with organizations that are involved in disaster response. As mentioned in the media relations section, this is also the time to foster relationship with the media so that you understand each other's needs when disaster does strike. Also, open a dialogue with the public because this fosters trust and helps to engage them in preparedness efforts.

Develop a Communication Plan

The preceding section presented the tools needed for a successful communication strategy. Now your organization needs to develop a plan to implement the tools—both in its day-to-day activities (for instance, while engaging in precaution advocacy) and during a crisis. Use the following outlined functions to assess your organization's existing capacities and to identify gaps. The functions that need to be carried out by your organization will vary based on its size and mission. A basic plan should address the following domains:[9]

- **Likely scenarios:** The plan should outline well thought out contingencies for various scenarios.
- **Leadership endorsement:** The plan should be endorsed (and signed) by the organization's director.
- **Assigning responsibility:** The plan should: (1) describe staff roles and designate responsibility (by name) for different emergency scenarios; (2) break down emergency communication activities into the tasks for the first 2, 4, 8, 12, 16, 24, and 48 hours in the form of a checklist; and (3) designate

- who will lead the communication response;
- the lead spokesperson and whether this changes for different scenarios;
- the public information officer (PIO);
- who needs to be consulted during the each phase of the communication process;
- who needs to be kept informed; and
- who is responsible for implementing various actions described in the plan.

■ **Organizational clearance:** The plan should include (1) procedures for information verification, clearance, and approval; (2) agreements on releasing information and on who release what, when, and how; and (3) policies and procedures regarding employee contacts from the media (train employees regarding these).

■ **Logistics:** The plan should include procedures to obtain the necessary human, financial, logistic and physical support, and resources (such as staff, space, equipment, and food) for communication operations during a short, medium, and prolonged emergency event (24 hours a day 7 days a week if needed).

■ **Coordination with partners:** The plan should: (1) include procedures for coordinating with important stakeholders and partners (for example, with other health agencies, law enforcement, and elected officials); (2) include day and night contact lists for partners (check these regularly and update them); (3) include day and night contact lists for media (check these regularly and update them); and (4) identify subject-matter experts (e.g., university professors, state epidemiologist) willing to collaborate during an emergency, and determine their perspectives in advance (you do not want any on-air surprises).

■ **Communications audiences, channels, materials, and protocols:** The plan should: (1) identify target audiences; (2) identify how media requests will be tracked (and include a tracking sheet if using); (3) identify preferred communication channels (for example, telephone hotlines, radio announcements, news conferences, Web site updates, and faxes) to communicate with the public, key stakeholders, and partners; (4) identify the standard components for your organization's press kit; (5) contain holding statements (messages prepared in advance) and key messages; (6) contain fact sheets, FAQs, talking points, and other materials for potential scenarios; and (7) contain procedures for posting and updating Web site information.

■ **Exercise and evaluation strategy:** The plan should: (1) include a schedule for testing the plan (both alone and as part of larger preparedness planning activities); (2) discuss employee training needs; and (3) contain an evaluation strategy and measurable, actionable procedures for evaluating, revising and updating the media communication plan on a regular basis.

PHASE 2: INITIAL PHASE

Ideally, if a crisis occurs and your organization is involved, you should break the story before someone else does. This gives you the opportunity to shape the news coverage rather than playing catch up and trying to correct misinformation later. When a crisis occurs, many organizations are hesitant to say something until all the facts are in, but the public responds best when organizations are quick to announce a problem.[46] Any information released can include the caveat that it may change as more facts come in.[9] However, waiting until all the facts are in will result in a missed opportunity to shape the news coverage, and may make your organization seem slow to respond, which could undermine the public's trust.

During the initial phase of a crisis, the media will first try to determine if something newsworthy has happened. Secondly, the media will try to gauge how big the story is.[17] If, for example, there are unusual cases of illness, are they innocent or were they caused by sinister agents? Are they isolated incidents, or do they portend something bigger, like an epidemic? When a crisis occurs, the media will try to learn the facts of the situation—the who, what, where, when, why, and how. With a camera phone seemingly in every pocket in America, large, public incidents (explosions, mass casualties, etc.) will most certainly appear on the Internet as they happen. With this in mind, the media will not have long to break a story, so while gathering facts and solid leads, they will also act quickly so that their competitors do not break the story first.[17] This is the phase where your organization will begin to field media calls and you will have to act quickly to provide them with the information you are able to release. You want to avoid answering with "no comment," because this will give the impression that you are hiding something and that your organization is unwilling to meet the media's needs. Implement a system for tracking calls, be it paper-based or electronic, and assign responsibility for following up.

If your organization plans to operate a public hotline, now is the time to call up and staff the hotline and publicize the phone number.[47] If you have completed template news releases, fact sheets, and FAQs, now is the time to fill in the final details and disseminate them.

Review your organization's key messages and be sure that spokespeople are familiar with them. Prior to granting interviews or holding press conferences, be sure that spokespeople are familiar with the following guidelines:[9]

1. **Convey empathy:** Express empathy within the first 30 seconds of an on-air message.

2. **State key messages:** Convey key messages in the 27/9/3 format using positive language.

4. **State supporting facts:** Use three facts to support each key message.

3. **Repeat key message:** Reemphasize your key message (remember primacy/recency).

5. **State next steps:** List the next steps and sources for further information.

During the beginning of a crisis, your organization's caring, commitment, competence, and openness[14] will determine your trustworthiness, and this will determine your ability to communicate with the public to effectively protect their health.

PHASE 3: CRISIS MAINTENANCE PHASE

The media will want updates on the situation. If the crisis at hand is an epidemic, media may experience casualties and be short–staffed.[17] Keep in mind that a report of no change (for instance, of no new cases of illness) is still worth sharing with the media. If the crisis is lengthy, consider scheduling daily briefings to keep the media apprised of any new developments.[43] Continue updating your organization's Web site, hotline scripts, and FAQs with information as it is available.

PHASE 4: RECOVERY PHASE

As the crisis winds down and the obvious stories diminish,[17] the media and public will begin to examine who is to blame and how effective the crisis response was. In addition to communicating recommendations to the public during recovery (for instance, concerning safety when reentering homes following flooding), communication may also need to focus on addressing the media's analysis of your organization's response. This is the point at which your organization should begin assessing which aspects of your communication strategy worked and which could be improved. Your communication plan should be updated with the findings in mind.

Conclusion

Communicating with the public via the media is a critical component of disaster preparedness, response, and recovery. The purpose of this chapter was to highlight important theories underlying effective risk communication, provide guidance on incorporating these theories when developing materials and interacting with the media, and, finally, to explore the ways in which these approaches can be implemented throughout the lifespan of a public health emergency. Successful risk communication through the media can mitigate what would otherwise become a public health disaster, and we hope we provided some essential tools to help with this goal.

Suggested Readings and Resources

1. Hyer RN, Covello VT. *Effective Media Communication During Public Health Emergencies.* Geneva: World Health Organization; 2005.
2. Nelson DE, Brownson RC, Remington PL, Parvanta C, eds. *Communicating Public Health Information Effectively: A Guide for Practitioners.* Washington, DC: American Public Health Association; 2002.
3. Wallack L, Woodruff K, Dorfman L, Diaz I. *News for a Change: An Advocate's Guide to Working with the Media.* Thousand Oaks, CA: Sage Publications, Inc.; 1999.

References

1. Pollard WE. Public perceptions of information sources concerning bioterrorism before and after anthrax attacks: an analysis of national survey data. *J Health Commun.* 2003;8(3):93–103.
2. Select Bipartisan Committee to Investigate the Preparedness for and Response to Katrina. *A Failure of Initiative—Final Report of the Select Bipartisan Committee to Investigate the Preparedness for and Response to Katrina,* Washington, DC: U.S. Government Printing Office; 2006. Report 109–377.
3. Brodie M, Weltzien E, Altman D, Blendon R, Benson JM. Experience of Hurricane Katrina evacuees in Houston shelters: implications for future planning. *Am J Public Health.* 2006;96:1402–1408.
4. Eisenman DP, Cordasco KM, Asch S, Golden JF, Glik D. Disaster planning and risk communication with vulnerable communities: lessons from Hurricane Katrina. *Am J Public Health.* 2007;97(suppl 1):S109–115.
5. Sandman PM. Crisis communication best practices: some quibbles and additions. *J Appl Commun Res.* 2006;34(3):257–262.
6. Glik DC. Risk communication for public health emergencies. *Annu Rev Public Health.* 2007;28(1):33–54.
7. Reynolds B, Seeger M. Crisis and emergency risk communication: an integrative approach. *J. Health Commun.* 2005;10:38.
8. Fischhoff B. Risk perception and communication unplugged: twenty years of progress. *Risk Analysis.* 1995;15:137–Z142.
9. Hyer RN, Covello VT. *Effective Media Communication During Public Health Emergencies.* Geneva: World Health Organization; 2005.

10. Glass TA, Schoch-Spana M. Bioterrorism and the people: how to vaccinate a city against panic. *Clin Infect Dis.* 2002;34(2):217–223.

11. Covello VT, Peters RG, Wojtecki JG, Hyde RC. Risk communication, the West Nile Virus epidemic: responding to the communication challenges posed by the intentional and unintentional release of a pathogen in an urban setting. *J. Urban Health: Bull. N.Y. Acad. Med.* 2001;78:382–391.

12. Bennett P, Calman K, eds. *Risk Communication and Public Health.* New York: Oxford University Press; 2001.

13. Covello V, Minamyer S, Clayton K. *Effective Risk and Crisis Communication during Water Security Emergencies.* Washington, DC: U. S. Environmental Protection Agency; 2007. Publication EPA/600/R-07/027.

14. Peters RG, Covello VT, McCallum DB. The determinants of trust and credibility in environmental risk communication: an empirical study. *Risk Analysis.* 1997; 17(1):43–54.

15. Reynolds B, Galdo JH, Sokler L. Crisis and emergency risk communication. October 21, 2008. http://www.bt.cdc.gov/cerc/. Accessed October 22, 2008.

16. Beaton R, Stergachis A, Oberle M, Bridges E, Nemuth M, Thomas T. The sarin gas attacks on the Tokyo subway—10 years later/lessons learned. *Traumatology.* 2005;11(2):103–119.

17. Masci JR, Bass E. *Bioterrorism: A Guide for Hospital Preparedness.* New York, NY: CRC Press; 2005.

18. Gigerenzer G, Gaissmaier W, Kurz-Milcke E, Schwartz LM, Woloshin S. Helping doctors and patients make sense of health statistics. *Psychological Sci Public Interest.* 2007;8(2):53–96.

19. Fischhoff B. Risk: a guide to controversy. In: National Research Council, ed. *Improving Risk Communication.* Washington, DC: National Academy Press; 1989:211–319.

20. Terry WS. Serial position effects in recall of television commercials. *J Gen Psychol.* 2005;132(2):151–163.

21. Glik DC, Drury A, Cavanaugh C, Shoaf K. What not to say: risk communication for botulism. *Biosecur Bioterror.* 2008;6(1):93–107.

22. Aldoory L, Van Dyke MA. The roles of perceived 'shared' involvement and information overload in understanding how audiences make meaning of news about bioterrorism. *Journalism Mass Commun Q.* 2006;83(2):346–361.

23. Rudd RE, Comings JP, Hyde JN. Leave no one behind: improving health and risk communication through attention to literacy. *J Health Commun.* 2003;8(suppl 1): 104–115.

24. Kutner M, Greenberg E, Jin Y, Paulsen C. *The Health Literacy of America's Adults Results From the 2003 National Assessment of Adult Literacy.* Washington, DC National Center for Education Statistics; 2006. Publication NCES 2006483.

25. Zarcadoolas C, Pleasant A, Greer DS. Understanding health literacy: an expanded model. *Health Promot Int.* 2005;20(2):195–203.

26. Zarcadoolas C, Pleasant A, Greer DS. Elaborating a definition of health literacy: a commentary. *J Health Commun.* 2003;8(suppl 1):119–120.

27. Rudd RE. Clear and to the point: guidelines for using plain language at NIH. Harvard School of Public Health: Health Literacy Studies Web site. http://www.hsph.harvard.edu/healthliteracy/how_to/clear.html. Accessed October 12, 2008.

28. McLaughlin GH. SMOG grading: a new readability formula. *J Reading.* 1969;12 (8):639-646.

29.   How to write in plain English. Plain English Campaign Web site. http://
       www.plainenglish.co.uk/files/howto.pdf. Accessed September 22, 2008.

30.   Wray R, Rivers J, Whitworth A, Jupka K, Clements B. Public perceptions about
       trust in emergency risk communication: qualitative research findings. *Int J Mass
       Emergencies Disasters.* 2006;24(1):45-75.

31.   Checklist for Developing Culturally Competent Health Communication
       Programs. Centers for Disease Control and Prevention Web site. CDCynergy
       Heart Disease and Stroke Prevention Edition version 2.1. http://www.cdc.gov/
       DHDSP/CDCynergy_training/Content/activeinformation/resources/CV-
       cross.cult.tool2.pdf. Accessed November 20, 2008.

32.   Wallack L, Woodruff K, Dorfman L, Diaz I. *News for a Change: An Advocate's Guide to
       Working with the Media.* Thousand Oaks, CA: Sage Publications, Inc.; 1999.

33.   Nelson DE, Brownson RC, Remington PL, Parvanta C, eds. *Communicating Public
       Health Information Effectively: A Guide for Practitioners.* Washington, DC: American Public
       Health Association; 2002.

34.   Garrett L. Understanding media's response to epidemics. *Public Health Rep.*
       2001;116:87-91.

35.   New York Times to cut size 5 percent; Keller says paper better off smaller. *The
       New York Observer.* July 17, 2006.

36.   Lacy S, Blanchard A. The impact of public ownership, profits, and competition
       on number of newsroom employees and starting salaries at mid-sized daily
       newspapers. *Journalism Mass Commun Q.* 2003;80(4):949-968.

37.   Singer JB. Partnerships and public service: normative issues for journalists in
       converged newsrooms. *J Mass Media Ethics.* 2006;21(1):30-53.

38.   Sandman PM. Telling reporters about risk. *Civil Eng.* 1988;58(8):36-38.

39.   Oak Ridge Institute for Science and Education Emergency Management
       Laboratory. *Emergency Public Information Pocket Guide.* Oak Ridge, TN: Oak Ridge
       Institute for Science and Education; 2006. http://orise.orau.gov/emi/epi/files/
       epi-booklet.pdf. Accessed January 21, 2010.

40.   Sandman PM. *Simplification Made Simple.* The Peter Sandman Risk Communication
       Web site. http://www.psandman.com/col/simplify.htm. Accessed Novem-
       ber 1, 2008.

41.   Blake K. Media writing tips. http://mtsu32.mtsu.edu:11178/171/tips.htm.
       Accessed October 5, 2008.

42.   Blake K. Six rules for writing straight news leads. http://mtsu32.mtsu
       .edu:11178/171/leads.htm. Accessed October 5, 2008.

43.   Robinson SJ, Newstetter WC. Uncertain science and certain deadlines: CDC re-
       sponses to the media during the anthrax attacks of 2001. *J Health Commun.*
       2003;8(suppl 1):17-34.

44.   American Public Health Association. *Climate Change: Our Health in the Balance—
       NPHW 2008 Partner Toolkit.* National Public Health Week Web site. http://www
       .nphw.org/nphw08/NPHW%20toolkit%202008.pdf Accessed April 5, 2008.

45.   National Cancer Institute. *Making health communications programs work.* Washington,
       DC: U.S. Department of Health and Human Services; 2002.

46.   Covello VT. Best practices in public health risk and crisis communication. *J
       Health Commun.* 2003;8(suppl 1):5-8.

47.   APC. "Hello, how may I help you?"—creating and operating a Public Information
       Call Center. https://migrate.kingcounty.gov/App_Media/health/publichealth/
       documents/apc/hello_001.doc. Accessed September 2, 2008.

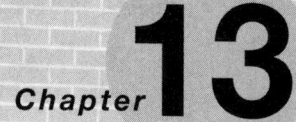

Chapter 13

Security and Physical Infrastructure Protections

Robert Michael Schuler, BGS, NREMT-P and

Veronica Senchak Snyder, MHS, MBA

Photo by Mark Wolfe/FEMA Photo

Learning Objectives

- Describe the protection of the healthcare delivery infrastructure to allow the system to continue operation and provide healthcare services under austere conditions.
- Implement the principles and practices of emergency management specific for security and physical infrastructure protection within your own hospital, healthcare system, facility, agency, and community.
- Discuss the barriers to healthcare facility security and potential solutions to the protection of patients, staff, and visitors as well as critical healthcare infrastructure.

Introduction

Healthcare delivery in the 21st century presents with significant and nontraditional security challenges. Traditionally, hospitals and medical clinics were generally perceived as safe havens; crimes were usually perceived as nominal and less harmful, limited to petty thefts. The catastrophic incidents that have occurred, from the terrorist attacks in the fall of 2001 to the earthquake in Haiti in early 2010, are indicative of a new paradigm: hospitals can be overwhelmed with mass casualties and fatalities; hospitals can become victims; hospitals can exhaust their resources and be rendered unable to provide care. Hurricane Katrina revealed startling realities that previously were never imagined. For example, sniper fire delayed the evacuation of Charity Hospital for almost a full day.

Security and physical infrastructure protection is a complex topic that includes and involves not only the daily operational security issues facing a fixed healthcare facility, but also includes protecting the physical infrastructure as well as the tangible and intangible resources and assets that allow it to continue operating and providing patient care during adverse incidents and under austere conditions. Any type of disaster, whether natural, man-made, or technological, could compromise the delivery of healthcare if comprehensive, integrated plans are not developed beforehand using a system-wide, all-hazards approach. It must also be considered that healthcare delivery can fail. This reality presents its own challenges that must be considered.

Definitions are provided to clarify key terms used in emergency management and Incident Command Systems. We offer a clear definition of the healthcare delivery system. We will then focus on the prehospital component of protection and how emergency medical services—such as first responders—public health, and primary care physicians play a role in the overall protection of a fixed healthcare facility. This shall be accomplished by addressing such areas as hazard vulnerability analysis and threat/risk assessments, the creation and integration of plans within the fixed healthcare facility, the use of triage, altered standards of care, and surveillance in the protection of receiving hospitals. The hospital/acute care component will focus on the physical security and emergency management issues facing hospitals today resulting from disasters. Specific security practices and procedures are included. An assessment and analysis of the legal issues and the lack of much-needed public policy to provide guidance to planners before, during, and after an incident or event are addressed. Both prehospital and hospital components will address these issues from an all-hazards standpoint while emphasizing the emergency management components of mitigation, preparedness, response, and recovery. The special circumstances of pandemic influenza and total hospital and complete campus evacuation are discussed separately. Finally, a case study is offered to apply and analyze the principles and practices in an effort to illuminate and assist the reader in understanding the multifaceted dynamics involved in emergency response.

The protection of the security and physical infrastructure of the healthcare delivery system is a laudable, desirable, and important effort. Homeland Security Presidential Directives 7 and 21 state provisions for the protection of the infrastructure and public health and medical preparedness.[1,2] While the government acknowledges the importance of protecting the nation's infrastructure, it is noted that generally accepted statistics indicate that between 85% and 90% of said infrastructures are privately owned. Perhaps the most significant challenges are financial resources and funding. Hospitals across the nation have been facing crises for years that are not just financial. Hospital emergency departments have been closing down, staff shortages lead to overworked personnel, and the lack of resources disallows the provision of services. Many hospitals cannot manage their day-to-day operating costs, let alone locate and secure the financial resources necessary to invest in costly security acquisitions and upgrades. Notwithstanding, there are two other crises that threaten the healthcare system: a seemingly imminent pandemic situation and terrorism. Hospitals are little prepared or outright unprepared for either crisis. This chapter offers strategies and solutions across the cost and feasibility spectrums that hospitals, health care, and emergency management responders may consider as viable tools for their security management and protection plans and implementations.

Definitions

Emergency management, the National Incident Management System (NIMS), and the Hospital Incident Command System (HICS) use clear and standardized language. It is important to understand the meanings of, and to differentiate between, the terms used to describe situations. For these purposes then, the following definitions apply.

An **event** is "a planned, nonemergency activity, such as a mass gathering or a national special security event." [3,4]

An **incident** is "an occurrence or event, natural or human-caused, which requires an emergency response to protect life or property. Incidents can, for example, include major disasters, emergencies, terrorist attacks, terrorist threats, wildland and urban fires, floods, hazardous material spills, nuclear accidents, aircraft accidents, earthquakes, hurricanes, tornadoes, tropical storms, war-related disasters, public health and medical emergencies, and other occurrences requiring an emergency response." Under the National Incident Management System, an incident is an unplanned occurrence; an event is preplanned. In healthcare, these two terms are often used interchangeably. [3,4]

An **emergency** in health care is "an event that a single hospital and a single prehospital emergency medical system can manage without help from other hospitals and emergency medical systems. Everyday emergencies differ from disasters both in qualitative and quantitative senses. In emergencies, organizations do not need to quickly relate to more and unfamiliar groups, adjust to losing part of their autonomy and freedom of action, apply different performance standards, or operate within closer-than-usual public and private sector interfaces as they do in disasters." [3,4]

A **disaster** in health care is "an event that produces casualties beyond the number and severity for which a single hospital or prehospital emergency medical system can plan. A disaster affects whole communities and regions. By contrast, an emergency is an event that a single hospital and a single pre-hospital emergency medical system can manage without help from other hospitals and emergency medical systems." The World Health Organization (WHO) defines **disaster** as "an occurrence that causes damage, ecological disruption, loss of human life, deterioration of health and health services on a scale sufficient to warrant an extraordinary response from outside the affected community area." Thus, the healthcare delivery infrastructure participates with the community during disasters by serving as a receiving hospital or site of care. It is also possible that the physical infrastructure can become a victim itself, as was tragically realized with Hurricane Katrina in 2005.[3,4]

A **catastrophic incident** is, "any natural, man-made, or complex incident, including terrorism, which results in extraordinary levels of mass casualties, damage, or disruption severely affecting the population, infrastructure, environment, economy, national morale, and/or government functions. A catastrophic event could result in sustained national impacts over a prolonged period of time; almost immediately exceeds resources normally available to state, local, tribal, and private-sector authorities in the impacted area; and significantly interrupts government operations and emergency services to such an extent that national security could be threatened. All catastrophic events are incidents of national significance."[3,4]

HEALTHCARE DELIVERY SYSTEMS

The healthcare delivery system is composed of numerous individual components that provide patient care to the communities they serve. Traditional definitions look at the components of financing, insurance, delivery, and monetary remittance. From a true systems standpoint, we are looking at the continuum of healthcare services that are no longer confined to hospitals or physicians' offices. The healthcare delivery system is composed of those components that provide any form of care to the community both prehospital (emergency medical services, public health, primary care physicians) and hospital (acute care and long term). (See Table 13-1.) The EMS *Agenda for the Future*[5] recognizes EMS as an integral part of the system providing out-of-facility care, thus making it one of the first

Table 13-1	
Components of the Health Care Delivery System	
Types of Health Services	**Delivery Settings**
Preventative	Public health programs, community health
Primary care	Physician office or clinic, alternative medicine
Specialized care	Specialist provider clinic
Long-term care	Long-term care facility, home health
Subacute care	Special subacute units (hospitals), outpatient surgical centers, home health
Acute care	Hospitals
Rehabilitative care	Rehabilitation departments (hospitals), outpatient rehabilitation centers
End-of-life care	Hospice services
Out-of-facility care	Emergency medical services

components of a healthcare delivery system. Acknowledging and accepting this definition, and understanding and affording integration with other components such as hospitals, physician offices, and public health offices, are essential to the systems approach to protecting the infrastructure of the healthcare delivery system.

According to the statistical reference edition of 2008 created by the American Hospital Association (AHA), there were 5,747 hospitals in the United States in 2006 with a bed capacity number of 947,412. Admissions during this same period were 37,188,775. Healthcare entities registered by the AHA are classified according to capacity within eight categories ranging from 6-24 beds to 500 or greater beds.[6] These statistics indicate that a facility's security needs will vary widely. Larger organizations are likely to have a department for security and emergency management services. Generally, hospitals with fewer than than 100 beds do not have a security department. Smaller facilities may have only one staff individual providing security services during the peak first shift of operations. While the range is considerable, the standard principles and best practices should remain the same, allowing scalability according to the hospitals' needs.

Emergency Management

The emergency management cycle consists of four key elements or components: mitigation and prevention, preparedness, response, and recovery. The processes of mitigation, prevention, and preparedness are often interdependent upon one other. After an incident or event occurs, the preparedness phase is over and the response phase is activated. Thus, it is vitally important to prepare and plan before an incident.

The majority of American hospitals already have a type of security plan. If your facility has a security plan, it is recommended that the plan be reviewed, analyzed, revised as appropriate, shared as appropriate, and tested through drills and exercises. The Joint Commission standards for 2009 require an accredited hospital facility to activate its Emergency Operations Plan twice a year, and thus conduct at least two emergency response exercises per year, with at least one exercise including involvement and participation with a communitywide functional to full-scale exercise.[7] In this compliance, the community and the hospital(s) will know and understand how each entity responds to incidents and information, thus allowing the shared knowledge of available resources, assumed leadership roles, and associated responsibilities.

Security Procedures

ASSESSING THREAT, RISK, AND VULNERABILITY

Healthcare delivery systems must assess their own individual vulnerabilities, threats, and risks, and upon identification, apply a remedy as needed. These assessments must also be shared with, and fully integrated into, the overall community healthcare delivery system plan. Healthcare facilities accredited through The Joint Commission are required to conduct a hazard vulnerability assessment following specific accreditation requirements. The hazard vulnerability analysis will identify potential emergencies that could affect the ability to provide services as well as define mitigation activities in order to reduce the risk of, and potential damage from, a disaster.[7]

The categories encompassing hazards are natural disasters, man-made disasters, and technologic disasters. Information technology falls under the technologic disasters category; however, information security is not discussed in this chapter. The hazards that most threaten the healthcare delivery system and hospital physical infrastructure are natural disasters and human disasters. Specific types of situations and scenarios are identified in the following list:

- severe storms and weather
- fire, internal and external
- transportation
  - motor vehicle accidents
  - airplane and helicopter crashes
  - train and transit systems
  - hazardous materials spills and releases

- loss of utilities
  - HVAC
  - water
  - sewer failure
  - generator failure
  - natural gas failure
  - steam and sterilization failure
- terrorism
- bomb threat
- forensic admissions
- civil disturbance

The major vulnerability and threat facing hospitals is the open and easy access to the public. The challenge for security and emergency management planners is to allow a comfortable and welcoming environment while implementing security measures to provide a safe and secure facility.

As part of the overall hazard vulnerability analysis effort, a dedicated security threat and hazard vulnerability analysis as well as a high-risk security survey should be conducted and reviewed annually.

PREPAREDNESS

Hospital and healthcare organizations cannot prepare and plan in a vacuum, nor is it appropriate to render the task to one individual. Therefore, the first step is to assemble a team. Specific to hospitals, the team is usually identified as the Emergency Management Committee. The objectives of the committee are to develop appropriate procedures and ensure that appropriate resources are identified to deal with potential emergency and disaster incidents that may affect the entity. Committee membership should be diverse and include representation from senior leadership, administration, medical staff—including physicians and nursing—and the support services, which generally includes security. Security and emergency management coordinators can provide valuable consultative information and guidance to the committee.

Hospitals have traditionally held a competitive-based perception toward care delivery, viewing neighboring hospitals and clinics as competitors rather than partners. While proprietary information is expected to be respected, there must be allowances and support from senior leadership to encourage collaborative efforts among the communities. Establishing a community committee for regional healthcare delivery is an effective way to establish and develop relationships with others in your community. Membership and participation in regional task forces is also strongly encouraged.

Healthcare Delivery Systems Planning

Healthcare system planning focuses on agency-specific planning and includes incident-specific plans or annexes that address the unique challenges these organizations encounter when managing a terrorist-related incident or natural disaster.

AGENCY-SPECIFIC PLANS

Each organization affected by the comprehensive emergency management plan will have specific responsibilities outlined in said plan. These responsibilities are usually defined by procedures and policies specific to the appropriate agency or group.

INCIDENT-SPECIFIC PLANNING

The comprehensive emergency management plan serves as the organization's blueprint for preparing for, and responding to, emergencies in general. Said plan contains the intentions and concepts for response and provides the cornerstone for more in-depth planning. The second type of planning is the incident-specific planning process, which is activated to organize the response to an actual incident with a measurement of any magnitude. There are several considerations when determining the magnitude of an incident, including the use of the incident complexity analysis. The incident command organization must be able to rapidly recognize the potential for an incident to escalate and become more complex, thus allowing the appropriate adjustment of plans and action. The incident commander or unified command and key staff must quickly gain situation awareness to accurately gauge the complexity of the incident and determine the resources and organization that will be required for successful management.[8]

Five Phases of Incident Planning

The incident planning process usually progresses through five distinct phases and is described in the incident action plan. Planning phases include understanding the situation, establishing objectives and strategy, developing the plan, preparing and disseminating the plan, and executing the plan while assessing progress.

Hospital Planning

As of January 1, 2009, emergency management has been removed from the Environment of Care chapter within The Joint Commission's accreditation manual, and now stands as its own chapter as a result of the Standards Improvement Initiative. In 2008, The Joint Commission set forth guidelines specific to the planning process and identified six critical areas to emergency management: communication, resources and assets, safety and security, staff responsibilities, utilities management, and patient clinical and support activities. The specific requirements have been revised and the standard of disaster volunteers has been added for 2009.[7] These critical areas, while written for healthcare facilities, are also applicable to EMS, public health offices, clinics, and physician offices. Acceptance of these critical areas specific to emergency management allows the creation of comprehensive plans that can be integrated more readily into the hospital and overall healthcare delivery system plans. The authors acknowledge that not all hospitals are accredited; notwithstanding, the following practices can be applied to all organizations in the planning phase. The critical areas are briefly discussed while emphasis has been applied to safety and security. It is noted that the elements of performance go into more depth than presented here because the focus of this chapter is on security and protection. We refer readers to the appropriate chapters within this text for further discussions.

As part of its Emergency Operations Plan, the organization will prepare for managing the following critical areas during emergencies, disasters, and catastrophes:[7]

1. **Communications:** This area defines how the organization will communicate. Upon initiation of emergency response measures, the organization will notify external authorities of the action. During the incident, the means of communicating with external agencies, hospitals, and other healthcare organizations will be maintained. Securely communicating patient and victim information to third parties (such as the state departments of health and law enforcement, including police and the Federal Bureau of Investigation) must also be preplanned.

2. **Resources and assets:** This area defines how the organization will manage resources and assets. Depending on the climate and circumstances of incidents, security may be required to protect resources and assets. Protection may be in the form of physical guard or escort of resources and assets if said resources and assets are required to be transported off-site.

3. **Security and safety:** This area defines how the organization will manage safety and security. The safety and security of personnel, patients, and visitors are prime responsibilities of the healthcare system during an emergency. As emergency situations develop and parameters of operability shift, healthcare organizations must provide a safe and secure environment for their patients and staff.

4. **Staff responsibilities:** This area defines how an organization manages staff. During emergencies and disasters, especially those that are not confined to the organization and involve the community, it is vital to keep critical staff focused on response and

performance. It is natural for staff to be concerned about their families. Staff assured beforehand that their organization has a plan to respond to their family needs are more likely to stay at work, at shift, and beyond shift obligations during an actual emergency.

5. **Utilities management:** An organization is dependent on the uninterrupted function of its utilities during an emergency. The supply of key utilities, such as power, potable water, ventilation, and fuel must not be disrupted or resultant adverse effects may occur. Alternative provisions must be pre-identified for the following: electricity, water, fuel, medical gases, and medical devices. If a facility's lockdown system is reliant on automatic locks powered by electricity and/or computer servers, then a redundant means of operations must be considered in the event of a partial or full loss of power.

6. **Patient clinical and support activities:** The clinical needs of patients during an emergency are of prime importance. The healthcare system must have clear, reasonable plans in place to address the needs of patients during extreme conditions when the system's infrastructure and resources are taxed.

7. **Disaster volunteers:** Specific to accredited hospitals, this area is concerned with granting disaster privileges to practitioners holding licenses to practice. Refer to Chapter 10 on managing volunteers for further information.

Incident Command Systems for Hospitals

Hospitals and healthcare entities must adopt an Incident Command System. The current national trend specific for hospitals is the adoption of the Hospital Incident Command System (HICS IV). The HICS was developed by the state of California Emergency Medical Services Authority and is in alignment with the National Incident Management System.

The security structure of HICS falls under the operations section chief. The security branch director manages and coordinates the activities of the following unit leaders:

- Access Control Unit
- Crowd Control Unit
- Traffic Control Unit
- Search Unit
- Law Enforcement Interface Unit

HICS documents are available from the California Emergency Medical Services Authority, Disaster Medical Services Division's Web site at: http://www.emsa.ca.gov/HICS/default.asp.

ISSUE IDENTITY BADGES

As mentioned in the preceding hazard vulnerability discussion, the openness of hospitals and clinics is likely the most significant threat facilities face. There are several security measures and practices that can mitigate the threat.

Staff and personnel should be easily identified. Decades ago, nurses donned the classic white cap and white uniform. Doctors wore long white lab coats. Housekeeping wore distinguishing uniforms. This dress code practice made personnel more easily distinguishable. Today, anyone dressed in scrubs is assumed to be a part of the healthcare and/or medical staff. Not only does the nursing staff wear colorful scrubs, so too do the environment services staff. Thus, confounding and rendering identification difficult for patients and visitors in regard to the actual identity of the medical staff and the nonmedical staff. Small organizations, such as clinics and hospitals with a census of fewer than 100 beds, are likely to know all of their staff members. The larger hospitals and healthcare systems, however, may find it impossible to know and identify all personnel. This is especially true for entities that experience high employee turnover.

To easily identify staff, it is recommended that an ID badge be issued to every employee, who must wear the badge on a clearly visible area.

ISSUE VISITOR PASSES

Visitors are a constant presence in healthcare. There are many legitimate reasons for visitors to be in facilities: they are visiting admitted patients; they accompany others requiring emergency department services; they escort others to outpatient or clinic appointments.

From a security perspective, it is desirable to have an easy way to identify and differentiate between individuals. It is for the individual hospital to decide its policy in regard to visitor passes. Some facilities have adopted a policy that all persons seeking access to the building are required to register and don a visitor pass; others require passes only for restricted and high-risk areas. Regardless of the daily operations policies, every hospital should have, at a minimum, a plan to issue visitor identification passes during times of heightened threat or alert. Said passes must be absolutely distinguishable from employee and staff identification badges.

ISSUE VENDOR BADGES AND PASSES

Vendors can also be a constant presence in hospitals. Companies and services range from outside maintenance contractors, to floral deliveries, to express package deliveries. Affording identifiable access to legitimate vendors can be accomplished in several ways. Vendors that conduct repetitive and frequent business with the hospital can be issued hospital-created badges. It is important to hold the vendor accountable and liable for the security of the badges. Infrequent vendors should be issued vendor passes. The passes can be as simple as paper tags that change color on a daily basis and provide specific information such as vendor name, destination, and time in. Individuals presenting with deliveries and visits from unknown and unscheduled vendors should be required to sign in and register their presence and the purpose of visit. Upon conclusion of business, badges must be returned to the appropriate issuing office.

Deterrence Practices

Deterrence is a key concept in risk management. According to an Israeli counterterrorism expert, the construction of the West Bank wall that serves as a means of separation between the Israeli and Palestinian terrorists is credited with reducing the number of suicide attacks in Israel. The simple strategy of increasing the time needed to traverse the wall seems to be serving its purpose as a deterrent. Tight controls on entrances, such as embassies and dance clubs, also serve as strategies to increase the time needed from the start of an operation to its execution and is likely to reduce the number of individuals affected. For example, an explosion outside of an emergency department will have fewer injuries and mortalities than one occurring within a crowded waiting room. Obviously, it is neither practical nor desirable to build physical walls around hospitals and their campuses. What these examples do demonstrate, however, is that passive physical and active deterrence measures can be applied to the protection of the healthcare infrastructure. Theoretical walls, however, can be installed. Landscaping and the creation of walkways and pathways is a simple way to control and route foot traffic on campuses.

SURVEILLANCE CAMERAS

Strategically placed surveillance cameras can serve multiple purposes. Cameras mounted clearly and visibly can become deterrents for would-be petty thefts and acting out with undesirable behaviors. The electronically watching eye can also provide evidence in assessing the proof or disproof of claims and disputes.

Covert camera monitoring operations should be reviewed and evaluated for their cost-value in relation to their return on investment. Patients have a right to expect that certain privacy levels are respected and maintained for them. Monitoring cameras can be considered appropriate in restricted and high-risk areas, such as pharmacies, nuclear medicine, access doors to labor and delivery, and nurseries. Other areas to consider are the dock areas, such as receiving and food service.

SECURITY STAFF TRAINING

Healthcare security officers are increasingly facing more dangerous situations. Danger is no longer considered an urban problem. Gang members and drug dealers find the seclusion and perceived safety of the rural areas attractive and have been taking up residence and opening illicit business operations in these areas at an alarming rate. Forensic (prisoner) patient visits are increasing and hospitals are faced with providing care to an ever-increasing violent offender population. Situations can quickly go bad because hospital visits are not only an opportunity to receive care, they are opportunities for escape. For example, on Monday, October 12, 1987, a corrections officer was assigned, along with three other corrections officers, to escort a prisoner patient receiving treatment at a medical center in Pennsylvania. The officers were ambushed by two men attempting to assist in the escape of the inmate. The .44 caliber weapon that was used to open fire upon the officers struck one officer, killing him instantly. Newspaper accounts report that, according to the security manager, no better precautions could have been had, because this was an ambush.[9]

Hospital security staff are generally not armed police forces. The majority of services provided by security personnel are security escorts for employees, pharmaceuticals, forensic/prisoner escorts, simple investigations, and other similar duties. Nonetheless, hospitals should consider identifying and screening appropriate personnel to be trained in elevated defense and deterrent tactics for the safety and security of staff, patients, and visitors. The following list offers some training topic suggestions.

- Act 235: Lethal Weapons Training Act of 1974, P.L. 705, No. 235 (Pennsylvania)
- Taser®
- Oleoresin Capsicum pepper spray Training (OCAT)
- Handcuffing and restraint techniques
- Hazmat technician level
- N95 respirator mask fit testing

GENERAL STAFF TRAINING

The security policies and procedures developed and implemented to protect the healthcare organization must be communicated to staff so they can be aware of the information and respond appropriately to an emergency management or security incident. This can be accomplished through classroom or online training sessions for all current staff and continued during the orientation process for new employees.

Staff who will likely have an active role in emergency response should be identified and trained, at a minimum, in Incident Command IS100, IS200, IS700, and the Hospital Incident Command System. Other key staff who will be participating in both the internal and the external response should also complete IS800. For hospitals, a few individuals may participate at a higher incident area command or unified command level. These key actors should secure IS300 and IS400. It is important to properly identify staff who may serve in these roles because the time commitment is substantial and costs may be borne by the hospital if the community emergency management agency or other public entity does not open enrollment to hospitals and clinics.

FACILITY LOCKDOWN

Certain incidents will cause hospitals to consider locking down the facility and strictly controlling both ingress and egress. A public health emer-

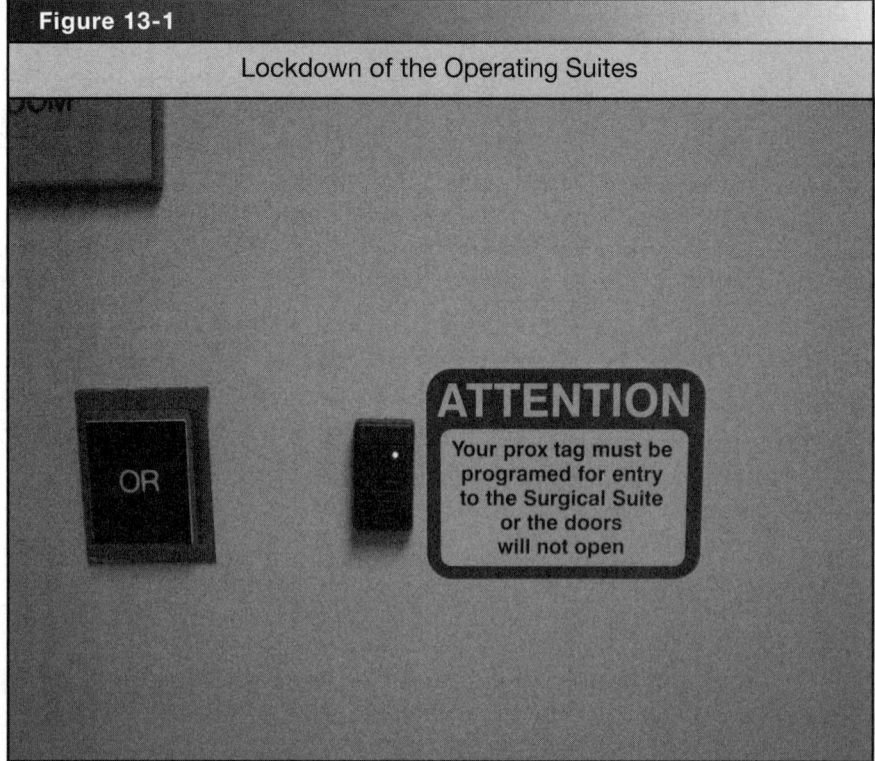

Figure 13-1

Lockdown of the Operating Suites

ATTENTION

Your prox tag must be programed for entry to the Surgical Suite or the doors will not open

Courtesy of Geisinger Health System

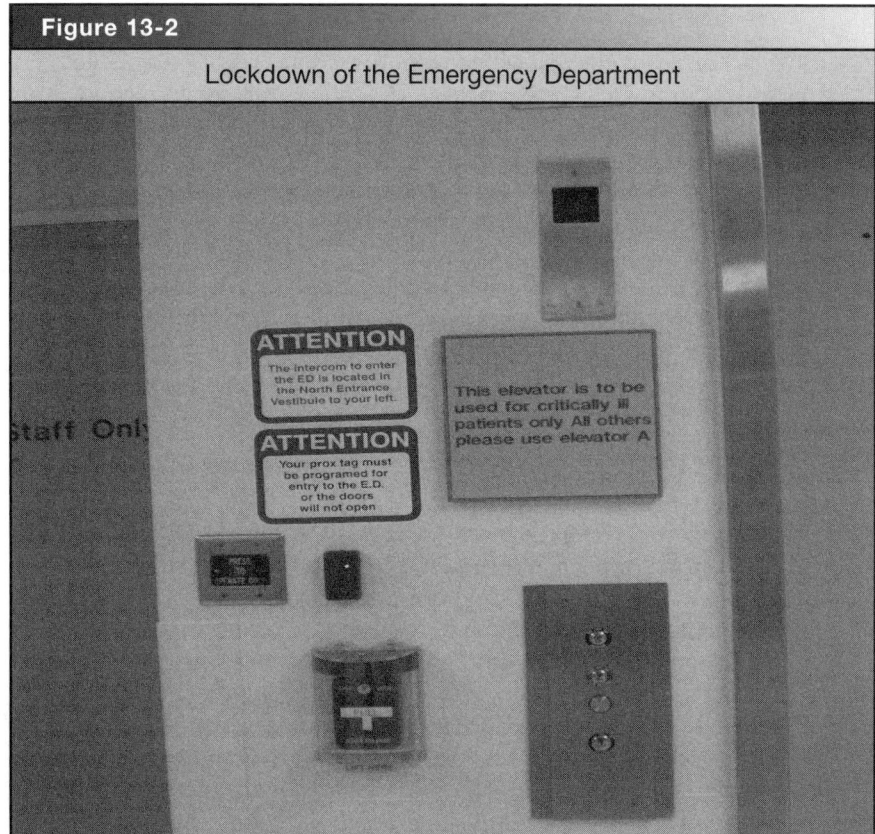

Figure 13-2

Lockdown of the Emergency Department

Courtesy of Geisinger Health System

gency such as a pandemic situation is a good example. Fear and panic among the public will quickly overwhelm the emergency department and become stressors on available medical services and resources. The lockdown of any healthcare facility is a serious decision and should be contemplated and prepared for before any incident. Lockdown can be applied for normal operations as well, thus providing in-place, prearranged mitigation and preparedness efforts. Figures 13-1 and 13-2 represent the lockdown and lockout access of the emergency department and the operating suites currently in service at a rural healthcare system.

It is critical to understand national, state, and commonwealth laws regarding lockdown. While appropriate to control, limit, and restrict the access to a facility under disaster and austere conditions, it is more than inappropriate to lock people in, because this practice may lead to serious regulatory agency and legal violations at best and may jeopardize the safety of all present within the facility and lead to undue injury and/or fatality at worst. The authors highly recommend legal council in the planning process of locking down the facility.

INTERACTION WITH LAW ENFORCEMENT

A hospital's interaction with law enforcement has been redefined in a post 9/11 world. Medical personnel, while familiar with traditional aspects of treating victims and the forensic processing of evidence potentially involved in suspected crimes, may not be aware of what constitutes unexpected and nontraditional identification, preservation, and processing of potentially forensic situations.

The Hospital Incident Command System avails the position of the law enforcement interface leader under the management of the security branch director. The interface position directs responsibility for coordination of the security of a hospital with external law enforcement agencies.

Legal Issues

According to the *Risk Management Handbook for Health Care Organizations*,[10] health care is one of the most regulated of all the sectors of commerce. This is true for normal operations; however, under austere conditions there is a tremendous lack of policies and laws available to guide health care in planning and responding. Currently, no national standards exist, merely guidelines. The authors advise referencing The Health Lawyers' Public Information Series, *Emergency Preparedness, Response & Recovery Checklist: Beyond the Emergency Management Plan*, which can be accessed from http://www.healthlawyers.org/Resources/PI/InfoSeries/Documents/Emergency%20Preparedness%20Checklist.pdf. Additionally, the authors recommend that conversations and consultation occur with in-house or other appropriate external legal council.

The Hospital Incident Command System avails the medical/technical specialist positions within incident command of legal affairs and risk management. These two positions bring risk-management and loss-prevention expertise, as well as active provision of legal counsel and guidance, to the planning committees and incident command and section chiefs. It is also advisable to include the hospital administration specialist as well as the clinic administration specialist.

Shelter and Defend in Place

Shelter in place is "The process of staying put and taking shelter, rather than trying to evacuate in an emergency situation. This action is recommended to protect people by keeping them inside a building with windows and doors closed and external ventilation systems shut off until the hazardous situation has resolved. Because many chemical and radioactive materials may rapidly decay and dissipate, remaining indoors may protect people from exposure."[11] When faced with an emergency or disaster, hospitals will traditionally defend in place. This practice is considerably safer for patients.

Surge Issues

"What you do in advance of a disaster is more important than what you do after."

Michael O. Leavitt, U.S. Secretary of Health and Human Services

RESPONSE

America's healthcare system is ill prepared to manage large numbers of patients that could result from a natural or man-made disaster. The Government Accountability Office has released several reports on the state of the nation's preparedness status. Not since the Spanish Influenza Pandemic of 1917–1919 has this country witnessed such widespread illness and death. The healthcare system, in both urban and rural areas, is at or near capacity with little capability to expand to meet the needs of a large scale incident. Said incidents could potentially result in an overwhelmingly large number of casualties. Additionally, during disasters of great magnitude, many emergency departments activate diversion, disallowing the acceptance of patient/victim arrivals and inpatient admissions. Economics drive the situation because financial budgetary restrictions have resulted in the closure of entire wards.[12] Sudden impact disasters and an influx of the walking "worried well" lead to disruption, injuries, disease, and deterioration of existing medical conditions, placing increased demands on the healthcare delivery infrastructure services.[13] The previously mentioned states are definitive areas that need to be considered prior to an incident in order to effectively lessen deleterious impact. Creation of a comprehensive surge capacity plan demands a focus on staffing, supplies and resources, and structure within the community and regional system.

Prior to addressing surge capacity, hospitals need a clear understanding of the impact and dynamics of what true *surge capacity* actually means. Defined by the Agency for Healthcare Research and Quality (AHRQ), surge capacity is "a health care system's ability to rapidly expand beyond normal services to meet the increased demand for qualified personnel, medical care, and public health in the event of a bioterrorism or other large-scale public health emergencies or disasters [sic]."[14] The Centers for Disease Control and Prevention additionally define surge capacity as "the ability of obtaining additional resources when needed during an emergency."[15] Either definition is acceptable and helps orient hospitals to prepare to meet the increased demand for services.

Triage should be one of the first issues understood and incorporated into a surge capacity plan. The basic concept of triage is to do the greatest good for the greatest number of casualties.[16] While this concept is loosely used prehospital, triage in the hospital setting looks at treating the most critical victims first. Disasters with mass casualties require hospitals to look at the *overall picture*, giving care to as many as possible, rather than focusing on each and every individual. This concept is counterintuitive to the universal physician and medical philosophy of *providing care and treatment to all*. Thus, it is imperative to educate staff members, who will be involved in mass casualty triage, and help them understand the austere dynamics of said counterintuitive treatment of victim patients. Triage should also be looked at as a resource management tool. Triage needs to be viewed as the organized evaluation of all disaster casualties to establish treatment and transport priorities. In addition, it involves the process by which casualties are rationally distributed among the available treatment facilities.[16] Without this firm understanding of what triage encompasses, addressing certain aspects of surge capacity is of little to no value.

The National Preparedness Goal has identified 36 target capabilities that are needed to help mitigate an incident. Under said capabilities, Medical Surge is listed as a priority and has associated critical tasks.[17] These tasks can be placed into three areas: staff, supplies and equipment, and structure. The Health Resources and Services Administration (HRSA) requires all states receiving funds under the Bioterrorism Hospital Preparedness Program to include these areas in their surge plans.[18]

Structure is extremely important in a surge plan. Structure includes facilities that would increase bed capability, decontamination, and isolation practices. According to HRSA, hospitals must have the capacity to expand bed capability to an additional 500 beds per every million of population (1:2000).[18] Meeting this requirement means that communities must assess current bed capacities and then escalate exploration to the identity of other options and contingencies. Said options and contingencies can include reopening shuttered facilities or closed wards, and using community health centers (CHC) or other sites of care. Regionalizing the requirement for additional beds can help lessen the strain placed on a single facility or community through the use of mutual aid agreements. When identifying alternative sites of care, public health officials should select facilities that can accommodate high-volume traffic and have the capacity for decontamination, showers, sewage systems, electricity, and parking.[14] One challenge will be the rate of expedition at which these facilities can be opened. One recommendation is the utilization of said alternative care facilities for use of triage and treatment. Tertiary facilities can consider, if feasible, the transfer of non-life-threatening, less critical medical/surgical patients to outlying facilities. Said facilities, in turn, can also consider, if feasible, the transfer of less critical patients to reopened shuttered facilities or alternative care facilities.[12] This practice may allow a tertiary facility, especially a Level 1 trauma center, to potentially meet the surge of a mass influx of patients/victims. Using *altered standards of care*, such as discharging patients early or cancelling elective surgeries, could also address the immediate need for additional beds. The authors strongly recommend legal consultation in the planning process for licensed hospitals that intend to provide treatment in any alternative site of care. Said sites may not meet the restrictions and limits imposed on the hospital operation's license.

Decontamination structures and increased isolation capability also need to be considered in the surge plan. While The Joint Commission requires those accredited hospitals to have the capability to decontaminate and isolate presenting patients resultant from a weapon of mass destruction incident, many facilities have not yet addressed the surge issue and demand. According to the Target Capabilities List, each participating hospital must have the capacity to isolate one patient in a negative pressure room and each hospital region must be able to accommodate at least 10 patients.[17] This is quite challenging in many areas of the country because it places additional demand on staffing and supplies. A major shortcoming of this requirement is that many rural areas lack a facility capable of self-sufficiency. Communities should consider a regionalized approach to meet the demands for increased capability, including isolation, dispatchment of security considerations, and pre-identification of the individual responsible for said security at the alternative site of care.

After the selection of an appropriate care site is made, the community or region must ensure that there is adequate staffing. Staff includes not only medical personnel, but also ancillary staff, such as coordinators for volunteers, logistics, and administrative staff. The challenge is to immediately be able to deploy direct patient care personnel.[19] Said facilities do have a recall system; however, there are associated drawbacks and downfalls. Such systems do not take into account issues such as natural human behavior. It is expected that some staff will fail to show up for work unless their safety and the safety of their families can be guaranteed. In times of crisis the concept of convergent volunteerism becomes an issue.[15] The propensity inherent in human nature of those trained to respond will compel them to converge on the scene or present at a facility without explicit orders from incident command. Staffing systems must account for the coordination of these volunteers, ensuring efficient utilization of these additional resources. Credentialing becomes an issue with additional staffing resources. The system must be able to confirm the credentials of staff, especially those rendering medical care. Some regions have Medical Reserve Corps, which can be utilized. Regionalizing staff resources would allow the proper placement of specialty providers as well as increasing a staffing pool that would be available during a disaster.

The Hospital Incident Command System activates the position of the support branch director, which manages the following unit leaders: employee health and well-being unit leader, family care unit leader, and labor pool and credentialing unit leader.

The final area for consideration is the availability of resources, such as additional medical supplies, personal protective equipment (PPE), and pharmaceutical cache. Studies have shown that a large number of casualties from sudden impact disasters are ambulatory and that they sustain similar types of injuries. Basic medical supplies, such as suture material, sterile saline for wound irrigation, splinting material, dressings, tetanus immunizations, insulin, beta-blockers, and common antihypertensives are among some of the supplies needed to treat a majority of casualties.[13] Specialized equipment, such as what is needed for treating pediatric patients, should be included in this cache of equipment. Communities must stockpile enough pharmaceuticals and equipment to provide prophylaxis for three days for hospital personnel, first responders, and their families. Agent-specific PPE must also be available to protect current and additional healthcare personnel.[17] Preparing for this, thus, demonstrates the intense challenges placed upon facilities, as said facilities are already suffering under the burden of financial crises. The closure of wards, emergency departments, and entire facilities bespeak the current negative trend. Notwithstanding, security personnel will likely still be demanded to ensure the security of said resources and cache.

Surge capacity is a broad topic where definitive guidance is limited. To lessen the strain and burden on local facilities, surge capacity should be viewed as a regional issue. This is especially critical when defining responsibility for security. For example, will local law enforcement assume responsibility or will hospital security departments dispatch to the scene or site? This concern is of obvious incident and jurisdiction dependency. Plans should be in place where the community or region can sustain itself for 24 hours or longer until additional resources can be made available.[13] By using the principle of triage properly and addressing the outlined areas, communities can create effective and efficient surge plans.

Public Health and Syndromic Surveillance in Protecting Infrastructure

An emerging threat facing our nation is a naturally occurring pandemic or other biologic incident. To better and more rapidly identify a disease outbreak or intentional release of a biologic agent, public health has taken the lead in developing syndromic surveillance systems to monitor these threats. The term syndromic surveillance applies to surveillance using health-related data that precede diagnosis and signal a sufficient probability of a case or an outbreak to warrant further public health response. Though historically syndromic surveillance has been utilized to target investigation of potential cases, its utility for detecting outbreaks associated with bioterrorism is increasingly being explored by public health officials.[20] Its use could help protect physical infrastructure by the early identification of possible surges of ill patients that may present to fixed facilities for treatment. Excessive surges could effectively cause the delivery system to fail as available bed capacity is diminished and the backlog of patients awaiting treatment increases.

Syndromic surveillance can only be successful if data collected is sensitive and timely. The integration of EMS data into the public health surveillance system can increase the ability to detect biologic events early. EMS is a unique component of the healthcare system because it is the interface between primary (prehospital) and hospital care. This component can be a source of epidemiologic and healthcare information that has thus far been historically underutilized in public health monitoring. This, however, appears to be changing. A comprehensive list of indicators can be collected from EMS that can be used to provide information on temporal and geographic distribution of illness. The collection of data from field reports, patient records, and dispatch information can help accomplish this goal.[21]

Clearly, the most compelling evidence into the integration of EMS into the public health syndromic surveillance system is the research conducted in New York City. A study was performed at the peak of influenza season at six New York City emergency departments to compare influenza-like illness (ILI) brought in via ambulance with other emergency department patients. Using a set of four identified EMS call types—sick adult, sick pediatric, difficulty breathing, and respiratory distress—a limited clinical evaluation has shown the effectiveness of such integration. The data collected in this limited clinical evaluation has demonstrated that those brought in by ambulance and placed into one of the four categories were sicker and older than those presenting to the emergency department on their own. Furthermore, the syndromic placement of these patients dictated that procedures such as chest radiography be performed, when this procedure might not have been ordered in those presenting on their own. The sensitivity of the study was found to be 58% with a predictive value positive (PVP) of 22%. The sensitivity of the emergency department visit was found to be 43% for ILI.[22]

Recovery

Recovery efforts are centered on returning the healthcare delivery system back to its pre-incident state. This includes a myriad of activities, such as demobilization with the replenishment and return of borrowed resources, restocking of in-house supplies and equipment, cleaning/sterilizing equipment and replenishing accessories, affording staff time off for recuperation, reopening the facility for repatriation of patients, and a return to pre-incident normal patient load. These tasks can appear enormous if a facility fails to plan for this in advance. Just like the goal of a controlled degradation of services, the goal in recovery is a methodic approach to bringing these considerations back online as patient services slowly return to normal.

Special Circumstances

An all-hazards approach in planning is appropriate for most disaster incidents. However, real-world professional experiences on the part of the authors have demonstrated that certain situations demand purposeful identification of the disaster dynamics. Two special circumstances are pandemic planning and the total hospital and complete campus evacuation. A discussion of pandemic follows. To secure additional information on total hospital and complete campus evacuation, please reference the author's ending note.

PANDEMIC

Of great concern to the United States and public health is the spread of influenza, especially an incident that escalates into pandemic. Historically, pandemics have taxed and deteriorated the healthcare delivery system to the point of failure through resultant staffing shortages, depletion of medical supplies and equipment, and bed space limitations within a facility. According to the U.S. Department of Health and Human Services (HHS), based upon extrapolated data from past pandemics, a pandemic in the United States could realize up to 9,625,000 hospitalizations, 18–42 million outpatient visits, and 20–47 million additional illnesses, dependent upon the attack rate.[23] In reiteration and reemphasis, this means that effective planning, exercising, and flexible and scalable implementation of said plans are all vital in maintaining the healthcare delivery system's ability to provide patient care under austere conditions. While there are numerous considerations that must be accounted for when preparing for a pandemic, there are several encompassing areas that are critical in protecting the healthcare facility as identified by HHS. The encompassing elements are triage, clinical evaluation, and admission procedures, as well as addressing facility access and security.[23] Ingress and egress of vehicular and pedestrian traffic affecting the hospital campus must be strictly controlled.

The Hospital Incident Command System avails the positions under the management of the security branch director. The leaders' positions in the Access Control Unit, Crowd Control Unit, and Traffic Control Unit should all be activated.

Unlike trauma triage, which involves physical injuries caused by disaster, triage during a pandemic is conducted to identify influenza-like illnesses; determine the need for isolation and quarantine; and determine patient hospitalization admission, homecare, and follow-up at a nonurgent facility. Furthermore, patients in a facility presenting with respiratory symptoms may require a separate evaluation area to limit the possibility of spread and to limit the number of hospital contacts.[23] It is likely that the situation shall deteriorate to a level where all patients presenting to a facility must be screened for ILI. The authors recommend an identification system such as badges that contain, at a minimum, the following information: simple color coding to indicate necessitated N95 mask use, destination in hospital, and time in and out. Donning a badge indicates to staff and personnel that ILI screening has been conducted. As mentioned earlier in the text, the badge must be easily distinguishable from staff identification badges.

Security of a facility will be important during a pandemic because a panicked population will likely present to an emergency department demanding treatment, antivirals, and vaccine. It is important to note that said vaccine will realistically be unavailable for many months. Nonetheless, this public reaction will quickly overwhelm the hospital system. Coordination between hospital security staff and local law enforcement will be necessary—although local police presence likely will be unavailable—because standards of care may change and wait times may increase in an effort to keep operations continuing in an orderly fashion.[23] Hospital security staff may need to limit access to the hospital by determining essential staff and those in need of treatment at the facility from nonessential persons. Facilities must develop access control procedures to aid security in this task, in addition to identifying access control points to limit access into the facility.

Case Study

Madrid Train Bombings
Applying the Principles to a Real-World Incident

On the morning of March 11, 2004, a bomb exploded on train 21431 in Atocha station at 7:37 A.M. Two additional bombs exploded at 7:38 A.M. within 4 seconds of each other. On train 17305, just outside the station, four bombs exploded in separate cars at 7:39 A.M. Almost simultaneously and along with these explosions, other trains were being attacked. At 7:38 A.M., at El Pozo del Tío Raimundo station, two more bombs exploded on train 21435, while another train, 21713, experienced a single blast concurrently.[24] These blasts resulted in 177 fatalities at the scenes, along with 2,062 injured victims.[25] The 112 emergency dispatch centers were inundated with telephone calls relaying reports of explosions on multiple trains. Based on this information, the incident was classified as extraordinary and rated a 3 on a scale of 0 to 4.[26] This classification was based on three categories of emergencies defined in the Spanish constitution. This emergency rating set off the activation of four groups:

1. Search and rescue: fire and emergency services

2. Security team: police and special investigators

3. Legal team: includes judges to authorize body [corpse] removal

4. Medical team: paramedics, doctors, and nurses

This constitutes the Spanish Emergency Services Catastrophic Emergency Plan. In all, 5,300 emergency services personnel, 3,500 police, 235 ambulances, 385 other emergency vehicles, 38 hospitals and other medical centers, and 317 psychological support staff were involved in the response. Emergency responders began arriving at the various scenes at 8:00 A.M., and by 8:30 A.M., a field hospital had been set up at a nearby sports facility. Hospitals were immediately notified to expect numerous casualties.[24]

Medical Consequences

Based upon the emergency classification and rating the incidents were given, the medical system in Madrid was activated. Thirty-eight facilities were utilized and a field hospital was set up. By 9:00 P.M., 1,430 casualties had been treated, 966 were taken to 15 public community hospitals. The two largest public hospitals in Madrid received 53% of the casualties.[25] Eighty-two casualties were reported as critical, and of these, 14 died from their injuries, bringing the overall mortality rate to 11%.

The hospital closest to the incidents was Gregorio Maranon University General Hospital (GMUGH). A 1,800-bed teaching facility, GMUGH is located near the Atocha train station. At 7:59 A.M., the first casualty from the explosions walked into the emergency department. Activation plans were initiated at GMUGH, which included cancellation of all non-life-threatening scheduled surgical interventions, the discharge of 161 patients, and the evacuation of 28 ICU patients to intermediate care facilities. The recovery room, with a capacity of 12 beds, was made available for critical patients. One-hundred-twenty-three patients were in the ED prior to the blasts and all but 10 had been discharged or transferred to other facilities by 9:30 A.M. The majority of the casualties were classified as walking wounded with minor to moderate injuries. The most frequent injuries were tympanic membrane perforations, chest injuries, shrapnel wounds, and fractures. A total of 312 patients were treated at GMUGH alone, with 272 treated between 8:00 A.M. and 10:30 A.M. Surgeries were performed on 32 patients and 5 patients expired upon arrival or shortly after arrival at the facility.[25]

Public Health System Analysis

The medical response to the Madrid bombings was extremely effective in field triage and transporting casualties to definitive treatment facilities quickly because of the immediate notification to hospitals. This quick action, however, has revealed certain weaknesses in the emergency health system. The first area that needs to be strengthened is staffing. The attacks happened on a midweek morning when most clinicians were on their way into work and night shifts were still on duty. Scheduled procedures had not yet started and operating rooms were relatively, if not completely, empty. This greatly and positively affected the medical response. Had the attacks happened an hour later, the situation would have been much worse.[25] Thus, hospitals absolutely do need to address *surge capacity*, not only in terms of accommodating large numbers of patients, but also in addressing the additional staffing requirements demanded by large-scale disasters. Another weakness in this particular response was *overtriage*, which is defined as the rate of noncritically injured victims being evacuated or hospitalized. Historically, this has been realized in large-scale disasters. Triage systems must become more efficient in placing the right patients at the right facilities in order to avoid overwhelming the medical facilities with noncritically injured patients. In a survey of members of a surgical association in the United States, it was made known that the level of preparedness among medical personnel and facilities needed to deal with large-scale terrorism incidents has many areas of weakness.[27]

Conclusion

Security is an important, responsible, and necessary aspect of protecting the healthcare delivery infrastructure and the hospital physical infrastructure. It is equally important to recognize and understand that hospitals are not airports, nor are they prisons. A balance must be reached between ensuring the compassionate and professional delivery of patient care while providing for the safety and security of all and the reality that hospitals are not exempt from security risks and threats. Regulatory bodies, such as The Joint Commission, OSHA, and the EPA, require hospitals to have a certain level of security plan already established and implemented. The current action suggested for health care is an assessment of existing plans with a concentration on identifying vulnerabilities and threats and then applying actions to mitigate and remedy said vulnerabilities and threats.

Financial constraints prohibit most hospitals from procuring and putting into operation the many high-tech security devices available on the market. Notwithstanding, there are several low- to no-cost options that can be incorporated into the daily practices of the healthcare delivery infrastructure. Awareness and education of staff in security and emergency management matters is one key component. The development of relationships within the first responder community and the sharing of response plans is also an essential element.

Authors Note: Address correspondence and reprint requests for the non-published document, Evacuating the Campus: A Rural Level One Trauma Center's Total Hospital and Complete Campus Evacuation Preparedness and Planning Experience, to Veronica Senchak Snyder, Emergency Management Coordinator, Emergency Management Services, Geisinger Health System, Geisinger Medical Center, M.C. 01-44, 100 North Academy Avenue, Danville, Pennsylvania 17822 (e.mail: vssnyder@geisinger.edu).

Acknowledgments: The authors wish to express sincere and genuine appreciation to Mr. Christopher E. Snyder and Ms. Laura Elizabeth McAloose, for their understanding patience and intelligent feedback in review of the manuscript. Thank you so very much.

References

1. Bush GW. Homeland Security Presidential Directive 7: Critical Infrastructure Identification, Prioritization, and Protection. Federation of American Scientists Web site. http://www.fas.org/irp/offdocs/nspd/hspd-7.html. Accessed November 3, 2008.

2. Bush GW. Homeland Security Presidential Directive 21: Public Health and Medical Preparedness. Federation of American Scientists Web site. http://www.fas.org/irp/offdocs/nspd/hspd-21.htm. Accessed November 23, 2008.

3. Biby Associates, LLC. Disaster Dictionary Web site. http://www.disasterdictionary.com/. Accessed April 5, 2009.

4. Disasters. World Health Organization Web site. http://www.who.int/topics/disasters/en/. Accessed April 6, 2009.

5. EMS Agenda for the Future. National Highway Traffic Safety Administration Web site. http://www.nhtsa.dot.gov/people/injury/ems/agenda/. Accessed October 20, 2008.

6. Health Care Statistics & Hospital Directory: AHA Data. American Hospital Association Web site. http://www.ahadata.com/ahadata/html/AHAGuide.html. Accessed November 30, 2009.

7. PPV: understand new Joint Commission scoring systems, symbols, and chapters for 2009. HCPro Inc. Web site. http://www.hcpro.com/HIM-226075-859/PPV-Understand-new-Joint-Commission-scoring-systems-symbols-and-chapters-for-2009.html. Accessed January 5, 2009.

8. Texas Engineering Extension Service. Medical preparedness and response to bombing incidents course, 2008. See http://www.teex.org for current courses.

9.   Fallen Officers. Correctional Peace Officers Foundation Web site. http://www
    .cpof.org/fallen_officers/. Accessed April 6, 2009.

10. Carroll R, ed. *Risk Management Handbook for Health Care Organizations.* 5th ed. Hoboken,
    NJ: Wiley Higher Education; 2009.

11. Suburban Emergency Management Project. Disaster Dictionary Web site.
    http://www.semp.us/publications/disaster_dictionary.php. Accessed April 1,
    2009.

12. *Reopening Shuttered Hospitals to Expand Surge Capacity.* Rockville, MD: Agency for
    Healthcare Research and Quality; 2006. AHRQ Publication No. 06-0029.

13. Stratton SJ, Tyler RD. Characteristics of medical surge capacity demand for
    sudden-impact disasters. *Acad Emerg Med.* 2006;13(11):1193–1197.

14. Koh HK, Shei AC, Bataringaya J, et al. Building community-based surge capac-
    ity through a public health and academic collaboration: the role of community
    health centers. *Public Health Rep.* 2006;121(2):211–216.

15. Kaji A, Koenig KL, Bey T. Surge capacity for healthcare systems: a conceptual
    framework. Acad Emerg Med. 2006;13(11):1157–1159.

16. Auf der Heide E. Triage. In: Auf der Heide E. Disaster Response: Principles of
    Preparation and Coordination. St. Louis, MO: Mosby; 1989.

17. U.S. Department of Homeland Security. *Target Capabilities List.* Washington, DC:
    U.S. Department of Homeland Security; 2005.

18. *Optimizing Surge Capacity: Regional Efforts in Bioterrorism Readiness.* Agency for Healthcare
    Research and Quality; 2004. AHRQ Publication No. 04-P009.

19. *Hospital Surge Capacity Performance Standards and Indicators.* Suburban Emergency
    Management Project; 2005. SEMP Biot #172.

20. Syndromic Surveillance: An Applied Approach to Outbreak Detection. Centers
    for Disease Control and Prevention Web site. http://www.cdc.gov/ncphi/
    disss/nndss/syndromic.htm. Updated January 3, 2008.

21. Krafft T, Garcia Castrillo-Riesgo L, Edwards S, et al. European Emergency Data
    Project (EED Project): EMS data-based health surveillance system. *Eur J Public
    Health.* 2003;13(suppl 3):85–90.

22. Greenko J, Mostashari F, Fine A, Layton M. Clinical evaluation of the Emergency
    Medical Services (EMS) ambulance dispatch-based syndromic surveillance sys-
    tem, New York City. *J Urban Health.* 2003;80(2 suppl 1):i50–i56.

23. HHS pandemic influenza plan supplement 3 healthcare planning. U.S.
    Department of Health and Human Services Web site. http://www.hhs.gov/
    pandemicflu/plan/sup3.html. Accessed January 23, 2010.

24. Madrid Train Attacks. BBC News Web site. http://news.bbc.co.uk/2/hi/in_
    depth/europe/2004/madrid_train_attacks/. Last updated February 14, 2007.
    Accessed March 18, 2010.

25. Gutierrez de Ceballos JP, Turegano Fuentes F, Perez Diaz, D, Sanz Sanchez M,
    Martin Llorente C, Guerrero Sanz JE. Casualties treated at the closest hospital
    in the Madrid, March 11, terrorist bombings. *Crit Care Med.* 2005;33(suppl 1):
    S107–S112.

26. Day of horror. DISPATCH Magazine On-line Web site. http://www.911dispatch
    .com/conference/apco2004/thursday.html. Accessed October 10, 2006.

27. Ciraulo DL, Frykberg ER, Feliciano DV, et al. A survey assessment of the level of
    preparedness for domestic terrorism and mass casualty incidents among Eastern
    Association for the Surgery of Trauma members. J Trauma. 2004;56(5):1039–
    1041.

Chapter 14

Hospital Decontamination and Worker Safety

Michael J. Reilly, DrPH, MPH, NREMT-P

Photo by Michael J. Reilly

Learning Objectives

- Identify the elements of a comprehensive hospital decontamination program.
- Discuss the equipment and personnel resources needed to conduct effective hospital decontamination operations.
- Describe the reasons for performing decontamination of contaminated patients at hospitals following a hazardous substance incident.
- List the potential outcomes of a hospital becoming secondarily contaminated by victims of a hazardous substance incident.

Background

For many years, the standard level of preparedness for most hospitals in the case of a patient with a hazardous substance exposure has been the ability to perform a cursory decontamination of the individual in the emergency department. Many hospitals have a dedicated "decon" or "HAZMAT" room, which has a shower and some equipment to perform this function, but it likely serves as an equipment closet or storage area most of the time. Although most hospitals have considered the need to perform emergency decontamination of victims from a hazardous substances incident, many reports have underscored the lack of hospital preparedness for victims from a hazmat-related event.[1-8]

Not including the daily incidence of industrial accidents and traffic accidents resulting in the unintentional exposure of persons to hazardous materials, there have been several man-made or terrorist incidents since the mid 1990s that have emphasized the importance of hospitals not only preparing for the single patient with an accidental chemical exposure, but for the possibility of multiple patients contaminated with a hazardous substance. Some of these events include the 1995 sarin attack in the Tokyo subways, where numerous victims self-referred to the closest hospital following the incident, resulting in 23% of the hospital staff becoming contaminated with nerve agent;[7] the terrorist attacks on the World Trade Center in New York City on September 11, 2001, where victims self-evacuated from lower Manhattan (many via mass transit to Connecticut, New Jersey, and the NYC suburbs) and self-referred to local community hospitals with symptoms resulting from the exposure to and contamination with silica, asbestos, solid and liquid waste, fuel, concrete dust, and multiple other chemicals and unknown substances; and the 2001 anthrax attacks in the United States that resulted in many hospitals throughout the country having to hastily draft procedures on how to handle patients presenting to their hospitals with symptoms resulting from an exposure to a "suspicious white powder."

Exposure and Hazardous Substances

A hazardous substance can be defined as any substance that is capable of causing harm to life, health, or property. Examples of hazardous substances include toxic industrial chemicals, such as chlorine, cyanide, or sulfuric acid; toxic industrial materials, such as radioisotopes or infectious materials; and weapons of mass destruction. Hazardous substances have various effects and are generally classified by their health effects, flammability, and reactivity. Hazardous substances can produce no health effect as a result of exposure or can cause immediate incapacitation and death. Hazardous substances may not burn or may readily ignite at room temperature. And hazardous substances may be relatively stable when interacting with other substances or may react violently and detonate when encountering certain environments. Any of these three categories can cause a substance to be deemed "hazardous." All hazardous materials that are used in industry; transported by ground, rail, air, or vessel; or are stored must comply with federal regulations on labels, placards, and provision of material safety data sheets (MSDS) with information for workers about the properties and hazards associated with the substance. This information may be made available to responders at a scene; however, if the name of the chemical is known, most MSDS can be found on the Internet.

When considering the potential effects of hazardous substances on patients, it is important to consider the first law of toxicology: The dose makes the poison. This can be interpreted in several ways, but what is important to understand is that proximity to the release, in the case of an airborne or vapor hazard, is an essential rate-limiting factor to determine dose. Generally, the closer a person is to the site of release of a hazardous substance, the higher concentration they will be exposed to, and the greater dose they will absorb. This is why areas adjacent to, or downwind from, hazardous materials releases are evacuated following an incident—to protect the public from the risk of exposure to a dose of the agent that may make them ill. We can assume that if a person was 10 feet from the release of a hazardous chemical, the amount of agent (or dose) they were exposed to is higher than an individual who was in an office building 1 mile from the incident. The higher the dose, the more significant the health effect, and the greater the chance of illness or death as a result of exposure to the hazardous substance.

It is also important to discuss the difference between exposure to a hazardous substance and contamination. A patient who has been *exposed* to an agent of interest has been close enough for it to be absorbed, inhaled, or ingested into his or her body. Based on the quantity of the agent, the duration of exposure, and the susceptibility of the individual, the victim may or may not show a health effect following exposure. A person who has been *contaminated* by an agent must have the hazardous substance or material physically present on his or her body. These individuals are always exposed because they have the substance on their skin or clothes. All contaminated patients have been exposed, but not all exposed patients are contaminated. An example of this is driving past a skunk. Most people can readily identify when they have been near a skunk because of its characteristic odor. This represents exposure to the skunk's self defense mechanism. However, if you are actually sprayed by a skunk, not only have you been exposed to the odor, but you are now contaminated with the offending substance. Contaminated patients require decontamination to remove all traces of the substance from their person and to ultimately stop continued exposure to the agent of concern.

Referral Patterns of Patients Following a Hazardous Substance Incident

Following any type of disaster, including a hazardous substance incident, victims will arrive at hospitals either on their own (self-referral) or via emergency medical services (EMS) in an ambulance. Research that has looked historically at different types of disasters across the globe has shown that approximately two thirds of victims will present on their own (self-referred) at hospitals seeking medical attention following an event and only one third will arrive at hospitals in ambulances.[8–9] The victims who self-refer to hospitals following an incident do not consider which hospitals have the best specialty care, received the most preparedness grant money, or have the best trained decontamination teams; these victims usually go to the closest or most convenient hospital to the event. Many of these victims will extricate themselves from the incident scene and wander to the closest medical facility. As a result, hospitals may receive no warning that an event has occurred until patients are literally at their doorstep.

Patients will typically present to a hospital following a disaster in one of three general groups or categories: symptomatic, non-symptomatic-exposed, and non-exposed "worried well."

The first category of patient is the victim who has the character-istics signs or symptoms of an illness secondary to an exposure from an agent of concern. These victims will meet the case definition of illness or injury, and be exhibiting the outward signs of illness, includ-ing the anticipated prodromes, exanthems, and sequelae of the disease process. These patients may be contaminated with a hazardous sub-stance, but have certainly been exposed to a sufficient dose for a du-ration of time necessary to cause illness. These patients may or may not require decontamination, but will definitely require treatment and/or admission for their condition.

The next category of patient will appear to be unaffected by the exposure or contamination. In fact, they may not even be complaining of symptoms of illness when they present to the hospital. These non-symptomatic patients have been exposed to the agent of concern, but have not developed the signs of illness yet. They may have accompanied a symptomatic friend, family member, or loved one to the hospital; or they may have been counseled to go to the hospital because of a poten-tial occupational or enviromental exposure to an agent of concern. These patients also need a medical examination and medical treatment for the illness, such as vaccination or postexposure prophylaxis (in the case of a biological or radiological agent exposure) prior to being discharged.

The final group of individuals who will present to the hospital fol-lowing an incident are non-exposed victims more commonly referred to as the "worried well." These patients may be complaining of symptoms caused by their psychosomatic manifestation of illness, or may be non-symptomatic but anxious and insistent that they receive medication or treatment because of a perceived exposure that did not occur. These "worried well" patients generally represent the largest percentage of patients who may converge upon healthcare facilities following an incident and can overwhelm the available resources of a hospital or emergency department.

Unfortunately, it is difficult to sort patients who may be legitimately symptomatic of illness requiring treatment from the patients with an acute stress reaction or anxiety-based need for medical care due to the physiologic changes caused by the autonomic response to stress. Patients in the "worried well" category may be sweaty, have increased heart rate, faster respiratory rates, elevated blood pressure, and other symptoms that may mimic illness caused by an agent of concern. What the "worried well" may not have is a reliable exposure history. These victims may not have been present in the area of the released hazardous substance; may not have any occupational or environmental ties to the area of the release; or may not have household contacts who have been exposed or are ill. Despite this, "worried well" will also require an examination by a healthcare provider to rule out illness, complicating the ability to care for the actual victims of the event.

Initial identification of the hazardous material may be impossible until scene responders contact the hospital with the specific nature of the substance. There are, however, ways to determine the general type of substance, based on the signs and symptoms reported by victims. Chemical agents are usually associated with an acute or rapid onset of symptoms consisting of irritation or burning of the eyes, mouth, and nose; dizziness or light-headedness; shortness of breath; altered mental status; or loss of consciousness. The rapidity of symptom onset in these victims is the key that will usually point to chemical exposure. Additionally, the history of present illness will give clues to the nature of the exposure, such as what the victim was doing when the symptoms began. Victims may report they were at work or in a traffic accident when the symptoms began, suggesting an occupational or accidental exposure.

Biological agents typically are associated with a gradual onset of symptoms that worsen over time. These patients will typically complain of symptoms such as fever, weakness or malaise, cough, a rash, etc. Many patients who are presenting to hospitals and healthcare facilities will typically be presenting with the same group of symptoms or "syndrome." Health officials may conduct syndromic surveillance of these patients and develop specific criteria of what is considered to be the illness. This determination is called a *case definition*.

Victims of a high-level radiological agent exposure may present with symptoms of acute radiation syndrome. This condition results from a high-level exposure to ionization radiation. There are two phases of illness: the prodromal phase and the latent phase. Immediately following a high dose of radiation, the individuals begin the first, prodromal, stage, which is characterized by significant nausea, vomiting, and weakness lasting for approximately 24 hours. Following this phase, the symptoms will dissipate and the patients will seem to recover on their own, even without medical treatment. As the victims of acute radiation syndrome enter the second, latent, phase, it will take approximately 2-6 weeks for the victim to develop the next stage of symptoms. Typically, these include anemia, immunocompromise, gastrointestinal bleeding, and fluid loss. At this time, hospitalization is warranted and medical treatment should begin if it has not already been initiated.

Decontamination Responsibilities of the Hospital—Building Capacity

Why should a hospital prepare to perform decontamination? Why is it the hospital's job to perform mass casualty decontamination following a hazardous substance incident? These questions have been asked repeatedly by hospital chief executive officers (CEOs), nursing administrators, and hospital emergency managers. Some hospitals have not yet accepted that it is their responsibility to perform mass patient decontamination following a major incident. Many CEOs and administrators believe that this is a function of first responders and hazmat teams and that the role of the hospital should be to treat the victims from an incident following the victims' decontamination by trained professionals, not to provide these services themselves. In a sense, these administrators are correct (but keep reading!). Public safety agencies and hazardous materials response teams have the duty to respond to the site of a release, contain the incident, decontaminate casualties, and transport the ill or injured victims to appropriate medical care facilities. Although these teams are well trained, equipped, and proficient in performing their duties, ill or injured ambulatory victims of hazardous materials emergencies do not always wait around on-scene for first responders to arrive, set up decontamination, characterize the nature of the release, perform mass decontamination, triage casualties, and provide treatment and transportation to emergency departments. As discussed earlier, two thirds of victims will leave the scene on their own, bypassing all scene controls, and seek medical attention by self-referring to hospitals. Many of these victims may be contaminated with a hazardous substance and pose a definite risk of harm to the individuals they encounter. These victims present a significant threat to the safety and security of the hospital, as well as a potential health risk to existing patients, staff, and visitors. *Hospitals do have the duty to protect their facility from contamination by victims of a hazardous materials emergency*; to prevent staff, patients, and visitors from coming in contact with these victims; and remaining open to serve the medical needs of the community. In order to do this, hospitals need to be able to respond to the threat and eliminate the potential hazard to their facility by performing emergency decontamination for patients seeking medical attention following a hazardous substance emergency.

Why should a hospital learn how to perform decontamination? If victims are likely to leave the scene and go to the hospital on their own, why not send the fire department or hazmat team right to the hospital to set up decontamination? This is another common question by hospital administrators. The answer is simply that the resources are not available. First responder and public safety agencies have a duty to respond to the site of the release, set up scene controls, limit the spread of the substance, terminate the release, perform decontamination of the victims on-scene, facilitate evacuation of the public, and respond to normal emergency call volume. Local or regional public safety agencies that are not responding directly to the scene have duties to provide station coverage and backfill deployed assets, to provide mutual aid and support to agencies that have committed resources to the incident, and to keep their personnel available to replace the initial responding units if the incident continues for several hours or days. For this reason, *hospitals cannot rely upon fire departments or hazmat teams to respond to the hospital to perform emergency decontamination.* Hospitals must develop the capacity to perform this function on their own, with limited outside assistance, for up to 96 hours. This fact has been echoed by regulatory and professional agencies as well, particularly the Occupational Safety and Health Administration (OSHA) and The Joint Commission on the Accreditation of Healthcare Organizations (JCAHO).[1,10–11]

Where do hospitals get the expertise to even begin to build the capacity to set up a mass decontamination program? If a hospital does have a good working relationship with its local fire department or hazmat team, inviting them to a planning meeting may allow you to identify training resources available to you to assist in beginning your program. Although first responder agencies may not be available to you during an actual event, you may find that they are willing to assist you in planning or training to perform decontamination. Another recommendation is to obtain the OSHA *Best Practices for Hospital-Based First Receivers of Victims from Mass Casualty Incidents Involving the Release of Hazardous Substances* guidance document.[1] This guidance document, released by OSHA in January 2005, discusses in detail the steps a hospital emergency planner should take to begin to set up a hospital-based decontamination program. The document discusses training requirements and competencies, equipment selection, team building, procedures, and emergency planning.

What should incentivize a hospital to be prepared to perform decontamination and maintain a constant state of readiness? There is no tangible return on investment for hospital decontamination preparedness. However, in the setting of a hazardous substance emergency or bioterrorism event, having a protective mechanism in place to ensure that the facility may remain "open for business" as opposed to having to close because of secondary contamination or the illness of staff members, may be what sets the prepared hospital apart from others in the community. As seen in the severe acute respiratory syndrome (SARS) outbreak in Toronto, some hospitals did become overwhelmed with highly infectious patients and needed to essentially close to normal hospital operations.[12] In the US healthcare system, the ability to maintain continuity of operations and remain open for revenue-generating activities may be the true return on investment for a comprehensive emergency preparedness plan that includes the capacity to perform emergency decontamination. Think of it this way; no one wants to be known as the "smallpox hospital."

Regulations and Guidelines

U.S. DEPARTMENT OF LABOR, OCCUPATIONAL SAFETY AND HEALTH ADMINISTRATION

The general duty clause of the Federal Occupational Safety and Health Act states that an employer must provide a hazard-free workplace for its employees.[1] There are numerous regulations set forth by OSHA, as well as state occupational safety and health agencies, designed to keep workers safe from exposure to hazards or environments that could be harmful. In addition to the OSHA standards for general industry (29 CFR 1910), OSHA has published several guidance documents that summarize federal requirements and recommendations to protect healthcare workers from illness, injury, or death from an occupational hazard or exposure. Hospital emergency managers should consult these publications and regulations when considering policy development to ensure that standard operating procedures reflect the current best-practices in occupational safety and health.[1,13–16]

Some of these documents and publications include: *Principal Emergency Response and Preparedness: Requirements and Guidance* (OSHA 3122-06R, 2004); *Pandemic Influenza Preparedness and Response Guidance for Healthcare Workers and Healthcare Employers* (OSHA 3328-05, 2007); *Guidance on Preparing Workplaces for an Influenza Pandemic* (OSHA 3327-05R, 2009); *OSHA Guidance Update on Protecting Employees from Avian Flu (Avian Influenza) Viruses* (OSHA 3323-10N, 2006); and the OSHA *Best Practices for Hospital-Based First Receivers of Victims from Mass Casualty Incidents Involving the Release of Hazardous Substances* (OSHA 3249-08N, 2005).[1,13–16]

THE JOINT COMMISSION FOR ACCREDITATION OF HEALTHCARE ORGANIZATIONS (JCAHO)

The Joint Commission has long advocated for hospitals to posses the capacity to perform decontamination. In 2003, it published a document called *Health Care at the Crossroads: Strategies for Creating and Sustaining Community-wide Emergency Preparedness Systems.*[2] In this document, JCAHO discusses the importance of decontamination capabilities in hospitals, particularly to "preserve the ability of the organization to provide care."[2] Additionally, in the revised emergency management standards for 2008, JCAHO discusses the requirement for hospitals to have plans that reflect the capability to perform decontamination.[10]

JCAHO has also discussed hospitals' lack of internal expertise to establish decontamination capacity.[2,10–11] JCAHO has advocated for federal and state government agencies to provide additional guidance and oversight of planning, training, and equipment for hospitals to begin building decontamination capacity and developing sustainable hospital decontamination programs.

The Hospital Decontamination Preparedness Process

A hospital or medical center cannot develop the capacity to perform single-patient or mass-casualty decontamination overnight. The process of developing this capability takes time, effort, and funding. It is easier for hospitals to initiate planning for hazardous substances emergencies when a full-time emergency manager is employed by the healthcare organization; however, this is often the exception rather than the rule in healthcare emergency management. Although the modern hospital emergency manager is often a member of the nursing, facilities, security, or environmental health and safety staff with other responsibilities, the process for developing a hospital decontamination program is the same regardless of the planner's day-to-day role.

The process of comprehensive hospital emergency planning is a four-phase process that begins by performing a hazard vulnerability analysis (HVA), drafting an emergency plan, conducting training, and then evaluating progress through the conduct of drills and exercises. In this chapter, we will discuss only the comprehensive emergency management planning process as it related to decontamination and hazardous materials emergencies.

The hospital emergency manager should review an updated HVA to determine what the likely threats would be to the hospital if a hazardous substance emergency occurs in the community. For example, perhaps the hospital is near a rail line that transports tanker cars filled with chlorine, a port where fuel oil is offloaded, or a manufacturing facility where toxic chemicals such as cyanide are utilized. This information is helpful in planning for incidents with a higher than normal likelihood of occurring compared to a random release of an unknown substance in the community.

The next step is the creation of the written decontamination plan. The OSHA *Best Practices for Hospital-Based First Receivers of Victims from Mass Casualty Incidents Involving the Release of Hazardous Substances* document discusses elements of decontamination planning and hospital emergency managers should include the decontamination plan as an annex to the hospital's overall emergency operations plan. Engaging community stakeholders during this process can assist in creating a sound operating plan. Community stakeholders include the local hazardous materials response team, the local office of emergency management, the health department, private companies that use toxic industrial chemicals or materials, and others as appropriate.

Essential elements of the decontamination plan should include the following information:

- Notification procedures for staff to take initial steps if information becomes available that patient decontamination may need to be performed
- How to contact members of the decontamination team and assemble the staff trained to perform decontamination
- Site security procedures to lock down the hospital and secure entrances to ensure that all victims who may present to the hospital are routed to a single entrance to minimize the risk of facility contamination
- Location of decontamination site set-up and appropriate criteria for determining when to set up tents and other equipment
- The appropriate type of personal protective equipment (PPE) and respiratory protection to be used to perform decontamination
- Triage procedures
- Functional roles of team members and relevant Job Action Sheets
- Training requirements of team members and general hospital staff
- Medical surveillance policies and procedures for team members
- Communications procedures
- Staffing configurations and shift rotations for decontamination staff
- Integration of the team Incident Command System (ICS) structure into the overall Hospital Incident Command System (HICS) structure
- Demobilization procedures
- Clean-up and site restoration plans

TEAM SELECTION

In selecting personnel to staff your hospital decontamination team, it is important to consider several factors. First, you need to have staff available to set up and perform decontamination on all three shifts. Disasters do not always occur from 9:00 A.M. to 5:00 P.M. Monday through Friday, even through our drills and site visits typically do! The OSHA guidelines discuss staffing models with anywhere from 2 to 12 persons during a decontamination operation. Actual staffing requirements will depend on the type of decontamination set-up you intend to deploy and the number of patients needed to be decontaminated.

If your hospital has the ability to set up a scalable decontamination process with a single patient ambulatory and nonambulatory procedure, this may be operational with only two team members in full PPE. If your hospital's plan calls for the erection of a decontamination tent and the operation of a multilane decontamination operation, you may need as many as 10 to 15 members in full PPE in order to operate this decontamination scenario. In addition, workers in full Level C PPE will likely need to be rotated out of the decontamination line after about 30 to 45 minutes of work for rehabilitation (rest, rehydration, nutrition, etc.) and replaced with the same number of personnel in order to continue decontamination operations.

Individuals selected for the decontamination team should come from a variety of departments within the hospital, both clinical and nonclinical. The majority of staff will be nonclinical because they will be involved in site set-up, security, assistance with PPE donning and doffing, safety, and the actual washing of contaminated victims. Departments that can provide staff will typically come from security, facilities management, environmental services, environmental health and safety, food services, etc. A few personnel, however, should be clinicians (nurses, physicians assistants, or EMTs/paramedics) because triage will need to be performed both prior to decontamination and then immediately following decontamination.

Predecontamination triage is necessary because your decontamination operation can only support so many patients at once. A clinical provider wearing full PPE needs to screen patients to determine which patients need to be decontaminated first based on acuity and available resources. This initial triage decision is based on the patient's symptoms of illness compared to all the other victims waiting for decontamination. In performing mass casualty decontamination, we triage with the understanding that we need to use our resources to treat the most patients with the greatest chance of survival. This is different than conventional triage, which allocates resources to the sickest patients first. In a disaster or mass casualty event, we want to maximize the number of victims saved and need to allocate our scarce resources to those who can benefit from them the most. An experienced triage nurse or paramedic should fill this role because they will be required to make triage decisions based on limited physical assessment while wearing PPE that limits their ability to communicate and elicit sensory input.

Postdecontamination triage is performed by a clinician as well, in order to determine when this patient should receive treatment compared to all other decontaminated victims, conventional patients in the ED waiting room, and the current ED patient census. Postdecontamination triage will be more detailed than predecontamination triage because the clinician is not required to be wearing PPE to assess a patient following decontamination.

Decontamination team members should be asked to volunteer, as opposed to being compelled to join the team. Using volunteers will typically give you personnel who are more motivated to participate in drills and training, and who have a positive attitude about participating in a hospitalwide team. Team members should be given time off for training, drills, etc., while on duty; if they come in on days off, they should be provided with "comp time" from their normal schedules. Most hospitals do not pay team members extra for participating on the decontamination team, but sometimes provide nominal incentives or rewards for participation, such as gift cards, T-shirts, or hats, and employee recognition, such as mention in the hospital newsletter.

Team members need to meet specific training requirements, such as ICS and National Incident Management System (NIMS) as well as decontamination-specific training at the operations-level or higher as discussed in the OSHA *Best Practices for Hospital-Based First Receivers of Victims from Mass Casualty Incidents Involving the Release of Hazardous Substances* guidance document. These training requirements are not optional and are based on the Hazardous Waste Operations and Emergency Response (HAZWOPER) standards found in 29 CFR 1910.120(q).[1,13] Additionally, team members need to undergo medical surveillance and be medically cleared by employee/occupational health to participate in decontamination activities, specifically wearing PPE and respiratory protection for extended periods of time. Decontamination team personnel should be physically fit, not claustrophobic, able to lift up to 50lbs, able to work under intense physical and psychological stress, and willing to attend trainings and drills as a condition of team membership. Record keeping of medical clearance, fit testing (when appropriate), and training compliance needs to be kept by the hospital emergency management coordinator.

Several health-centric hazmat training programs have suggested functional roles/titles for decontamination team members, but the following specific roles are essential to all decontamination operations and should be staffed when possible:

■ **Decontamination Team Leader**: This individual serves as the decontamination operation supervisor and directs staff in their respective functional roles. Additionally, this person would communicate to the hospital command center regarding progress with decontamination and resource needs for both personnel and equipment.

- **Decontamination Safety Officer**: This individual is responsible for monitoring and ensuring the safety of all workers in the decontamination operation. He or she has the authority to stop all decontamination operations if unsafe conditions exist, and ensures safe and proper use of PPE by workers.
- **Predecontamination Triage Officer**: This person is a clinician who wears full PPE and screens patients who require decontamination to determine which individuals should be decontaminated first, based on clinical priority.
- **Postdecontamination Triage Officer**: This clinician medically assesses all patients after they have been decontaminated and triages them to the appropriate care areas within the emergency department or hospital, based on their level of acuity.
- **Decontamination Area Security**: These workers are in full PPE and are responsible for perimeter security, ensuring that contaminated patients do not enter the hospital through any entrance other than the decontamination corridor. They keep patients calm and orderly while waiting to proceed through the decontamination lanes.
- **Scrubber/Washer**: These members of the decontamination team are responsible for assisting ambulatory patients with the removal and bagging of contaminated clothing and performing decontamination, as well as performing the decontamination on all nonambulatory victims.
- **Set-up Staff**: These members of the decontamination team are responsible for the rapid deployment of decontamination equipment and positioning of supplies, such as the decontamination tent; supportive equipment; water supply; heating, ventilation, and air-conditioning (HVAC); and control of contaminated runoff.
- **PPE Valet**: These members of the decontamination team are specifically tasked with assisting the other members with the donning and doffing of their PPE.

EQUIPMENT

Funding to purchase equipment for decontamination and personal protection has been easier with the creation of the federal Hospital Preparedness Program grants through the Health Resources and Services Administration (HRSA). This program has provided money to states to disperse to local hospitals to assist in developing plans, conducting training, and purchasing equipment to support overall hospital preparedness programs. Additional capital is sometimes available through other sources of state or local grant funding.

Specific types and kinds of equipment will vary based on the hospital's size and location, as well as the anticipated volume of patients to be decontaminated. Most hospitals have a decontamination tent that is inflatable or has a rigid skeleton that can be set up by trained staff in several minutes. These tents are typically custom-designed for each facility and have the option of integrated heat and ventilation, a reservoir for holding contaminated runoff, integrated shower heads and spray nozzles, and privacy curtains. Additional equipment, such as lighting, water heaters, signage, fencing, barrier tape, drums, hoses, etc. can also be purchased and these accessories often can be demonstrated on-site by most major vendors.

The most cited deficiency in hospital equipment and supplies has been personal protective equipment (PPE).[3–6] The OSHA *Best Practices for Hospital-Based First Receivers of Victims from Mass Casualty Incidents Involving the Release of Hazardous Substances* document discusses PPE selection and criteria. Most of this equipment is evaluated and/or certified for use in hazardous environments by the National Institute for Occupational Safety and Health (NIOSH). Hospital decontamination teams can operate in PPE Levels B, C, or D, depending on the type of decontamination procedures being performed and the level of chemical protective clothing and respiratory protection available to the decontamination personnel. It is recommended and generally accepted that Level C PPE should be utilized by hospital decontamination personnel. This consists of a plasticized or laminated HAZMAT suit with integrated hood and booties, multiple layers of gloves such as nitrile and butyl-rubber, and chemical protective over-boots all sealed with a chemical-rated tape around seams, etc. Respiratory protection typically consists of an air purifying respirator (APR) or powered air purifying respirator (PAPR), which offers a full-face mask or hooded option. This ensemble is generally sufficient and recommended in the OSHA *Best Practices for Hospital-Based First Receivers of Victims from Mass Casualty Incidents Involving the Release of Hazardous Substances* document to protect the hospital decontamination worker from becoming contaminated by a victim of a hazardous substance emergency. Various brands and types of suits and respirators, which comply with all federal occupational safety and health standards and requirements, are available from vendors.

TRAINING

Training for decontamination team members involves several important topics. These include Incident Command System (ICS) training,

National Incident Management System (NIMS) training, first receiver operations-level training, equipment-specific training, and functional role training. First-receiver operations training is required for all staff working in the hospital decontamination zone as defined in the OSHA *Best Practices for Hospital-Based First Receivers of Victims from Mass Casualty Incidents Involving the Release of Hazardous Substances* document. This includes members of the decontamination team.

ICS and NIMS training is required of all decontamination team members by the federal government (Federal Emergency Management Agency/Department of Homeland Security) and many states, to ensure that emergency response personnel can easily integrate into a larger event-specific Incident Command System. Decontamination team members should be trained to the ICS 200 level with individuals acting as team leaders to the ICS 300 level. NIMS introductory-level training is required at the IS-700 level.

When conducting hospital-specific functional role training, instructing personnel on how to perform their designated duties according to the hospital's decontamination plan, training should emphasize this three-phased process:

1. Familiarization with the agency/facility emergency response plan

2. Identification and recognition of their individual roles during an emergency response

3. Demonstration of proficiency/competency in performing their assigned roles during mock disaster drills and exercises

Presenting worker education and training in a three-phase approach has several advantages. In particular, it allows the worker to receive repeated exposure to the material because reinforcement is a critical element in adult learning models. Creating a training and education program that consists of three distinct and cumulative stages of learning will increase the likelihood that the material will be retained over a period of time.[17] For example, the first phase may be a brief computer-based self-study assignment or a short presentation given during a new employee orientation, which would introduce the worker to the rationale behind the training and would allow the student to learn the fundamentals of the institutional response plan. This initial introductory exposure to the principles of the public health emergency response plan allows the worker to experience an affective form of learning. The second phase may consist of department in-service training focused on specific occupation roles during the emergency response. This phase of training would build on the worker's previously acquired foundation of knowledge and add specific job-oriented tasks that are consistent with the objectives of the disaster plan. This phase allows the worker to experience cognitive learning, by teaching tangible skills that can be used during an event. Finally, the third phase, which would take place during an exercise or drill, allows the worker to develop the psychomotor and hands-on skills relevant to their specific job tasks and individual roles during the event. This final phase involves the integration of their affective, cognitive, and psychomotor learning, and establishes the worker's baseline level of competency for public health preparedness and response.

DRILLS AND EXERCISES

Conducting drills and exercises will enable the preparedness planner to assess if the goals and objectives of the decontamination plan are being achieved. Additionally, from an education and training standpoint, it gives us the opportunity to see if the students are able to adequately integrate the affective, cognitive, and psychomotor learning objectives during their performance in the mock incident response.

Conducting decontamination drills and exercises is an important step in assessing the overall success of the decontamination plan and the training program. First, drills and exercises are designed to assess where planning can be improved and where planning has succeeded. Next, we can evaluate staff performance based on their designated functional roles and determine if performance is successful or if it requires modification of training programs. Finally, we can evaluate our equipment readiness and determine if our resources are sufficient to sustain decontamination operations and effectively meet the objectives of decontaminating patients and preventing contamination of hospital facilities.

It may be helpful to have an evaluation team from outside the organization conduct the actual exercise and evaluate the success of the drill. This will allow the hospital emergency manager to observe and take independent notes during the exercise, and examine those of a third, neutral party during the postevent analysis. Lessons learned from drills and exercises can be turned into improvement plans, upon which planning revisions and programmatic changes can be monitored and tracked in order to improve the hospital's overall ability to effectively perform emergency decontamination procedures.

References

1. U.S. Department of Labor, Occupational Safety and Health Administration. *Best Practices for Hospital-Based First Receivers of Victims from Mass Casualty Incidents Involving the Release of Hazardous Substances*. Washington, DC: OSHA; 2005. OSHA publication 3249-08N.

2. The Joint Commission on Accreditation of Healthcare Organizations. *Health Care at the Crossroads: Strategies for Creating and Sustaining Community-wide Emergency Preparedness Systems*. Oakbrook Terrace, IL: JCAHO; 2003.

3. U.S. Department of Health and Human Services. Health Resources and Services Administration. *A 2002 National Assessment of State Trauma System Development, Emergency Medical Services Resources, and Disaster Readiness for Mass Casualty Events.* Washington, DC: Health Resources and Services Administration; 2002.

4. U.S. General Accounting Office. *Hospital Preparedness: Most Urban Hospitals Have Emergency Plans but Lack Certain Capacities for Bioterrorism Response.* Washington, DC: U.S. General Accounting Office; 2003. Publication GAO-03-924.

5. Rubin JN. Recurring pitfalls in hospital preparedness and response. *J Homeland Security.* January, 2004. http://www.homelanddefense.org/journal/Articles/rubin .html. Accessed August 5, 2009.

6. Ghilarducci DP, Pirallo RG, Hegmann KT. Hazardous materials readiness of United States Level I trauma centers. *J Occup Environ Med.* 2000;42(7):683–692.

7. Institute of Medicine. *Chemical and Biological Terrorism: Research and Development to Improve Civilian Medical Response.* Washington, DC: National Academy Press; 1999.

8. Reilly MJ, Markenson D. Hospital emergency department referral patterns in a disaster. *Prehosp Disast Med.* 2009;24(2):s29–s30.

9. Reilly MJ. Referral patterns of patients in disasters—who is coming through your emergency department doors? *Prehosp Disast Med.* 2007;22(2):s114–s115.

10. Joint Commission Resources. Emergency management standards. *Environ Care News.* 2007;10(12):2–8.

11. Joint Commission Resources. Preparing for catastrophes and escalating emergencies. *Environ Care News.* 2008;11(1):1–3,11.

12. U.S. General Accounting Office. *SARS Outbreak: Improvements to Public Health Capacity Are Needed for Responding to Bioterrorism and Emerging Infectious Diseases.* Washington, DC: U.S. General Accounting Office; May 7, 2003. Publication GAO-03-769T.

13. U.S. Department of Labor, Occupational Safety and Health Administration. *Principal Emergency Response and Preparedness: Requirements and Guidance.* Washington, DC: OSHA; 2004. OSHA publication 3122-06R.

14. U.S. Department of Labor, Occupational Safety and Health Administration. *Pandemic Influenza Preparedness and Response Guidance for Healthcare Workers and Healthcare Employers.* Washington, DC: OSHA; 2007. OSHA publication 3328-05.

15. U.S. Department of Labor, Occupational Safety and Health Administration. *Guidance on Preparing Workplaces for an Influenza Pandemic.* Washington, DC: OSHA; 2009. OSHA publication 3327-05R.

16. U.S. Department of Labor, Occupational Safety and Health Administration. *OSHA Guidance Update on Protecting Employees from Avian Flu (Avian Influenza) Viruses.* Washington, DC: OSHA; 2006. OSHA publication 3323-10N.

17. Silberman M, Auerbach C. *Active Training: A Handbook of Techniques, Designs, Case Examples, and Tips.* 2nd ed. San Francisco, CA: Jossey Bass/Pfeiffer; 1998.

Chapter 15

Pharmaceutical Systems Management in Disasters

David S. Markenson, MD, FAAP, FACEP, EMT-P

Photo by Marvin Nauman/FEMA

Learning Objectives

- Describe the important role pharmaceutical agents play in hospital operations and emergency preparedness.
- Determine the pharmaceutical needs of a hospital in a disaster situation.
- Determine how to plan for and address the delivery of pharmaceuticals from stockpiles.
- Develop plans for addressing the pharmaceutical needs of staff including prophylaxis and vaccination.
- Plan for staff requirements to support pharmaceutical needs during a disaster.

Overview

This chapter will cover the emergency preparedness considerations for hospitals relating to pharmaceutical agents. As anyone involved in health care knows, a significant part of daily operations of healthcare institutions involves the acquisition, storing, dispensing, and accounting for pharmaceuticals, including the staffing considerations for these functions. In times of disaster the needs for these pharmaceutical-related functions continue, but are modified by loss of access to supply chains, increased need for pharmaceutical agents caused by different disease and injury patterns, increased volume of patients, and limitations on available qualified staff. In addition to the challenge of maintaining pharmaceuticals for hospital operations based on usual needs, in a time of disaster one must also account for the needs of persons seeking care who have either lost their needed medications or lost access to primary care physicians for prescribing them, the needs of staff for their personal medications, and the needs of staffs' families. Lastly, whether considering bioterrorism or public health emergencies, any hospital planning for disasters must also account for vaccination and distribution of prophylactic medications or antidotes before or after the event.

Case Study

The Centers for Disease Control and Prevention (CDC) has reported to hospitals that they expect a novel strain of influenza to affect the population this fall, leading to a possible pandemic. In addition, state and local health officials are advising hospitals to prepare for a pandemic. Both federal and state officials advise that some, but not all, of the current antivirals may work against the novel strain and there will be a vaccine against the novel strain. Lastly, they state that they will be able to provide additional dosages of antivirals from the state stockpile if hospitals develop shortages.

1. What would be your plans for ensuring that there are enough pharmaceuticals to handle the increased volume of patients?

2. How would you handle staff vaccinations?

3. How would you decide which type and how many doses of antiviral to keep on hand?

4. What would be your threshold for requesting resources from the stockpile and how would you accept and handle them?

Introduction

Pharmaceutical supplies and the staff to support the distribution, cataloging, dispensing, and accounting of pharmaceuticals are essential to the daily operations of a hospital and, as such, are an essential service to maintain during disaster operations. Ongoing research by the federal government and pharmaceutical industry attempts to address medication needs, uses, and problems in disasters. In addition, reports in the literature demonstrate recurrent trends regarding pharmaceutical supplies during disaster response.[1] As more research into disasters is done, hopefully, mechanisms that have the ability to predict more precisely the pharmaceutical needs and utilization will be developed. This data may be used to develop models to guide effective hospital pharmaceutical needs and staffing for disasters.[2] One has to also recognize that hospitals will need to know when their own supplies and systems will be exhausted and they will have to rely on external resources. When planning for these external resources, the plans must also include the time lag from disaster impact to receiving supplies and the logistics and costs of maintaining and using these external resources. As improved methods of rapid, systematic, and accurate hospital emergency preparedness assessment are developed, a targeted supply approach to pharmaceutical distribution will enhance disaster response and will improve patient care.

Determining Pharmaceutical Needs

Sudden reductions in available medical resources commonly occur after disasters. Following Hurricane Andrew, one report of 1,500 patient encounters in a field hospital found that all supplies of tetanus toxoid, antibiotics, and insulin were depleted within 24 hours. Replacement of basic pharmaceutical supplies and refill medications were the most pressing medical care problems.[3] After Hurricane Iniki struck Kauai, Hawaii, in September 1992, disaster medical assistance teams found that the largest treatment categories were injuries (40.4%), illnesses (38.6%), and preventive services (9%). The conclusions were that, in this setting, teams need to be prepared for the provision of primary health care extending beyond the impact phase of a hurricane.[4] Similar patterns have been reported following hurricanes Frederick, Elena, Gloria, Hugo, Andrew, and Georges, and seem to be holding true for Katrina and Rita.[5] The need for basic medical care after any type of disaster that reduces local medical resources or destroys the medical infrastructure is the mainstay of medical disaster relief efforts.[6] The disaster itself may lead to only a modest increase in direct injuries. Pharmaceutical inventories of relief supplies should be directed toward meeting this goal of provision of primary care.

Disasters may require the mass evacuation of people from their home region, thereby denying medical care to victims and leaving them dependent on relief help. During Operation Fiery Vigil, more than 20,000 military dependents were evacuated from Clark Air Base in the Philippines to Guam following the eruption of Mount Pinatubo. Of the 20,000 evacuees, approximately 2,500 needed medical care during the evacuation. Some medical problems, such as sunburn, dehydration, and motion sickness, were associated with the evacuation operation. However, most pharmaceutical agents dispensed were for routine and chronic medical diagnoses.[7]

In addition, there are multiple sources for clinical recommendations regarding the treatment of casualties of events involving biologic, chemical, or radiologic weapons. In addition, many have tried to determine the quantity of regularly used pharmaceuticals a hospital should have on stock for disaster situations and potential loss of supply chains. The public health consequences of disasters should also guide emergency planners in assessing the pharmaceutical and medical equipment needs of their communities.[8] Several medical equipment and supply lists exist and can provide examples from which emergency planners may select and begin developing an inventory that is appropriate for their populations and threat analysis. For example, the World Health Organization (WHO) has published and developed an essential drug list that identifies those pharmaceuticals that should be available at any given time in appropriate amounts and formulations. The WHO essential drug list has been adopted by numerous international agencies that supply pharmaceuticals within their healthcare programs and is being used to evaluate the appropriateness of drug donations.[9] While this list is for international relief planning, it still can be used as one reference for hospital preparedness.

Several factors influence the pharmaceutical needs of a hospital in a disaster; these needs should be based on normal patterns and the hospital's hazard vulnerability analysis. These include the following examples:

- Type and phase of the disaster often dictate what medicines are needed.
- Epidemiological patterns of diseases of the region should be considered.
- Conditions influencing or enhancing communicable diseases are also important considerations.
- Hazardous materials are a potential problem during disasters; treatments may be needed if specific hazards, such as chemical manufacturers or nuclear plants are in the region. Ideally, known antidotes, treatments, and protective agents should be stockpiled in advance.

In the recovery phase of a disaster, victims may have difficulty accessing physicians and pharmaceutical services for ongoing medical care because of the loss of the medical infrastructure. At the same time, pharmacists and physicians may not have access to patients' medical records. Primary care of acute and chronic conditions is the mainstay of health care relief efforts during the recovery phase of any type of disaster.[3] Epidemiologic surveillance programs will assist in fine-tuning the need for specific pharmaceutical agents, but the key need will be patients' chronic medications.

One must also consider that in disasters, even during the recovery phase, there will be changes in the types of pharmaceuticals needed, although some basic concepts will remain the same. For example, pathogens expected in a region after a disaster are generally the same as those before the disaster because new organisms rarely emerge.[10] A population may be more susceptible to the usual pathogens after a disaster because of factors such as malnutrition, environmental stress, injuries, interruption of treatment of chronic diseases, contamination of water supply and food storage facilities, and crowding leading to increased exposure to respiratory pathogens. However, new pathogens have been introduced to regions by relief workers following disasters. Soft tissue injury is a prominent complaint following many disasters. Many of these injuries occur during recovery operations. Diphtheria and tetanus vaccines are in high demand, and the local stocks are often quickly depleted. This was one of the most commonly used pharmaceutical items on St. Croix following Hurricane Hugo and in Oklahoma City following the bombing.[11] In addition, antibiotics for these soft tissue injuries and other infections will be needed. Antimicrobial agents considered as first-line agents include penicillin, macrolides, first-generation cephalosporins, and trimethoprimlsulfamethoxazole. Following the destruction of St. Croix by Hurricane Hugo in September 1989, disaster medical assistance teams found dicloxacillin to be the most commonly prescribed outpatient antibiotic, and parenteral cephalosporin was the most commonly prescribed inpatient antibiotic. Antibiotics were the most frequently mentioned supply problem during the Bosnia and Croatia conflict from 1994 to 1995, with cephalosporins being mentioned most often among the antibiotics. Intramuscular administration is preferred because intravenous infusion requires equipment that is not always available.

Immediately following the impact of a disaster, each hospital, at a minimum, must depend on its own resources. Usually, drugs sent for the rescue phase of a disaster do not arrive until days to months after the recovery period begins. Blood and plasma products from outside sources usually arrive too late. Even very rapid aid from outside the disaster zone will have a minimal effect on early deaths and casualties. The local or regional area must supply the pharmaceutical agents that are used for the rescue phase of most disasters. This may be through either state, regional, or in some cases, local stockpiles. Disasters in more populated, developed regions usually do not overwhelm the regional supplies for the rescue phase. In fact, most hospitals are not likely to run short of all essential pharmaceutical agents early in a disaster response if it is a contained event. This may not hold true with a nationwide public health emergency when all hospitals need access to the same agents. It takes a minimum of 24 to 72 hours for organization, transport, and distribution to the disaster site, and then it will often take an additional 24 to 48 hours to be distributed to hospitals.

Pharmaceutical Storage

Drug stability and storage requirements are issues that need to be addressed when considering drugs for use in disasters. This includes both those kept for routine usage and those stockpiled by the hospital for disasters. While frozen storage with thawing before use is commonly practiced with certain pharmaceutical agents in U.S. hospitals, multiple freeze-thaw cycles are unacceptable for many drugs. Frozen stability information is readily available. The method of defrosting and the timing must be part of disaster plans. In addition, instructions that can be followed by those not usually in the pharmacy but brought on as disaster surge staff should be readily available.

In certain areas, the extremes of temperature, such as humidity or cold temperatures, may alter pharmaceutical stability. While in most cases pharmaceutical storage areas have environmental controls, these may be lost during disasters or pharmaceuticals may have to be moved to alternative locations without these controls. Instructions for nontraditional pharmacy staff on the effects of environment changes on the pharmaceuticals also need to be readily available.

Identification of Pharmaceutical Agents

The identification of drugs is essential for their usefulness in a disaster. As part of disaster planning, it is important to plan for pharmacy operations to be supported by nontraditional pharmacy staff. The identification of medications in simple and easily understood methods is essential. Proper packaging will help ensure that the labels remain on the items and that they are not defaced or damaged beyond recognition. Identifying a medication and its usage, among the thousands of products available, each with multiple names, is a tremendously difficult task that will be further compounded by the fact that untrained persons may be sorting and dispensing.

The identification of proper drug indications is essential for appropriate use, and, when it is lacking, patients may be harmed. Appropriate references or readable product package inserts should accompany international donations. Readily available reference works, such as the American Hospital Formulary Service (AHFS) drug information that is updated annually, should be included in each box of pharmaceutical supplies. Pharmaceutical agents cannot be used to help the intended disaster victims if they cannot be accurately identified in a timely manner.

Dispensing Pharmaceutical Agents

Some difficulties in dispensing medications following a disaster are unavoidable. Three problems typically seen in regions struck by natural disaster are the lack of electric power, appropriate stocks of medications, and narcotic security. The lack of electricity and telephone service will put a modern pharmacy out of normal operation, but these technical problems will also impede the operation of even the most technically advanced pharmacy. Pharmacists may be unable to contact physicians to authorize orders or to access patient records to refill current medications.

In previous domestic disasters, such as floods, hurricanes, and tornadoes, pharmacists have used professional judgment to dispense sufficient quantities of medication to patients until the records and prescribers could be accessed. Lists of medications dispensed should be kept, compared, and added to patient records as soon as possible. Narcotics dispensing should be kept to a minimum. When pharmacies are physically damaged or are in temporary locations, narcotics need to be relocated to secure areas.

The relocation of a pharmacy to a temporary site in the hospital or the deployment of a pharmacy in an alternate location requires compliance with state laws. Such requirements should be part of the planning procedure for each organization. The physical requirements for a pharmacy during a disaster (such as running water and temperature control) need to be addressed. Packaging and labeling requirements may also be difficult to meet after a disaster. Small zipper-lock plastic bags with labels that can be written on with pen or pencil are helpful for dispensing individual prescriptions, especially when computers or other equipment may not be available. These bags are easy to pack and transport, they are lightweight, and occupy less space than traditional containers.

Personnel Considerations

Personnel available during disasters will vary significantly among countries and disasters. Individuals with pharmacy or medical training may facilitate the sorting of donated pharmaceuticals in large disaster relief efforts. Hospitals should make provisions for and clarify the status of license requirements for the various pharmacy functions to determine the type of individuals who can help and what functions must be performed by licensed individuals.

In domestic disasters, such as Hurricane Andrew, and in the aftermath of tornadoes and floods, using pharmacists with the legal flexibility to use professional judgment and provide needed medications, as well as lifting the requirements for written labels, is recommended.[12] Pharmacy personnel have proved to be a valuable resource, and they should continue to be included in disaster planning and response.

When dealing with a crisis, we often do not have the luxury of certainty of cause, effect, or resolution. Despite this characteristic lack of definition, pharmacy management can enhance the department's response to such events through encouraging staff participation in the growing number of public health emergency simulation exercises being conducted across the country. Institutional pharmacy practitioners need to be "plugged-in" to the overall city, state, and regional public health emergency response planning activities. In addition, they need to avail themselves of training opportunities from hospital associations, pharmacy professional organizations, and pharmacy colleges.

The American Society of Health-System Pharmacists (ASHP) released the ASHP Statement on the Role of Health-System Pharmacists in Emergency Preparedness, which suggests that hospital administrators, "Encourage and enable pharmacy personnel employed by the institution to participate in local, state, regional, and federal emergency preparedness planning and to volunteer for community service in the event of a disaster." Hospital pharmacy directors, likewise, need to promote the involvement of staff members at all levels (clerks, technicians, students, pharmacists, and managers) in their communities' public health emergency response planning, disaster drills, and, when needed, actual events. Although it is acknowledged that staff members owe their primary allegiance to their employer, when the institution's disaster plan is activated, there is considerable room and numerous scenarios whereby staff members can effectively participate in their community response without neglecting the needs of their employer institutions.

Stockpiles

Centralized or decentralized stockpiles of medical supplies and equipment may be considered as an option for disaster preparedness. Certain biologic threat agents will require prophylaxis of persons responding to the event. Prepositioned stockpiles can reduce the time to prophylaxis for first responders and provide a sense of security for their welfare. Medical stockpiling may be one option for treatments that must be given within minutes to hours after an event and often much sooner than federal assistance can arrive. Communities with specific technologic risks, such as chemical storage depots or nuclear power plants, may consider the stockpiling of specific antidotes or treatments as part of their disaster plan.

The US government took steps for a targeted supply distribution network in 1999 when Congress created a system for stockpiling pharmaceutical agents and medical supplies. In 1998, the Centers for Disease Control and Prevention (CDC) received funding under an anti-bioterrorism initiative to develop the Strategic National Stockpile (SNS) program to assist states and communities in responding to public health emergencies, including those resulting from terrorist attacks and natural disasters. Congress charged the Department of Health and Human Services (DHHS) and the CDC with establishing the National Pharmaceutical Stockpile (NPS). The goal of the NPS was to provide medicines and supplies on short notice to domestic localities during natural or man-made disasters. After the terrorist attacks in 2001, the Department of Homeland Security briefly assumed control of the NPS before returning the responsibilities to the DHHS and CDC under the new name, Strategic National Stockpile (SNS).

The SNS program ensures the availability of medicines, antidotes, medical supplies, vaccines, and medical equipment necessary for states and communities to counter the effects of biologic pathogens, chemical nerve agents, radiologic events, and explosive devices. If a public health emergency overwhelms the local authorities, they can request federal help with disaster management. After activation by federal officials, pharmaceutical agents and supplies can be deployed within 12 hours to any location in the United States. Each state has received special training on receiving and distributing the medications and supplies. These items are meant to supplement and resupply the local areas affected by the disaster. The SNS program is designed to deliver medical assets to the site of a national emergency within 12 hours of a federal decision to deploy medical assets. Medical assets available within the SNS program include antibiotics, chemical nerve agent antidotes, intravenous fluids, intravenous administration supplies, bandages, burn ointments, analgesics, antiemetics, sedatives, antiviral medications, antitoxins, and vaccines. The SNS can respond to different types of needs. The 50-ton push packages contain pharmaceuticals and medical supplies needed quickly for general resupply after widespread disaster. The medications and supplies are useful for airway support and IV fluid and medication administration. They include antibiotics and chemical antidotes used for treating certain types of chemical and radiation exposure. The push packages do not contain pharmaceuticals for primary care (e.g., hypertension, diabetes). Push packages are positioned in strategically located, secure warehouses, ready for immediate deployment to a designated area.[13] If a specific man-made threat is known, the SNS can deploy Vendor Managed Inventory (VMI) supplies, which contain medications and antidotes for the known agents. In addition, follow-up VMI deliveries can be made to a disaster area with additional pharmaceuticals and supplies.

A 12-hour response time for delivery of chemical nerve agent antidote is not optimal for the initial care of casualties. In addition, many hospitals carry only limited stocks of chemical nerve agent antidotes.[14] These antidotes have variable shelf lives, and replacing them is costly and may impact a community's ability to respond. Therefore, the SNS program is currently executing a nationwide forward deployment of chemical nerve agent antidotes under its CHEMPACK project. Through this project, emergency medical services and hospitals will have access to chemical nerve agent antidotes for immediate use during an event.

The SNS is designed so that it is the responsibility of the state and local authorities to coordinate staging, distribution, and dispensing of the supplies. From there, it will often fall on the hospital to determine how to receive, organize, triage, and dispense these supplies. As such, a key aspect of hospital preparedness planning is to develop a plan for receipt of stockpile assets from stockpiles such as the SNS, but may also include state, county and even local stockpiles. Beyond the financial concerns of stockpiling medical supplies and assets, there are multiple logistical and clinical considerations for states, communities, or hospitals to consider. A major component of stockpiling medical assets is determining the storage locations. Pharmaceuticals should be stored in a secure temperature-controlled environment. An inventory system should be incorporated into any stockpiling program that allows up-to-date access on available products, notice of impending expiration of product, controlled access to restricted pharmaceuticals such as narcotics, and tracking of distributed products or assets. A centralized storage system of medical assets must be combined with an efficient and secure distribution system. Medical assets should be considered that have longer expiration dates and require no specialized storage needs or ancillary supplies. Clinical considerations include assessing products for duplicity of use. Products that can be used to respond to multiple agents or events can reduce the number of pharmaceuticals purchased. Decisions regarding the formulations of products should consider special populations, such as antibiotic suspensions for children or those persons who cannot swallow pills. Appropriate sizes of medical equipment for children should be considered.[15] Medical personnel in charge of stockpiles used to address biologic, chemical, or radiologic agents will need to regularly review their formularies for inclusion of improved vaccines, newer treatment modalities, and changes to a drug's approval status by the U.S. Food and Drug Administration (FDA).

Pharmaceutical agents used in disasters from stockpiles will vary among the different stockpiles. Using drugs that are familiar to the local providers is important for providing optimal care and preventing medication errors. While the individual agents used may vary by source, the same therapeutic categories are usually contained. Antibiotics, tetanus toxoid, insulin, analgesics, cardiac medications, anticonvulsants, rehydration fluids, cold preparations, and contraceptives are commonly mentioned. In addition to the stockpiles, additional pharmaceuticals may be part of disaster medical assistance team formularies, including advance cardiac life support, antidiarrheal agents, antiemetics, antihypertensives, anti-inflammatory agents, bronchodilators, intravenous solutions, oral electrolyte solutions, baby formula, muscle relaxants, and steroids.

Hospital Staff Pharmaceutical Needs

In addition to the needs of patients, one must also consider the needs of staff when planning for pharmaceuticals in an emergency. These needs come from multiple sources, each requiring a specific plan. The needs can be categorized as follows:

- Prophylaxis and vaccination
- Treatment following exposure
- Personal medications
- Family medication needs

For certain events, there may be a vaccination available that will provide individuals with protection from the agent. This most likely will occur in the setting of a biologic agent, either naturally occurring such as a pandemic or artificially through an act of bioterrorism. In these instances, a high priority will be to protect healthcare workers because they are at increased risk of exposure and there is a societal need for them to be protected so they can continue working and caring for patients. Such hospitals need to have preplanned mechanisms to ensure that available vaccinations can be administered to all hospital staff. In addition to vaccination, there may be a need to provide prophylaxis to staff prior to an event if indicated and provide prophylaxis to staff who may be exposed, either by a break in exposure control after an event or the lack of exposure control before the event is identified.

In addition, the staff working during a disaster will be faced with the same issues in obtaining their personal medications as the rest of the public, which includes being away from home for a period of time, destruction of their homes that have the medications, lack of access to local pharmacies, and lack of access to their primary care provider to prescribe refills of the medications. In order for hospital workers to be able to keep working as needed for hospital operations, the hospital disaster plan, with regard to pharmaceuticals, must account for the need to provide staff members with refills of their personal medications.

Lastly, staff will always be concerned with the health and welfare of their families and this concern will often take precedence over reporting to work and staying at work. As a result, an essential part of ensuring that hospital staff report and stay at work during a disaster is to assure them that hospital preparedness plans account for staff's families with regard to prophylaxis, mass distribution, vaccination, and supply of personal medications. In some cases, this may be mandated, as is the case in several of the federal hospital preparedness grant guidance recommendations. In all cases, it is a good practice to maximize staff willingness to report to work and stay at work during a disaster.

Alteration in Hospital Pharmaceutical Dispensing, Formulary, and Triage of Scarce Pharmaceuticals

During a disaster, one must recognize that despite appropriate planning and use of resources, there may occur a time when the need for pharmaceutical agents will exceed the available supply. This could be a transient phenomenon while awaiting further resupply or a long-term shortage. This will require all hospitals to have a preplanned mechanism to monitor all pharmaceuticals to anticipate a time when a pharmaceutical agent shortage either actually has occurred or possibly could occur. The actions that will be needed include a combination of alterations in dispensing practices, changes in hospital formulary either transiently or permanently, and potentially imposing new restrictions on the agent's usage. As with the majority of emergency preparedness, if one can use normal operational mechanisms during disasters, it often provides solutions with the least amount of barriers. In the case of a medication shortage while using a hospital's existing pharmacy, the therapeutics committee and hospital administrative procedures are often the best mechanism to handle shortages along with the mechanisms available through the Hospital Emergency Operations Center and/or Hospital Incident Command System. These mechanisms already allow for change in dispensing, alterations in indications within the hospital, and the placement of restrictions. What may need to be different for disaster situations is the ability to make these decisions and pass them through the approval process in a shortened time, which in some cases may be hours. This may require those involved in the process to be available or alteration in the approval process during disasters. In addition, you may need the ability to bring into these decisions additional people, such as senior leadership, ethicists, clergy, etc., because restriction of pharmaceutical agents may be an alteration of typical operations and the normal standard of care. Despite the need to alter the standard in some cases, the goal should be to ensure that despite the scarcity of pharmaceutical agents in disasters, all patients still receive the best care with the available resources.

Conclusion

Pharmaceutical supply and donation remain critical elements of disaster medical relief. Historically, disasters attract large pharmaceutical donations, both solicited and unsolicited, often in proportion to media coverage of the event. Difficulties with drug donations are frequently encountered, including massive quantities and improperly labeled, packaged, expired, and unsorted pharmaceutical agents. Serious problems of identification, sorting, and logistics are often encountered. Items are often inappropriate for the type or phase of the disaster and the endemic diseases of the region. Local health care providers may have no knowledge of the appropriate uses for many of the donated pharmaceutical agents. Many of the agents may not be replaceable when relief supplies are exhausted. Narcotics handling and dispensing may be problematic. Education regarding the problems and solutions concerning the use of pharmaceutical agents during disasters should be a standard part of the disaster healthcare provider's curriculum. Better anticipation of needs on the basis of epidemiologic data of experiences and improved field disaster assessment will provide enhanced medical care during future disasters.

References

1. Lesho EP. Planning a medical relief mission. *J Am Osteopath Assoc.* 1995;95(1): 37–44.
2. Noji EK. Disaster epidemiology: challenges for public health action. *J Public Health Policy.* 1992;13(3):332–340.
3. Alson R, Alexander D, Leonard RD, Stringer LW. Analysis of medical treatment at a field hospital following Hurricane Andrew, 1992. *Ann Emerg Med.* 1993;22(11):1721–1728.
4. Henderson AK, Lillibridge SR, Graves RW, et al. Disaster medical assistance teams: providing health care to a community struck by Hurricane Iniki. *Ann Emerg Med.* 1994;23(4):726–730.
5. Centers for Disease Control and Prevention. Needs assessment following hurricane Georges—Dominican Republic, 1998. *MMWR.* 1999;48(5):93–95.
6. Roth PB, Vogel A, Key G, et al. The St. Croix disaster and the national disaster medical system. *Ann Emerg Med.* 1991;20(4):391–395.
7. Shalita EA, Samford JE. Pharmaceutical services to evacuated U.S. military dependents. *Am J Hosp Pharm.* 1992;49(10):2474–2476.
8. Noji EK. The public health consequences of disasters. *Prehosp Disaster Med.* 2000;15(4):147–157.
9. *The Use of Essential Drugs: Eighth Report of the WHO Expert Committee.* Geneva: World Health Organization; 1998:1–77.
10. Aghababian RV, Teuscher J. Infectious diseases following major disasters. *Ann Emerg Med.* 1992;21(4):362–367.
11. Hogan DE, Waeckerle JF, Dire DJ, et al. Emergency department impact of the Oklahoma City terrorist bombing. *Ann Emerg Med.* 1999;34(2):160–167.

12. Scott S, Constantine LM. When natural disaster strikes with careful planning, pharmacists can continue to provide essential services to survivors in the aftermath of a disaster. *Am Pharm.* 1990;11:651.

13. Centers for Disease Control and Prevention. Strategic National Stockpile (SNS). Centers for Disease Control and Prevention Web site. http://www.bt.cdc.gov/stockpile/. Accessed August 28, 2005.

14. Keirn ME, Pesik N, Twum-Danso NA. Lack of hospital preparedness for chemical terrorism in a major US city: 1996-2000. *Prehosp Disaster Med.* 2003;18(3): 193–199.

15. American Academy of Pediatrics, Committee on Environmental Health and Committee on Infectious Diseases. Chemical-biological terrorism and its impact on children: a subject review. *Pediatrics.* 2000;105(3 Pt 1):662–670.

Chapter 16

Laboratory Preparedness

Ramon Rosal, PhD

Photo by Marvin Nauman/FEMA

Learning Objectives

- Describe the role of the clinical laboratory in emergency preparedness for disasters, terrorism, and public health emergencies.
- Discuss the roles and responsibilities of the laboratory response network.
- List actions a hospital or clinical laboratory may take during a potential chemical terrorism event.

Introduction

The role of laboratory testing in the management of emergency incidents will continue to be of paramount importance in the future of hospital and health system emergency management. From lessons learned in the 2001 anthrax attacks to the latest incident of melamine in infant formula/milk, never has it been more critical for hospital facilities to not only understand the role of the public health laboratories (PHLs) and the testing they do, but, more importantly, to work more closely with the public health laboratories in emergency preparedness. The need for hospital facilities to collaborate more closely with PHLs has never been so critical in order to protect the public against diseases and other health threats, including terrorism.

Role of the Laboratory in Emergency Preparedness

Public health laboratories, which are run by state and local municipalities, operate as a first line of defense in protecting the public in collaboration with other branches of the nation's public health system to provide diagnostic and surveillance testing in support of federal, state, and local preparedness initiatives. As new public health challenges arise, the effectiveness of the public health system's response will depend on the capability of PHLs and their close relationship with hospitals. It is important to note that state and local PHLs are distinctly different from private commercial laboratories that do similar testing. PHLs, not private laboratories, are the only type of laboratory authorized to work directly with federal agencies.

Beginning in fiscal year 2001, the CDC Public Health Preparedness and Response for Bioterrorism Cooperative Agreement, now called the Public Health Emergency Preparedness Cooperative Agreement, has funded activities to strengthen public health laboratories around the nation for efficient and effective response to potential acts of bioterrorism, infectious disease outbreaks, and related emergencies. Using these funds, most public health laboratories have renovated and expanded laboratory space, implemented rapid detection technologies, improved biosafety and biosecurity protection, hired and cross-trained additional personnel, and worked with law enforcement entities to develop screening and triage plans. With preparedness funding from the Centers for Disease Control and Prevention (CDC), public health laboratories continue to make progress in training, outreach, and collaborations with other partners, including hospitals.

Role of the Laboratory Response Network

As mandated by the National Response Plan, public health laboratories are intelligently integrated with the Laboratory Response Network (LRN). This global network was established by the CDC in 1999 in response to Presidential Decision Directive (PDD) 39 to strengthen the preparedness of the United States in order to prevent and respond to threatened or actual domestic terrorist attacks, major disasters, and other public health emergencies by requiring a national domestic all-hazards preparedness capability. The other founding members of the LRN are the Federal Bureau of Investigation (FBI) and the Association of Public Health Laboratories (APHL). In the event of terrorism-based incidents, the FBI will be the law enforcement entity to prosecute the perpetrators.

The LRN is in charge of maintaining an integrated network of state and local public health, federal, military, and international laboratories that can respond to bioterrorism and chemical terrorism as well as other public health emergencies. The LRN is a unique asset in the nation's growing preparedness for biological, chemical, and, in the future, radiation-nuclear terrorism. This conglomeration of state and local PHLs, which also includes veterinary, agriculture, military, and a water- and food-testing laboratory, is unprecedented. Since its inception, the LRN has played a vital role in enhancing public health infrastructure by assisting in increasing laboratory testing capacity, where PHLs are now better equipped with more advanced lab testing technologies, along with increased staff levels. This enhanced public health infrastructure also mandates that hospitals, with their associated healthcare system, integrate their emergency preparedness capabilities with PHL capabilities.

The LRN has been subdivided into divisions to respond to biological terrorism (BT), chemical terrorism (CT), and soon-to-be-developed radiation terrorism (RT). The main federal agency in charge of BT agent testing is the CDC, with the U.S. Army Medical Research Institute for Infectious Diseases (USAMRIID) and the Naval Medical Research Center (NMRC) serving as backup in the event of a high-surge testing situation. In addition to laboratories located in the United States, facilities located in Australia, Canada, and the United Kingdom serve as back-up laboratories abroad.

For BT incidents, the LRN continues to work with the American Society for Microbiology (ASM) and state and local PHLs to ensure that hospital microbiology and clinical laboratories are part of the LRN, also known as the LRN-B (biological component of the LRN). There are an estimated 25,000 private and commercial laboratories in the United States. The majority of these laboratories are hospital-based microbiology/clinical laboratories. PHLs are mandated by the LRN to work with hospital laboratories to better respond to public health emergency incidents.

Hospital-based units, including clinical and microbiology laboratories, are considered "sentinel laboratories" and play a key role in the early detection of biological infectious agents. These sentinel laboratories provide routine diagnostic services. They are considered the most vital part of the LRN response because they provide the first and critical step in the rule-out process, and more importantly, offer the key referral step in the infectious agent identification process. In a public

---

Figure 16-1

LRN Structure for Bio-Agent Response LRN-B

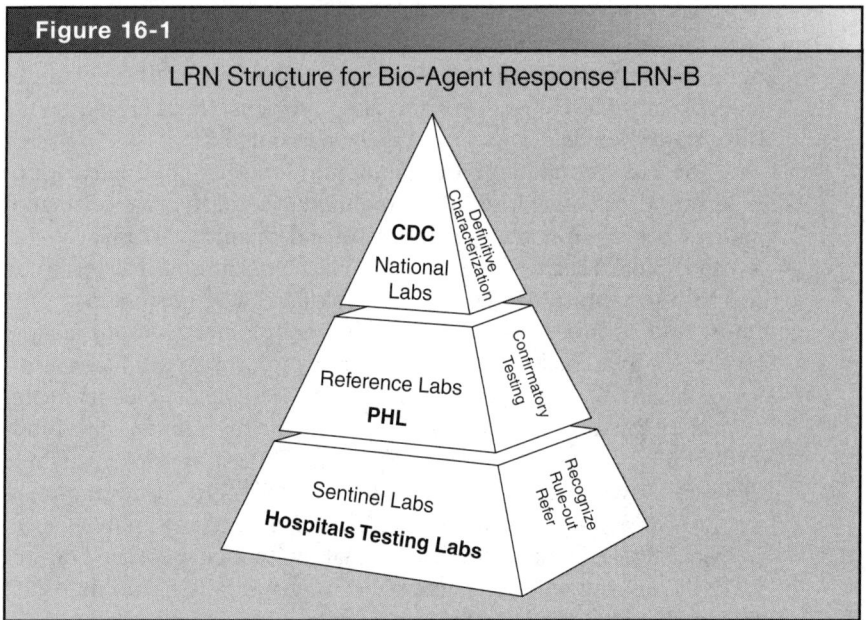

Source: Centers for Disease Control and Prevention, Laboratory Network for Biological Terrorism

health emergency involving infectious agents, either natural occurring ones such as West-Nile or pandemic flu or an intentional BT incident such as anthrax, it is expected that affected individuals will first make contact with hospital facilities emergency departments (ED) to seek medical care. It is, therefore, the hospital's clinical-microbiology laboratory that will first be able to perform testing on these patients. If the hospital laboratory finds a suspicious infective agent, either natural or terrorism in origin, then it is to refer the samples to its respective state or local PHL, which is also known as a reference laboratory for confirmatory testing. The PHL then performs LRN-approved testing methods to confirm the hospitals' results. As a third and final confirmatory procedure, the PHL will refer the samples to the CDC for final testing to assure the utmost accuracy.[1] (See Figure 16-1.)

Even as the LRN-B was created in 1999 to help laboratories in preparing and responding to acts of bioterrorism (BT), the emerging threat of chemical terrorism (CT) was also addressed. Today, the LRN is charged with increasing laboratory preparedness for handling chemical agents in clinical (blood and urine) specimens. The chemical component of the LRN (known as LRN-C) consists of three distinct levels of laboratory capability. Presently, there are 62 state, territorial, and metropolitan PHLs that are part of the LRN–C. All of these state, territorial, or metropolitan PHLs in the LRN-C have been designated by the CDC to have a numerical Laboratory Level designation signifying their chemical testing capability. The lowest laboratory testing designation, which is no testing capability, is a Level 3 PHL. Level 3 PHLs have several important functions. These include (1) working with hospitals in their jurisdiction; (2) the ability to properly collect and ship clinical (blood and urine) samples; (3) ensuring that specimens that could constitute forensic evidence are handled properly, including secured storage and chain-of-custody procedures; (4) familiarity with chemical agents and associated health effects; (5) training on anticipated clinical sample flow and shipping regulations; and (6) developing a coordinated response plan for their respective state and jurisdiction.

Out of the 62 laboratories, 38 are designated as Level 2 laboratories. These laboratories are capable of detecting exposure to a limited number of toxic chemical agents in human blood or urine, such as analysis of cyanide and toxic metals.

Six laboratories out of the 62 are designated as Level 1 laboratories within LRN-C. These laboratories are capable of detecting an expanded number of chemical agents in human blood or urine, including all Level 2 laboratory analytes, plus testing capabilities for mustard agents, nerve agents, and other toxic industrial chemicals. The CDC

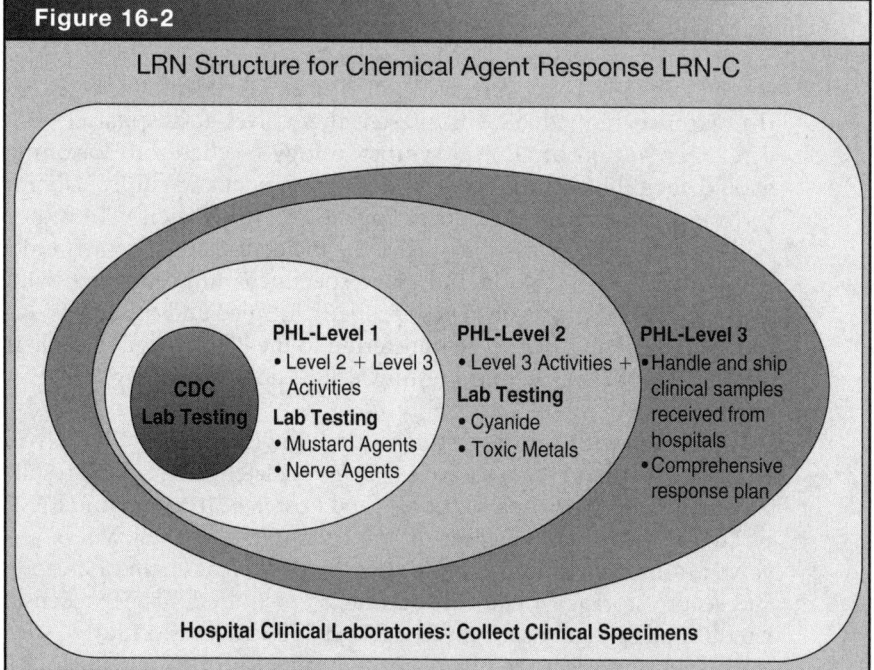

Figure 16-2

LRN Structure for Chemical Agent Response LRN-C

CDC Lab Testing

PHL-Level 1
• Level 2 + Level 3 Activities
Lab Testing
• Mustard Agents
• Nerve Agents

PHL-Level 2
• Level 3 Activities +
Lab Testing
• Cyanide
• Toxic Metals

PHL-Level 3
• Handle and ship clinical samples received from hospitals
• Comprehensive response plan

Hospital Clinical Laboratories: Collect Clinical Specimens

Source: Centers for Disease Control and Prevention, Laboratory Network for Chemical Terrorism

continues to develop new testing methods that make Level 2 and Level 1 laboratories almost similar in analyte-type capability. In a CT incident, the CDC is the central entity that monitors these testing events, ensuring that testing workload is distributed evenly among all Level 2 and Level 1 laboratories around the nation.[2] (See Figure 16-2.)

Actions of the Laboratory during a Chemical Terrorism Event

The main difference between the LRN-B (Figure 16-1) and LRN-C (Figure 16-2) is that in the LRN-B there is a need to confirm twice, once with the PHL and again with the CDC, to ensure laboratory testing accuracy. In the LRN-C, the testing is only done once, but the testing is shared between the Level 2, Level 1, and the CDC in the event of a large CT incident with clinical specimens possibly numbering in the hundreds or even thousands to be tested. If a PHL is only designated as Level 3 (LRN-C), then they will rapidly ship the specimens to the CDC (Atlanta, GA), where they will perform the laboratory testing immediately, providing test results within 36 hours after receiving the specimens. In the event that the CDC needs assistance in testing, it will send the clinical specimens to either a Level 2 or Level 1 PHL for backup assistance. The choosing of which Level 2 or Level 1 PHL chemical laboratory the CDC picks around the nation will depend on which laboratory is the most ready or capable for the unknown chemical analyte at the time of the CT incident.

In a chemical exposure event, such as a CT incident, it is expected that exposed individuals will present themselves at hospital EDs for care. Recognition of clinical symptomology of chemical poisoning should elicit the hospital's emergency department and clinical laboratories to first contact their local Poison Control Center, where they will confirm the terrorism nature of the incident. These hospital units should then collect blood and urine specimens in accordance with LRN-sanctioned protocols. These properly handled and collected clinical specimens are then to be transferred to the PHLs assigned to their jurisdiction, where chemical testing will be done according to the algorithm in Figure 16-2.

The lab results of the testing in both the LRN-B and LRN-C will be reported back to the respective PHL immediately, after which results will then be relayed back to the affected hospitals. In either an LRN-B or LRN-C activation when terrorism is suspected, the FBI will be involved immediately and forensic procedures such as chain of custody and secure storage of clinical specimens is required. Proper forensic handling of specimens for either a BT or CT incident is critical in successful court prosecution of terrorist assailants. Throughout either a BT or CT incident, the PHL involved will be in close contact with the hospital for results and updates and for follow-up testing after the incident for postevent monitoring with the CDC. Even though the role of both the LRN-B and LRN-C was developed primarily for BT and CT incidents, it was also designed to be able to address unintentional public health emergencies, such as emerging infections or an accidental chemical spill, where testing of many affected individuals is necessary.

In accordance with the latest National Response Plan that addresses emergency preparedness, specifically HSPDs 9, 10, 21, and 22 addressing public health emergencies, other federal agencies besides the CDC are now mandated to work together in responding to public health emergencies, including the Environmental Protection Agency (EPA), Food and Drug Administration (FDA), National Plant Diagnostic Network (NPDN), and the National Animal Health Laboratory Network (NAHLN). The EPA is developing its own network of laboratories similar to the LRN called the Environmental Response Laboratory Network (ERLN). The FDA has its well-established Food Emergency Response Network (FERN), while both the NPDN and the NAHLN have not yet formalized a name for their established networks of laboratories. All of these federal-based entities are now attempting to form the so called "Integrated Consortium of Laboratory Networks" (ICLN), thereby creating a homeland security infrastructure with a coordinated and operational system of laboratory networks that provide the most efficient testing capability for early detection and effective consequence management for acts of terrorism or other events requiring an integrated laboratory response.[3] (See Figure 16-3.)

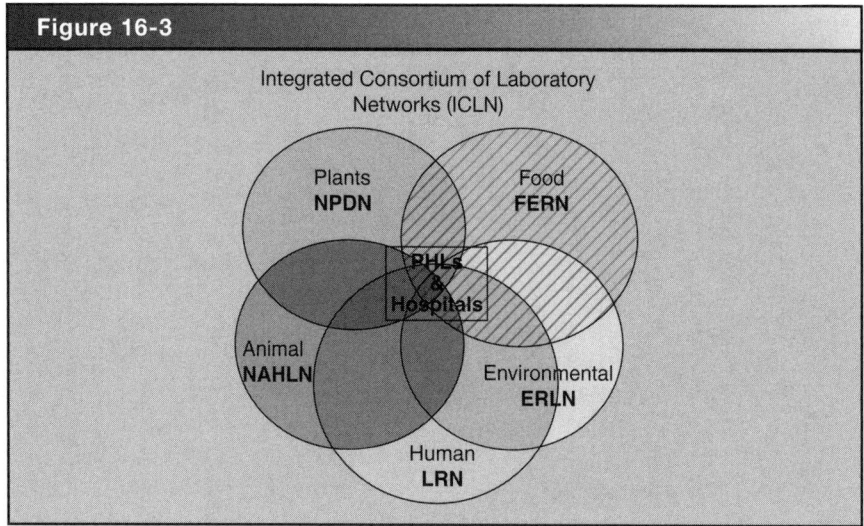

Figure 16-3

Integrated Consortium of Laboratory Networks (ICLN)

Plants
NPDN

Food
FERN

PHLs & Hospitals

Animal
NAHLN

Environmental
ERLN

Human
LRN

The LRN, including PHLs and hospitals, will take the forefront in an incident during a public health emergency involving affected individuals, with the other networks providing backup support laboratory testing of any part of the incident environment. Most state and local PHLs around the nation are active members of several of these networks already, especially with the LRN, FERN, and ERLN. And, because PHLs are the entities that are mandated to work closely with hospitals, PHLs will be the ones to provide all hospitals in the nation the only conduit to interconnect with the ICLN during any kind of public health emergency, where laboratory testing of any component of an incident can assist in the care of the affected individuals in hospitals.

Regardless of the type of public health emergency, whether terrorism or purely accidental in nature, hospitals play a vital role in carrying out the response so that lives are saved and damage to their environment is mitigated. More importantly, it is of extreme importance that hospitals maintain close relations with their respective PHL in their jurisdiction to not only provide the best clinical response, including being trained in shared protocols such as proper forensic clinical specimen handling with both the LRN-B and the LRN-C, but to be ready for any type of emergency incident requiring laboratory testing.

References

1. Centers for Disease Control and Prevention. Laboratory Network for Biological Terrorism. Centers for Disease Control and Prevention Web site. http://www.bt.cdc.gov/lrn/biological.asp. Accessed April 28, 2009.
2. Centers for Disease Control and Prevention. Laboratory Network for Chemical Terrorism. Centers for Disease Control and Prevention Web site. http://www.bt.cdc.gov/lrn/chemical.asp. Accessed April 28, 2009.
3. Integrated Consortium of Laboratory Networks. ICLN Portal Web site. http://www.icln.org/. Accessed April 28, 2009.

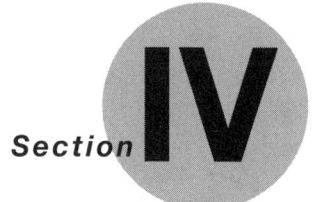

Clinical Considerations

Chapter 17

Principles of Disaster Triage

E. Brooke Lerner, PhD and Richard B. Schwartz, MD

Photo by Andrea Booher/FEMA News Photo

Learning Objectives

- ▦ Describe existing field triage schemes.
- ▦ Describe the SALT triage method.
- ▦ Discuss types of triage.

Overview

By definition, a disaster or any event with numerous casualties is chaotic. Mass casualty triage is a tool that responders can use to systematically bring order to the chaos while attempting to ensure the best possible outcome for the greatest number of people. This is primarily done by ensuring that people who need immediate aid receive care first and that resources are initially diverted away from those who are minimally injured or unlikely to survive. This process allows responders who do not have sufficient resources to treat everyone, to prioritize the care they provide, and to do the greatest good for the greatest number of patients. It is the process of organizing and ordering patients for treatment and/or transport. However, triage is a dynamic process that changes as available resources change, and the accuracy of triage improves with each subsequent evaluation.

The goals of this chapter are to discuss the process of triage throughout the course of a disaster response.

Case Study

You are visiting one of your local fire departments when you hear a loud explosion and watch as the bay door bows in from overpressure. You look outside and realize there has been an explosion at a nearby manufacturing plant. You respond with the fire crew to the scene. There is only one exit from the plant's compound and there are a couple of hundred people, who look dazed and shocked by what has happened, walking toward it. Someone in the crowd says that they had been told there was a propane leak and as they began to evacuate, the building exploded. The majority of people you see are not injured; you can visually identify many with obvious injuries and you know there must be more nonambulatory people inside the compound.

Your first instinct is to help people, but one of the fire officers places his hand on your shoulder and says to wait because there may be a secondary explosion or other hazards. The plant used a large number of chemicals, making the possibility of chemical contamination and the need for patient decontamination an additional concern. Then, the fire officer gets notified that the plant information on file with the city indicates that there is no risk of chemical contamination and other responders report that the scene is safe; there is minimal risk of a second explosion. Now the work of moving and organizing all of the victims begins. The responders begin telling people who can walk to go to a specific location in the parking lot. The responders then split up, with a handful headed out to the parking lot and the rest making their way to those more seriously injured people who were not able to extricate themselves from the plant's compound.

Once inside, you find that two people are not breathing. They are tagged as dead and left where they were found because this will assist law enforcement with its investigation of the incident. Another person appears to have a through and through shrapnel wound to his head, he is breathing three times per minute, unconscious, and does not have a palpable radial pulse. He appears to be unlikely to survive, given the available resources, and is tagged as expectant. He is temporarily left where he was found so that other patients can be evaluated. After more responders arrive, a provider will be sent to this patient to attempt resuscitation. Two people are found to be unconscious; they are tagged as immediate and sent first to the local trauma center. Another patient has a partial amputation of his right arm; the bleeding is immediately controlled with a tourniquet and he is triaged as delayed. You and the other initial responders continue to work through the remaining casualties. In the end, three people died at the scene, 44 were transported to local hospitals, and two of those were admitted to an intensive care unit.

After the event, you go back to the engine company's quarters, where many of the providers admit that it was their first real mass casualty experience. They marvel at how different it was from their previous drill experiences because the victims were not simply lying on the ground waiting to be assessed. The number of people who moved toward them waving and asking for directions and medical aid made the situation much more stressful.

This case study illustrates the realities of responding to a mass casualty event. The goal of responders is to bring order to a chaotic environment while ensuring the safety of everyone—the victims as well as the responders. Further, actual mass casualty events can be very different from drills and other community training exercises. In this chapter, we will discuss the process of bringing order to these situations. Specifically, we will discuss using mass casualty triage to sort and prioritize patients for transport to an appropriate treatment center and then further organize people throughout the phases of treatment.

Introduction

The first descriptions of triage date back nearly 200 years. Triage was primarily developed around the needs of providing care to injured soldiers on the battlefield. It was first described by Dominique Jean Larrey, Surgeon-in-Chief for Napoleon's army. Therefore, the word triage comes from a French verb, which literally translates as "to sort." It is the process of ordering patients for care so as to maximize patient outcome.

The principles of military triage have since been incorporated into civilian mass casualty care, but are also used daily in emergency departments and by prehospital care providers. Of course, in the non-mass casualty setting, the resources that drive triage are different from the resources in the mass casualty situation. When triage is used in a mass casualty setting, the goal is to do the greatest good for the greatest number of people. The available resources are not sufficient to treat everyone. Therefore, those who are minimally injured or unlikely to survive must wait for or forego medical care so that resources are used first by victims who have the most need and are the most likely to survive.

Triage is also used on a day-to-day basis, such as when a triage nurse in an emergency department selects who should be sent to a treatment room first and who can wait. Typically, during this process the nurse attempts to identify those patients with the greatest severity so that they can be seen first. This is because, in general, there are sufficient resources for everyone, but the resources are not available all at once. Likewise, when prehospital care providers triage trauma patients to the local trauma center, it is for the good of that single patient to get him or her to the facility that will provide the best care, while not overburdening the response system or the receiving trauma center.

Description of Triage Schemes

In 2008, a committee convened by the Centers for Disease Control and Prevention conducted an extensive review to identify all known mass casualty triage systems.[1] They identified nine systems, including two that were pediatric-specific (Exhibit 17-1). Each of these systems have been described in detail in another publication.[2] However, it is important to note that they are all relatively similar in that they use a coding scheme, with four or five categories, that is based on basic physiologic criteria.

Exhibit 17-1

List of Mass Casualty Triage Systems

Simple Triage and Rapid Treatment (START)[3]
JumpSTART[4]
Homebush[5]
Triage Sieve[6,7]
Pediatric Triage Tape (PTT)[8]
CareFlight[7]
Sacco Triage Method (STM)[9,10]
Military triage[11]
CESIRA

TRIAGE CATEGORIES

The coding system is frequently referred to as triage categories and the most common categories that are utilized are based upon those used by the U.S. military. Casualties are divided into five categories: immediate, delayed, minimal, expectant, and dead. These categories can be remembered by the mnemonic ID-MED.

Immediate casualties are generally those who need immediate medical attention because of an obvious threat to life or limb. Examples of immediate patients include those who have the following characteristics: unresponsive, an altered mental status, respiratory distress, uncontrolled hemorrhage, sucking chest wounds, unilateral absent breath sounds, or absent peripheral pulses.

Delayed patients are those who are in need of definitive medical care, but are unlikely to decompensate rapidly if care is delayed. Examples of injuries sustained by delayed patients include: deep lacerations with controlled bleeding and good distal circulation, open fractures, abdominal injuries with stable vital signs, amputated fingers, or hemodynamically stable head injuries with an intact airway.

Minimal patients are those with minor injuries that require medical attention, but this care can be delayed for days, if necessary, without an adverse effect. Examples of injuries sustained by minimal patients include: abrasions, contusions, and minor lacerations.

Expectant casualties are patients who have little or no chance for survival despite maximum therapy. Examples of injuries sustained by expectant patients include: 95% total body surface area burns or multiple trauma with exposed brain matter. In systems with only four triage categories, the expectant category is not used and these patients are triaged as either immediate or dead.

The final category is dead, which is used for those patients who are not breathing. Because of resource limitations, cardio-pulmonary resuscitation is not attempted during a mass casualty event. One exemption to this is the child, because cardiac arrest most commonly occurs from a respiratory cause rather than a cardiac one. With this in mind, if a child is found who is not breathing, the responder may attempt to give a few rescue breaths before declaring that the patient is dead. However, whether the patient is a child or an adult, the responder will need to provide only limited interventions before considering the patient to be dead; a full attempt at resuscitation is not recommended unless there are more resources at the scene than are needed.

REASSESSMENT

It is important to note that triage categories should not be considered static. After a prioritization category is assigned, that patient may not stay in that category for the duration of the incident. Assignment of a triage category may be affected by changing patient conditions, resources, and scene safety. As more resources become available, including more highly trained medical personnel, patients should be reassessed. Reassessment is important because a patient's condition may change and rapid initial evaluations may miss important and life-threatening injuries.

Further, it is important that you do not ignore the patients who are placed in the expectant category. The expectant category is a subjective category that indicates that in the best estimate of the person who performed the triage, that patient will not survive his or her injuries. However, if/when there are sufficient resources, these patients should receive comfort care or be resuscitated. Further, these patients should be reevaluated at regular intervals like any other casualty, because their condition may improve or they may further decompensate.

LIFESAVING INTERVENTIONS

During the triage process, it is important that you do not provide complex medical care such as intubation, chest tube insertion, or traction splinting. Care providers must keep sight of their goal during triage, which is to prioritize patients for treatment and/or transport. If a provider begins to provide extensive care to a single patient during the triage process, the provider may incorrectly apply resources to one patient when there is another patient who needs them more urgently.

However, there are some cases where simple rapid lifesaving procedures should be provided during the triage process. These are referred to as lifesaving interventions and Exhibit 17-2 provides examples. Lifesaving interventions should only be provided if they can be done rapidly, the equipment is immediately available, and the provider is properly trained to provide them. These interventions should be initiated rapidly and then the provider should move on to the next patient. As a general rule, any intervention that requires a provider to stay with the patient or requires a great deal of time should not be performed. For example, inserting an oropharyngeal airway would be acceptable, but attempting endotracheal intubation would not be acceptable because it takes a long time to insert and would likely require a provider to stay with the patient to provide ventilation.

Exhibit 17-2

Examples of Lifesaving Interventions

- **Control major hemorrhage**: Tourniquets or direct pressure.
- **Open the airway**: Use basic airway adjuncts or positioning.
- **Chest decompression**
- **Auto-injector antidotes**
- **Rescue breaths**: Provide only to children who are not breathing.

TRIAGE TAGS

After a patient is assigned to a specific triage category, some method must be used to communicate to other providers the category that has been assigned. This will save time because other providers will be able to easily identify the category the patient has been assigned without evaluating the patient themselves.

There are many methods for communicating the triage category that has been assigned to a patient. These include using commercial triage tags, marking the patient with some type of pen or marker, or placing the patient in a geographic area that has been designated for a specific triage category.

There are many types of triage tags available on the market. These range from folding cards that are placed in plastic envelopes and attached by a rubber band to the patient's wrist or ankle; bracelets that are placed around the patient's wrist or ankle; or simple cards, ripped to show which category has been assigned, that are attached to the patient. One of the simplest methods for communicating triage category is to write the category on the patient's forehead or hand with a marker. Finally, tarps or other methods may be used to identify geographic areas for a specific category of patients. As patients are assigned to a triage category, they are moved to the area that is designated for that category. The geographic method may also be used in combination with tags to further organize patients. There is no evidence to show that any of these methods is better than the others.

Regardless of the system used, triage labeling systems should account for the dynamic nature of triage and be easily modified for a single patient. Further, it is useful if color codes are used to assist providers in quickly recognizing the triage category that has been assigned. Exhibit 17-3 lists each of the triage categories and the typical color designation. Finally, when considering tagging systems, it is important to remember that patient tracking is an important aspect of mass casualty triage. Some tagging systems incorporate systems for patient tracking in the tags, such as barcodes. This might be a consideration when selecting a tagging system.

Exhibit 17-3
Typical Color Designations for Triage Categories

Immediate: Red
Delayed: Yellow
Minimal: Green
Expectant: Grey
Dead: Black

SALT Triage

The committee convened by the Centers for Disease Control and Prevention to review the existing triage systems found that there was insufficient evidence to support one system over the others. However, using aspects of the existing systems and the best evidence available, they developed a proposed national standard for mass casualty triage.[12] The proposed guideline is called SALT triage and is shown in Figure 17-1. SALT stands for: Sort, Assess, Lifesaving interventions, Treatment and/or Transport.

The process starts by globally sorting patients into three groups based on simple voice commands. The first command is "If you can walk, move over here." Victims who move to the designated area are prioritized as last for individual assessment because they are clearly able to follow commands and ambulate, indicating that the patient likely has adequate vital signs. The rescuer then says "If you need help, wave your hand or leg and I will come help you in a few minutes." The victims who remain still or have obvious life-threatening conditions, such as uncontrolled hemorrhage, are assessed first because they are the most likely to need immediate lifesaving interventions. Those who can follow the command to wave or are making purposeful movements are assessed second, followed by those who followed the command to walk out of the area.

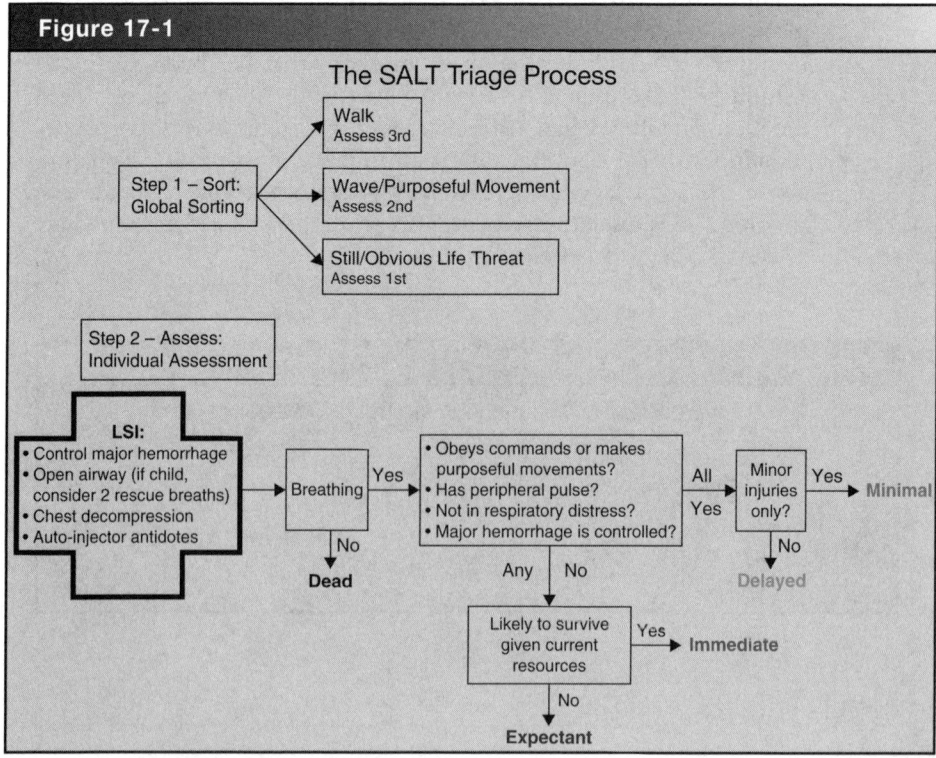

Figure 17-1

The SALT Triage Process

Centers for Disease Control and Prevention

After patients are sorted into these three large groups through voice commands, each casualty is individually assessed and further sorted into triage categories. Individual assessment begins by providing rapid life-saving interventions. These are shown in Exhibit 17-2 and should only be performed within the responder's scope of practice and only if the equipment is immediately available. Further, these procedures should be time limited and the provider should move quickly to the next patient without spending large amounts of time with any one patient during the triage process.

After lifesaving interventions are provided, the patient is assigned a triage category. The victim is first assessed to determine if he or she is breathing; if he or she is not breathing, even after one attempt to reposition the airway, then the patient is categorized as dead. Next, the provider must determine if the patient is not able to obey commands, does not have a peripheral pulse, is in respiratory distress, or has uncontrolled major hemorrhage. If the provider determines that, yes, one of these unfavorable conditions is true, then the patient is considered to be immediate. However, before making that designation, the provider must consider whether the victim is likely to survive, given his or her observed injuries and the available resources. If the patient appears to be unlikely to survive, he or she is triaged as expectant. If the patient is likely to survive, then he or she is triaged as immediate. If the provider determines that, no, none of the unfavorable conditions (not able to obey commands, does not have a peripheral pulse, is in respiratory distress, has uncontrolled major hemorrhage) are present, then the provider considers if the victim's injuries appear to be minor injuries for which a very long delay in care will not increase mortality. If a delay will not affect the patient, then the patient should be designated as minimal. Otherwise, the patient should be considered delayed.

Types of Triage

Several types of triage exist. In this chapter, we have focused exclusively on mass casualty disaster triage as it applies to acute incidents, such as a bombing or chemical event in the field. These same principles can be applied at the hospital if large numbers of people self-triage to the hospital or if an incident takes place on or near the hospital's campus. However, it is expected that patients will arrive at the hospital from the field via EMS already assigned to a triage category and the hospital staff will need to conduct secondary triage.

Secondary triage is the actions done after patients are grouped into large basic triage categories to decide which of the patients in a group get care first. Examples of secondary triage include deciding which immediate patient in need of the operating room goes first, or selecting the patient who will be placed on the ventilator if multiple patients need a ventilator but the number of ventilators is limited. These types of decisions are typically made based on altered standards of care. The issues surrounding altered standards of care are well addressed in a document produced by the Agency for Healthcare Research and Quality (AHRQ).[13] This document recommends that these decisions be fair and clinically sound; that the fair distribution of resources be considered and planned prior to an event; and that nonmedical issues, such as legal and financial issues, are considered as well.

Finally, population triage is applicable to infectious disease outbreaks such as pandemic influenza. In this case, there will likely not be a single scene with multiple patients, but instead patients will be distributed across a community and person-to-person contact will increase the spread of disease. In this case, rather than trying to bring order to a chaotic scene, public health officials are trying to control disease spread. This type of triage is conducted through public health announcements that are used to educate the population on when they should seek medical assistance or through 911 dispatch operators who follow protocols that keep mildly infected patients away from hospitals. These protocols are designed to minimize exposure and limit spread of the disease through emergency healthcare workers and hospitals.

Conclusion

Mass casualty triage is the process of trying to bring order to the chaos at a mass casualty incident. It is the process of attempting to use limited resources to do the greatest good for the greatest number of people. Patients are assigned to one of five triage categories: immediate, delayed, minimal, expectant, and dead. Key aspects of triage include (1) reassessment is essential and assignment to any one triage category is not static; (2) if needed, a properly trained medical professional who has the equipment readily available should rapidly perform lifesaving interventions prior to moving to the next patient; and (3) after a triage category is assigned, it must be communicated to other providers using tags or other methods.

There are several other methods of triage. Mass casualty triage is only the initial process of placing patients into one of five groups. After patients are put into the five triage categories, it might be necessary to use some method of secondary triage to further sort patients within each of the triage categories. Further, when there is no distinct "scene" for the event, such as during a pandemic flu, population triage will be used rather than mass casualty triage.

References

1. Lerner EB, Schwartz RB, Coule PL, et al. Mass casualty triage: an evaluation of the data and development of a proposed national guideline. *Disaster Med Public Health Prep.* 2008;2(suppl 1):S25–S34.

2. Jenkins JL, McCarthy ML, Sauer LM, et al. Mass-casualty triage: time for an evidence-based approach. *Prehosp Disaster Med.* 2008;23(1):3–8.

3. Benson M, Koenig KL, Schultz CH. Disaster triage: START, then SAVE—a new method of dynamic triage for victims of a catastrophic earthquake. *Prehosp Disaster Med.* 1996;11(2):117–124.

4. Romig L. *The JumpSTART Pediatric MCI Triage Tool and Other Pediatric Disaster and Emergency Medicine Resources.* The JumpSTART Pediatric MCE Triage Tool Web site. http://www.jumpstarttriage.com/JumpSTART_and_MCI_Triage.php. Published January 2, 2008. Accessed February 10, 2008.

5. Nocera A, Garner A. An Australian mass casualty incident triage system for the future based upon triage mistakes of the past: the Homebush Triage Standard. *Aust N Z J Surg.* 1999;69(8):603–608.

6. Hines S, Payne A, Edmondson J, Heightman AJ. Bombs under London. The EMS response plan that worked. *JEMS.* 2005;30(8):58–60, 62, 64–67.

7. Garner A, Lee A, Harrison K, Schultz CH. Comparative analysis of multiple-casualty incident triage algorithms. *Ann Emerg Med.* 2001;38(5):541–548.

8. Hodgetts TJ, Hall J, Maconochie I, Smart C. Paediatric Triage Tape. *Pre-hospital Immediate Care.* 1998;2:155–159.

9. Sacco WJ, Navin DM, Fiedler KE, Waddell RK 2nd, Long WB, Buckman RF Jr. Precise formulation and evidence-based application of resource-constrained triage. *Acad Emerg Med.* 2005;12(8):759–770.

10. Sacco WJ, Navin DM, Waddell RK 2nd, Fiedler KE, Long WB, Buckman RF Jr. A new resource-constrained triage method applied to victims of penetrating injury. *J Trauma.* 2007;63(2):316–325.

11. Wiseman DB, Ellenbogen R, Shaffrey CI. Triage for the neurosurgeon. *Neurosurg Focus.* 2002;12(3):E5.

12. SALT mass casualty triage. *Disaster Med Public Health Prep.* 2008;4(2). In press.

13. Agency for Healthcare Research and Quality (AHRQ). *Altered Standards of Care in Mass Casualty Events, Bioterrorism and Other Public Health Emergencies.* Rockville, MD: AHRQ; 2005. AHRQ Publication No. 05-0043.

Chapter 18

QUARANTINE

CONTAGIOUS DISEASE

Managing an Infectious Disease Disaster: A Guide for Hospital Administrators

Ariadne Avellino, MD, MPH

Centers for Disease Control and Prevention

Learning Objectives

- Describe how a healthcare institution should plan for a public health emergency involving an infectious disease.
- Identify specific elements involved in planning, containment, control, and treatment of an infectious disease.

Introduction

According to the World Health Organization (WHO), the danger posed by emerging infectious diseases has become greater since 2000. The World Health Organization further insists that the threat of an avian influenza pandemic is imminent.[1] Ultimately, and almost uniformly in the United States, hospitals are the front lines in providing health care to patients. Given the ominous warnings of impending threat, at any moment, a patient carrying a highly communicable disease imposed either naturally or through man-made intentions, could appear for treatment at any local hospital. These patients may require immediate emergent treatment; other patients may present in a more stable condition; even other people may present, fearful that they might have been exposed to the agent. For some of these individuals, the hospital emergency department may be the only place they have access to health care. Because of the looming threat of an infectious disease disaster, hospitals must accept their responsibility of being key players if a highly communicable illness presents in the community.

Administrators must prepare, act, structure, and maintain their institution's physical readiness as well as the continued training of employees, because hospitals in the United States, as institutions, carry a burden of helping public agencies and the government manage public health emergencies. Healthcare facility involvement, even in small communities, can help curb a communicable disease so that it does not evolve into a global pandemic. However, this responsibility requires several action steps. For example, prior to an actual event, partnerships between public health entities and local hospitals should be formed and strengthened.[2] Hospital administrators must be well-versed in the everyday practice of infection control and the common public health practices of isolation and quarantine. Additionally, hospital leaders must recognize and address the fact that the institution's healthcare providers and staff may also be at great risk of becoming ill.

If a highly communicable disease presents, hospitals are faced with many new challenges. In the end, an institution's ultimate focus of patient-centered care may need to be altered to a perspective in which the public's health is recognized as the utmost importance rather than the health of an individual. This transition of visions requires a dynamic change involving early recognition, planning, and preparation at every level within healthcare institutions and healthcare delivery.

Thinking Ahead

In effectively preparing a healthcare institution for a public health emergency involving an infectious disease, hospital administrators must address the following topics.

ACTIVATE AND FORM INTERNAL PLANNING COMMITTEES WITHIN YOUR INSTITUTION

There are several different individuals who must be members of these types of planning committees. Perspectives present at the meeting table should represent a variety of different interests in order to provide optimum planning. Members of planning committees within hospitals should include: hospital administrators, legal counsel, nurses, physicians (from the emergency department, intensive care, and psychiatry), physical therapists, respiratory therapists, and medical examiners, as well as staff specialized in infection control, disaster preparedness, public relations, human resources, facilities and engineering, central supply, environmental health, security, nutrition, pharmacy, information technology, laboratories, ethics, food services, and volunteer services.[3] Initially, the sheer number of people who should be involved with these types of planning committees may seem overwhelming. However, the participation of each member is critical because each may lend different views regarding necessary preparations for infectious disasters.

FORM PARTNERSHIPS AND DEVELOP GOAL-DRIVEN LOCAL PROTOCOLS

In addition to internal preparation within an institution, the National Association of County and City Health Officials (NACCHO) strongly suggests forming partnerships between local hospitals and public health officials. NACCHO stresses the advantages of planning a unified response as: the ability to provide a rapid and more effective response than either body could provide alone, being able to approach state and federal agencies with a unified voice, allowing the sharing of the burden of cost and resources, being able to coordinate training exercises and the purchase of equipment, and allowing better coordination and reduced redundancy of staff and volunteer deployments.[4]

NACCHO also provides general guidelines for forming effective partnerships among entities. Of particular importance is the need for partnering entities to develop clear and mutual goals of affiliation. In the partnership, the groups become stakeholders with common goals. If these objectives are well understood and trust is established, then the group will be more effective and the ability to achieve the common goal will be more easily attained.[4]

Further, NACCHO recommends that a Memorandum of Agreement (MOA) between partnering agencies be created. A MOA is a formal accord developed by legal representatives that specifies the protocols and coordination commitments between the entities in the partnership. In doing this, it is recommended that the partners appoint a senior administrator committed to managing the partnership and acting as the liaison between the attorneys of each organization.[4]

INTERNAL SURVEILLANCE SYSTEMS AND EARLY RECOGNITION OF THREATS

Early recognition of a highly infectious disease is the first step in battling potential disaster. In order to effectively detect a disease threat, such as pandemic influenza or other communicable disease, specific steps are advised by the United States Department of Health and Human Services. These recommendations include: establishing recognition methods to help with detection (such as visual alerts specifying symptoms of highly communicable diseases and patient care areas), having all patients and staff always respect the principles of "respiratory and cough etiquette" (Table 18-1), and having a triage officer who can direct patients with suspected communicable disease to separate triage and waiting areas for exposed and symptomatic patients of a particular communicable disease separate from the area in which other patients may be seeking care. Each of these items are critical steps in quickly and efficiently helping to identify and control potential patients who may be afflicted with highly communicable diseases while maintaining the goal of contaminating as few of the other patients and staff as possible.[3]

Further, it is critical that surveillance for highly communicable infections should not be limited to the emergency department. It is possible, although clearly unfortunate, that a patient with such a disease may already be admitted to a floor. This may occur because some institutions allow physicians to directly admit patients. This may also occur if the emergency department failed to recognize the patient's symptoms as potentially indicating a highly infectious disease. Regardless of the cause, it is critical that the medical staff on the patient floors also be educated to provide the tools necessary to recognize these conditions. The responsibilities of detection and recognition should not be limited to the emergency department.

In addition to these principles, there is an imminent need for the development of additional surveillance strategies. These strategies must be shaped to recognize a variety of infectious diseases, the focus of which should be determined by current and local guidelines as to the levels of threat of specific pathogens within the community.[5] Additionally, the importance of continued education of medical, nursing, and ancillary staff in recognizing symptoms of potential infectious diseases that may threaten patients cannot be stressed enough.

Table 18-1
Respiratory Hygiene and Cough Etiquette[10]
1. Provide continuing education of healthcare facility staff, patients, and visitors.
2. Post signs, in language(s) appropriate to the population, that provide patients and accompanying family members with instructions to recognize signs of potential communicable disease.
3. Provide source control measures that include covering the patient's nose and mouth with a mask or tissue.
4. Perform hand hygiene (thorough cleansing of hands) after contact with respiratory secretions.
5. Provide spatial separation (> 3 feet) of infected or potentially infected patients.

Surveillance and early recognition, while important, are not enough. If there is any question that a patient may have a communicable disease, measures should immediately be taken to isolate the affected patients and quarantine any exposed individuals. These methods of controlling infectious diseases will be discussed later in the chapter.

ENHANCE THE INSTITUTION'S COMMUNICATION CAPABILITIES

Being able to effectively communicate within the institution, as well as with entities outside of the hospital, is critical. Communication with all partners, as well as staff, is essential. Most disaster experts will agree that being able to effectively communicate before, during, and after a disaster is critical to a successful response and recovery. In most cases, action in any situation, but especially in public health emergencies, requires coordination that is only possible through clear and effective communication. Perhaps most importantly, in the United States, hospital administrators must be able to contact the Centers for Disease Control and Prevention (CDC) and make them aware of a potential outbreak. This notification must occur promptly; the message must get through. Additionally, NACCHO guidelines stress the importance of having a state-of-the-art communications system in which all stakeholders may connect in the event of a disaster.[4] The value of this investment, however, is not limited to these guidelines. Importantly, it should be recognized that this communication should not be limited to those within the partnership. The hospital and public health officials also carry the responsibility of being able to deliver messages to the public that may indicate warnings or messages of instruction to those who have been infected or exposed,[6] or perhaps provide directions as to how people should protect themselves from exposure.

In addition to being able to send information out of the hospital, it may be equally as important to be able to access information from outside sources. Hospital staff must have access to reliable guidance from outside public health agencies, as well as other officials. For example, in 2003, healthcare workers working in one Toronto hospital during the appearance of severe acute respiratory distress syndrome (SARS) reported difficulties in receiving updates on infection control precautions from outside public health officials.[7] Being unable to access dependable advisory information and current infection control guidelines may cause severe injury or even death to staff and other persons.

Because of the dynamic requirements of disaster situations, the importance of being able to establish direct contact with the Centers for Disease Control and Prevention and other public health entities is one of the most valuable tools in any disaster involving an infectious agent.

Hospitals must have this capability and should also be able to contact other local government agencies and be able to provide accurate and reliable information to other partners and the public.

STAFFING CONCERNS

In preparing for a potential infectious disease disaster, hospital administrators must be sensitive to staff-specific concerns. One study conducted in 2006, estimates that approximately half of the healthcare workers in the United States will not report to work if an influenza epidemic occurs.[8] The study cites the staff's reasons, such as fear of exposure and fear of spreading the illness to family members.[8,9] This consideration, in addition to the problematic likelihood of some staff members who are unable to work because of their own exposure or infection, leaves serious questions about how to provide enough staffing during infectious disease disasters.

Additionally, and without question, a decrease in the number of employees stresses not only the hospital as an institution, but also those workers who are available. Problematically, this adds additional physical and mental exhaustion to those workers.[9] For example, during the SARS outbreak in Toronto in 2003, healthcare workers reported increased fatigue caused by increased numbers and lengths of shifts, in addition to the extra time required during repeated donning and doffing of personal protective equipment[7] when seeing patients. Administrators should also not forget the importance of providing ongoing psychological care for staff dealing with the stresses and ramifications of treating patients in disaster situations; psychological services should be readily available for all staff at all times during a disaster situation. Because of this type of high pressure environment created during disaster situations, in order to propagate smooth workings of the hospital facility and properly support staff, hospital administrators must consider the possibility of providing additional incentives, supplementary and ongoing continuing education, as well as psychological services to employees[9] during times of disasters.

CONCERNS FOR THE "EVERYDAY PATIENT"

Dealing with patients on an everyday basis requires efficiency and planning. On the other hand, treating and managing multiple, even hundreds of patients infected with a highly communicable disease can be extremely difficult. When these two situations are combined, it can create an environment of chaos. Hospital administrators must remember that even though they may be presented with a situation in which they have to manage and treat many patients with a highly infectious disease, they still have the responsibility of treating the patients already in their facility and patients who may show up to the emergency department with complaints other than the infection. Those who are not infected with the disease, but who have other ailments, may already be very ill and, if exposed to the highly transmissible pathogen, are at great risk of catching and further spreading the infectious agent. Because of this combination, hospital administrators must consider the ongoing needs of already established patients. In order to do this, staff should consider isolating and cohorting the infected patients, as well as dedicating specific equipment to patient populations afflicted with similar illness. Additionally, in some cases, this may mean transferring ailing patients (who are not infected and have not been exposed to the infections in other healthcare facilities) and/or limiting new admissions to only afflicted persons. These actions, however, do not go without consequence. This may mean certain financial losses for the institutions, which do not go unnoticed, but hospital administrators must dutifully maintain dedication to the goal of ensuring public health.

Specific Planning for Hospitals in Containment, Control, and Treatment

UNIVERSAL PRECAUTIONS

Establishing everyday infection control practices in patient care areas is critical when treating any kind of infectious disease. General practices that aid in preventing exposure and contamination of infectious diseases include: prohibiting meals from being eaten or stored at nurses' stations, advising healthcare providers not to wear jewelry or apply make-up while on the wards, as well as strictly instructing providers not to chew their fingernails at work.[7]

In addition to providing and upholding these strict guidelines on an everyday basis, healthcare providers should also always use standard precautions when treating anyone suspected of having or having been exposed to highly infectious diseases such as avian influenza H5N1. These standard precautions combine the principles of universal precautions and body substance isolation into one practice. Standard precautions are based upon the principle that all body fluids may contain transmissible infectious agents; infected body fluids may include secretions (excretions except sweat), non-intact skin, and mucous membranes.[10] Standard precautions include the need for standard hand hygiene and use of personal protective equipment (gloves, gown, shoe covers, mask, eye protection, and face shield) for all patients, as well as utilizing safe injection practices. In everyday healthcare practice, but especially during the treatment of communicable diseases, it is essential that providers utilize hand hygiene practices—both hand washing and the use of alcohol-based products. Hand hygiene must always be performed between patient contacts after removing other personal protective equipment. It is crucial that healthcare facilities provide readily accessible and working hand-washing facilities, as well as hand disinfection products.[11]

Of particular note is the use of protective masks. This type of mask is designed to guard healthcare providers from respiratory illnesses. For example, NIOSH N95 masks are required to protect against tuberculosis. In providing these masks, hospital administrators must understand that it is not adequate to just have a supply available. Staff must also be trained and fit-tested for their appropriate use. Use of these masks without proper fit-test renders the protection ineffective. Because of these additional requirements for masks, studies have shown that their use is of moderate effect in that their success hinges upon their correct use, sizing, and level of compliance by healthcare workers.[12] Other supply items to take specific note of are bedsheets. Current guidelines require that the bedsheets of patients with communicable diseases either be reusable sheets or be regular cloth sheets that are then autoclaved or washed in hot water with bleach.

A study from 2006 suggests that healthcare providers who acquired SARS after being exposed to patients with the illness, were never formally educated regarding infection control practices or the appropriate use of personal protective equipment. In particular, physicians reported that their infection control training usually only consisted of the presence of informational posters throughout the patient floors.[7]

Enforcing universal precautions guidelines requires that an adequate number of necessary supplies be on hand and accessible to all healthcare workers in the facility, and are ready to be used at any moment. Having an increased supply likely requires additional onsite readily accessible storage capability and may necessitate additional funding. However, it is not just acquiring these supplies that will ensure staff safety against potentially lethal illnesses. Rather, staff (everyone from healthcare providers to housekeeping and maintenance staff) must be properly trained to use the equipment. This is typically a function of the hospital infection control practitioner or employee/occupational health.

RESPIRATORY HYGIENE AND COUGH ETIQUETTE

Upon entering a healthcare facility, any patient presenting for care with symptoms of a respiratory infection (which include coughing, wheezing, congestion, and malaise) should be advised to adhere to the respiratory hygiene/cough etiquette guidelines set forth by the Centers for Disease Control and Prevention.[10] (See Table 18-1.) These guidelines include source control measures such as wearing a mask over nose and mouth, hand hygiene, and spatial control measures (maintaining at least three feet of distance between persons). More specifically, these methods of infection control should be instituted when any patient is suspected of having influenza, Bordetella pertussis, adenovirus, rhinovirus, Neisseria meningitides, or in the early stages of infection with Group A streptococcus.[10]

ISOLATION

Isolation is defined as the separation of a person or a group of persons who is infected or believed to be infected with a contagious disease to prevent the infection from spreading. The practice of isolation, which in most cases is voluntary (but may be involuntary), is utilized when patients actually carry the infection or are contagious. Typically, if a person were placed in isolation, the patient's separation would last for the entire period of communicability of the illness, which varies upon the infectious agent as well as the availability of treatment.[13]

The practical application of creating isolated space in which to treat patients must include not only having the space and airspace dedicated to these patients. It must also include a clean zone for staff to be able to change in and out of street clothes and for recording healthcare workers' entrance and exit times. Additionally, there should be an intermediate zone in which staff can change into personal protective equipment. Finally, there should be a contaminated zone for entering isolation areas.[5]

Notably, isolation of patients involves not only physically separating patients into different rooms, but also isolating the air breathed, a term referred to as *air space isolation*. Air space isolation involves having visitors and healthcare providers wear fitted masks (NIOSH N95) when it is likely that they could breathe the same air, as well as housing the patients in a negative pressure room. By definition, negative pressure isolation rooms have, at a minimum, 6 to 12 air changes per hour; they share no joint circulation with other rooms, and their air is vented outside the building.[13] Additionally, patients placed in isolation must be treated and diagnosed using dedicated equipment, such that only when absolutely necessary is a patient brought out of isolation, thereby preventing cross-contamination of patients who may also need tests and treatment with the same equipment. Because of the requirement of isolation, hospital administrators must advocate and demand that these types of resources be available at a moment's notice.

It is crucial to recognize isolation and its components as an essential tool to implement in the event of an infectious disease. This being said, isolation, in and of itself, may not stop an outbreak of a highly infectious disease unless clinical diagnostic tools and treatment can be applied early.[12]

QUARANTINE

Quarantine, as opposed to isolation, refers to the restriction of activities or limitation of freedom of movement of those presumed exposed to a communicable disease in such a manner as to prevent effective contact with those not exposed. Quarantine of persons typically lasts as long as necessary to protect the public by providing care through immunizations and treatment and ensuring that quarantined persons do not actually carry the disease.[13] Its primary goal is to prevent the transmission of the virus from people who may not know that they have it, in addition to allowing easier accessibility to patients (because their whereabouts are known) with early symptoms of illness.

Most often, people think of quarantine in terms of restricting a person's movement to his or her home or other quarantine site. However, like isolation, hospitals may use the practice of quarantine to aid in preventing the spread of an illness. For example, if a patient in early stages of SARS is admitted directly to a specific floor of a hospital by his or her primary care physician who has missed the diagnosis, it is likely that other patients, as well as healthcare providers, will be exposed. In addition to isolating that patient, the hospital may then quarantine the patients and workers who were exposed and closely monitor them for signs of illness.

In 2005, the Centers for Disease Control and Prevention updated the list of communicable diseases that require quarantine. This list includes: yellow fever, diphtheria, small pox, cholera, infectious tuberculosis, viral hemorrhagic fevers, plague, severe acute respiratory syndrome, and some types of influenza.[13]

COHORTING AFFLICTED PATIENTS

In the event that a large group of patients presents to the same hospital for treatment of a communicable disease, the institution should consider cohorting patients and staff[3] in isolating the disease. Cohorting is defined as the act of physically grouping people together according to their illness, which helps to prevent the cross-transmission of illnesses such as respiratory viruses. For example, if 20 patients with avian influenza virus H5N1 presented to a hospital, the hospital could cohort these patients onto one specific floor, closing the area to patients with other conditions, and dedicate specific personnel to treating these patients. Because hospital staff themselves can act as a reservoir of transmission for some illnesses[14] having dedicated caregivers and ancillary support persons prevents any kind of cross-contamination. Further, having all of the patients in the same location allows illness-specific resources to be concentrated in this area, allowing more efficient treatment and use of resources.

PROVIDING ADDITIONAL AND DEDICATED EQUIPMENT

During any type of disaster, especially those involving an infectious agent, many resources are necessary and must continuously be resupplied. Specific medical equipment that will be most important during an infectious disaster includes: personal protective equipment (discussed earlier), oxygen delivery materials, intravenous fluids, intravenous pumps, and ventilators. Because some of this equipment may normally be in limited supply in one facility, Memorandums of Agreement may be useful to more efficiently share supplies between institutions.[15] As previously stated, if patients are in isolation or cohorted, it is critical to limit patient transport outside of these areas[3] unless there is some emergency requiring them to be moved. Therefore, in these situations, it is important to have dedicated equipment for those patients who have the same type of communicable disease. For example, hospital administrators should plan to have dedicated and portable X-ray and ultrasound equipment. This may mean that the hospital needs additional radiologic machinery in order to meet these needs.

CONCERNS OF SURGE CAPACITY

Surge capacity refers to the ability to expand services in response to a prolonged demand in order to care for hundreds to thousands more patients at the same time.[2,16,17] Being able to extend services and staff beyond normal limits during the time of a disaster can be incredibly stressful for both administrators and healthcare providers. Additionally, with the overall number of hospitals in the United States decreasing, leading to a quantitative decrease in hospital services and staff, the issues related to surge capacity are a serious concern for all institutions.

The Joint Commission on the Accreditation of Healthcare Organizations (JCAHO) specifies that during such situations, a great demand for hospital services will require additional beds, space, personnel, medical supplies, general medical equipment, and healthcare providers, in addition to ancillary and support staff. JCAHO provides formulas for hospitals to use in order to predict their surge capacity (Table 18-2). Specifically, the surge capacity of hospitals for noncritical patients during a highly transmissible respiratory infection, such as avian influenza H5N1, is related to the availability of radiology ser-vices at that facility. The surge capacity of a hospital in treating critical patients, regardless of the type of disaster, is related to the total number of operating rooms and staff available.[2]

Table 18-2	
Surge Capacity[2]	
Predicted capacity	**Determination**
Noncritical patients	Determined by the capacity of the radiology department. hospital capacity/hour = (# of X-ray machines) x (6 patients/hour)
Critical patients	Dependent on the number of available operating rooms with working staff.

The biggest question related to surge capacity remains—in reality, how does a facility deal with this added pressure? The best solution in dealing with this added stress is simply stated: the institution, hospital administrators, healthcare providers, and other staff must be flexible. While this solution is simply stated, its implementation can be extremely difficult. For example, healthcare providers may be forced to provide care to patients in areas that are not normally used—this may require the redesign of existing space to accommodate more patients as well as treating individuals in unlicensed or unstaffed beds.[15] This approach may be sufficient to meet the healthcare needs of patients, but, in the process, may compromise current privacy standards. Ultimately, in these types of disaster situations, health care should be delivered to patients, even if their privacy is somewhat compromised.[18] Dealing with surge capacity also may require closing the hospital to new admissions when capacity is reached and ceasing elective procedures in order to respond to the additional pressures of patients with a highly infectious disease.[15] Additionally, because surge capacity refers to not only having enough space to treat patients, but also enough staff to deliver care, hospitals should consider the possibility of recalling retired workers[15] or recruiting volunteer healthcare providers—doctors, nurses, pharmacists, and allied medical personnel—from outside agencies and the community.[18] As previously discussed, hospitals will also have to deal with the difficulties of staff becoming exposed to the agent and infected as well. It is hypothesized that healthcare workers can expect to become ill at the same rate as the general population, which could result in a 30% or higher absenteeism rate.[19] Another strategy to deal with surge capacity involves early discharge for all patients who are not severely ill.[15]

LIMITING VISITORS

Many patients have visitors—family members, friends, and co-workers—who come to the hospital to provide comfort to them. Unfortunately, during times in which patients carry highly transmissible diseases, allowing visitors may not be possible. Certainly, any patient with a communicable disease should only have a limited number of visitors, if absolutely necessary. If visitors do come, they should don the appropriate protective equipment. This being said, in handling situations where many patients are sick, it may just not be possible to allow patients to have visitors. This recommendation is not, however, to be taken lightly and hospital administrators should be sensitive to the emotional needs of ill patients and their family members who will want to be together. Therefore, these types of limitations should only be imposed when absolutely necessary.

SECURITY ISSUES

It is absolutely crucial that hospital administrators understand the importance of having adequate security in situations where there may be many patients being treated for highly communicable diseases. Unfortunately, it is likely that the public will be overwhelmed and perhaps even panicked during times of infectious disease disaster. At a hospital entrance, there may be a mob of people demanding access to the hospital for fear that they were exposed to the agent. Intermingled with these people, there may also be infection carriers who need to be isolated and admitted immediately. While this situation clearly demands a triage officer and separate waiting areas for infected patients (as previously discussed), security officers will be critical staff to be on hand to help manage and regulate who and what enters and exits the facility. Hospital administrators must take this requirement very seriously and prepare for these very specific, and perhaps additional, staffing needs.

Conclusion

In anticipation of an infectious disease disaster, hospital administrators must swiftly and efficiently address the daunting tasks involved with preparing their facilities. Many hospitals are already overwhelmed with existing and ever-expanding patient needs. In the event of an infectious disease disaster, hospitals must deal with existing patients as well as incoming infected patients. Because of the sheer number of patients who may need treatment, as well as the complexity of their conditions and treatment requirements, a thorough team-oriented approach to conquer this tremendous workload is essential. There is no question that numerous challenges present to hospital facilities during these events. Concerns regarding surge capacity, staffing capabilities, staff protection, isolation, and quarantine are difficult issues to confront. However, simple actions, plans, and agreements in preparation may lend solutions to a great deal of these anxieties. Partnerships with external entities, such as local public health departments, as well as utilizing state-of-the art communications systems are critical. Hospital administrators must now face these challenges head-on and prepare, practice, and continuously evaluate their strengths and weakness in dealing with potential infectious disease disasters, because if these issues are left unaddressed, at the time these events actually hit it will be too late.

Additional Resources

1. Centers for Disease Control and Prevention. Preparedness Resources for Hospitals Web site. http://emergency.cdc.gov/healthcare/hospitals.asp. Accessed March 6, 2009.
2. United States Department of Health and Human Services. Hospital Pandemic Influenza Planning Checklist Web site. http://www.pandemicflu.gov/professional/planningtools.html. Accessed March 31, 2010.

References

1. World Health Organization. World is ill-prepared for "inevitable" flu pandemic. *Bull World Health Org.* 2004;82(4):317–318.
2. The Joint Commission on Accreditation of Healthcare Organizations. *Health Care at the Crossroads: Strategies for Creating and Sustaining Community-wide Emergency Preparedness Systems.* Oakbrook Terrace, IL: JCAHO; 2003. http://www.jointcommission.org/NR/rdonlyres/9C8DE572-5D7A-4F28-AB84-3741EC82AF98/0/emergency_preparedness.pdf. Accessed March 6, 2009.
3. United States Department of Health and Human Services. HHS Pandemic Influenza Plan Supplement 4 Infection Control. http://www.hhs.gov/pandemicflu/plan/sup4.html. Published 2009. Accessed March 6, 2009.
4. National Association of County and City Health Officials. Teaming Up for Emergency Preparedness. http://www.naccho.org/topics/emergency/MRC/resources/upload/NACCHO-and-Health-Care-Orgs-JCR-2007-2.pdf. Published 2009. Accessed March 6, 2009.
5. Apisarnthanarak A, Warren DK, Fraser VJ. Issues relevant to the adoption and modification of hospital infection-control recommendations for avian influenza (H5N1 infection) in developing countries. *Clin Infect Dis.* 2007;45(10):1338–1342.
6. Barbera JA, Macintyre AG. The reality of the modern bioterrorism response. *Lancet.* 2002;360 Suppl:s33–s34.
7. Ofner-Agostini M, Gravel D, McDonald LC, et al. Cluster of cases of severe acute respiratory syndrome among Toronto healthcare workers after implementation of infection control precautions: a case series. *Infect Control Hosp Epidemiol.* 2006; 27(5):473–478.
8. Balicer RD, Omer SB, Barnett DJ, Everly GS Jr. Local public health workers' perceptions toward responding to an influenza pandemic. *BMC Public Health.* 2006;6:99.

9.   Wong T. Concerns, perceived impact and preparedness in an avian influenza pandemic—A comparative study between healthcare workers in primary and tertiary care. *Ann Acad Med Singapore.* 2008;37(2):96–102.

10.   Centers for Disease Control and Prevention. Standard Precautions (excerpt from the guideline for isolation precautions in hospitals). CDC Web site. http://www.cdc.gov/ncidod/dhqp/gl_isolation_standard.html. Published 2007. Accessed March 6, 2009.

11.   Collignon PJ, Carnie JA. Infection control and pandemic influenza. *eMJA supplement.* http://www.mja.com.au/public/issues/185_10_201106/col10881_fm.html. Published 2006. Accessed March 6, 2009.

12.   Pourbohloul B, Meyers LA, Skowronski DM, Krajden M, Patrick DM, Brunham RC. Modeling control strategies of respiratory pathogens. *Emerg Infect Dis.* 2005;11(8):1249–1256.

13.   Centers for Disease Control and Prevention. Controlling the Spread of Contagious Diseases: Quarantine and Isolation. http://www.redcross.org/preparedness/cdc_english/IsoQuar.asp. Published 2006. Accessed March 6, 2009.

14.   Salgado CD, Farr BM, Hall KK, Hayden FG. Influenza in the acute hospital setting. *Lancet.* 2002;2(3):145–155.

15.   Rebmann, T. Preparing for pandemic influenza. *J Perinat Neonatal Nurs.* 2008; 22(3):191–202.

16.   Asia-Pacific Economic Cooperation Health Task Force. Functioning Economies in Times of Pandemic: APEC Guidelines. http://aimp.apec.org/Documents/2007/HTF/HTF2/07_htf 2_004.doc. Published 2007. Accessed March 15, 2009.

17.   Centers for Disease Control and Prevention. Predict Casualty Severity and Hospital Capacity. http://emergency.cdc.gov/masscasualities/capacity.asp. Published 2009. Accessed March 6, 2009.

18.   Lam P. Avian influenza and pandemic influenza preparedness in Hong Kong. *Ann Acad Med Singapore.* 2008;37(6):489–496.

19.   Nap RE, Andriessen MP, Meessen NE, van der Werf TS. Pandemic influenza and hospital resources. *Emerg Infect Dis.* 2007;13(11):1714–1719.

20.   Centers for Disease Control and Prevention. Emergency Preparedness Tools for Hospitals. http://emergency.cdc.gov/healthcare/hospitals.asp. Published 2009. Accessed March 6, 2009.

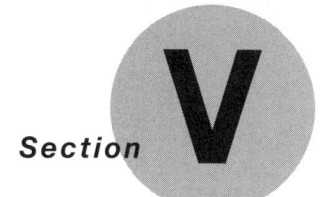

Section **V**

Special Topics

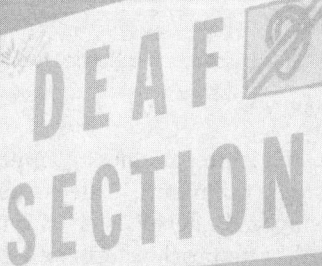

Chapter **19**

Vulnerable Populations and Public Health Disaster Preparedness

Elizabeth A. Davis, JD, EdM; Rebecca Hansen, MSW; and

Jennifer Mincin, PhD (ABD)

Photo by Andrea Booher/ FEMA

Learning Objectives

- Identify segments of the general population who have unique needs that require special consideration during disaster planning.
- Discuss how to include special and vulnerable populations in comprehensive emergency planning at a hospital or healthcare facility.
- Describe steps to improve the disaster readiness of a healthcare institution to handle special or vulnerable populations following a disaster or public health emergency.

Overview

This chapter will focus on vulnerable populations as they relate to emergency preparedness in hospitals and other healthcare facilities. This chapter also focuses on how healthcare facilities should incorporate vulnerable

371

populations into their preparedness planning and how they can best work with the larger community. Understanding the needs of vulnerable populations during and after disasters is critical to planning and preparedness so healthcare providers can better utilize available resources during a disaster.

This chapter begins and ends with a case study. Think about some of the challenges the case studies present as you read through the chapter. What did you learn? How might you have approached the disaster response differently? Remember, healthcare professionals play a vital role during disasters, especially when it comes to the care of patients and others with special needs who have been impacted by an emergency or disaster.

Case Study

Fire at Big Bear Valley, California

This case study is an excerpt from Booz Allen's *Technical Memorandum for Federal Highway Administration: Assessment of State of the Practice and State of the Art in Evacuation Transportation Management.*[1] During 2003, Southern California was besieged with 13 wildfires, one of which was called the Old Fire in the San Bernardino National Forest. The Old Fire affected many surrounding communities, including Big Bear Valley. Overall, the incident involved the voluntary evacuation of approximately 20,000–30,000 residents. Among the facilities ordered to evacuate was Bear Valley Community Hospital.

Facing a first-time evacuation of its patients, the hospital initiated its disaster plan. The evacuation of elderly patients was coordinated with the local fire department and emergency management office. Hospital staff assisted patients in packing their belongings and were also responsible for gathering and transporting medical records, as well as items for other clinical needs. A task force from American Medical Response (AMR) provided five ambulances to transport the 20 long-term residents located at the hospital. Two of the acute care residents were evacuated by air because of the lengthy ambulance trip. There were several successes of the evacuation:

- Leadership and tasks were delegated to staff. This went so well, in fact, that it only took approximately 3.5 hours to evacuate the hospital.
- Patients were boarded onto appropriate transportation vehicles along with their medical records and medications, reducing confusion later at the evacuation site.
- Because drills were conducted and plans were in place, staff members understood their roles and responsibilities and were able to respond quickly.

- The hospital had a good relationship with the local fire department and emergency management office. This established relationship proved helpful during the disaster because the evacuation was well coordinated and the hospital had continual communication and support from the first response community.

Although the evacuation was deemed a success, there were still lessons learned and challenges recognized.

Lessons Learned

- The hospital needed to develop an emergency contact information book that included not only staff information, but also that of surrounding resources, such as local nursing homes. The emergency contact list must also include a current list of emergency contacts for residents, patients, and staff.
- There is a need to have a written evacuation plan that is shared with the staff.
- There is a need to ensure there is a place to send residents/patients during an emergency.
- It is important to establish agreements with other facilities for the evacuation of patients/residents.
- It is important to pack emergency supplies that will last longer than three days, because residents were away from the hospital for five days.

Challenges and Study Questions

- While beds were found so patients could be relocated, they were scattered throughout the area. This raised concern over patients who may not be able to adjust to the new environment. Other concerns included confusion about directing family to loved ones and overly taxing staff because they would be working throughout a broader area.
  Study question: How would you address this?
- Agreements were not in place between the hospital and nursing homes.
  Study question: How would you deal with this situation and how would *you remedy it* in the future?
- While annual drills were conducted, the staff was not well exercised in evacuations.
  Study question: How would you better prepare staff for future evacuations?

Introduction

While the federal government, states, and localities have begun in earnest to better address special needs issues, debates still exist where best practices are concerned. This chapter may not answer all existing questions when it comes to special needs issues, but it will provide an overview of this population segment and highlight key ways to work with and engage those with special needs. This information may prove quite helpful to state and local entities, as well as hospital preparedness staff trying to address these issues. However, there is still debate among key planners at the national level over different components of the planning (e.g., the very definition of "special needs populations" is widely contested). Therefore, as local emergency planners and healthcare professionals, it is important to utilize national guidance and become familiar with the latest opinions and views on these issues; however, you will find that solutions come locally, through resources and participation in emergency management activities. Additionally, information on this topic is increasingly being made available within specific industry texts, manuals, newsletters, and so forth. For example, texts including chapters on disability and emergency planning are now available in the field of nursing.[2] It is important to immediately begin to take steps that will improve your community's overall capabilities to meet its emergency needs.

The catastrophic events of 9/11 and Hurricanes Katrina and Rita led to some advancement in greater integration of special needs issues as they relate to emergency management planning at the national level. Much advancement has been made that has yet to be seen. With hurricanes intensifying (as evidenced with the 2008 hurricane season) and man-made threats continual, now, more than ever, emergency professionals must be more prepared and ready to respond. Disasters will always exist and if we, as emergency managers and healthcare professionals, can work together with vulnerable populations to better prepare these communities, then more lives will be saved. While new guidance documents and revisions of existing plans, such as the National Response Framework and other federal activities, reflect a purposeful strategic approach for addressing special needs issues before, during, and after disasters, it is unclear how it will be presented to states and localities. For example, will it be presented as federal directives, mandates tied to funding, or guidance to assist communities? An example would be the 2009 funding of CDC Preparedness Research Centers, which required inclusion of special and vulnerable populations. As emergency managers and health professionals address special needs, it is important they continually keep updated on new and changing federal guidelines, mandates, regulations, and opportunities for funding. After the devastation caused by Hurricane Katrina, one important change on the federal level was the Post-Katrina Emergency Management Reform Act of 2006 (discussed later in the chapter).

Defining and Understanding Vulnerable Populations

Some emergency managers and public health professionals may consider all people who face crisis or disaster to be vulnerable, and certainly that is the case. Anyone who is facing the threat of a Category 3 hurricane, a sudden but extended power outage, or a widespread fire is indeed vulnerable. However, there are certain segments of the population who may be at an additional disadvantage compared to that of the general population.[3] While definitions of "vulnerable populations" differ, as do definitions of "special needs," it is ultimately up to each jurisdiction, hospital, and agency to determine who in their community will need additional assistance and specialized resources. The National Emergency Management Resource Center (NEMRC) asserts that while "much controversy exists within the emergency management and disability advocacy field over the term 'special needs' and who should be included . . . each jurisdiction has an obligation to conduct community assessments and identify people within their population who may need additional assistance and support" (NEMRC, 2008).

Vulnerable populations may include the following people:

- **People with acute medical conditions, chronic diseases, and the medically fragile/frail, including the full age spectrum, from pediatric to geriatric:** Those with acute medical conditions or chronic diseases may include people with temporary or episodic as well as chronic conditions, such as cancer, Alzheimer's, multiple sclerosis, cerebral palsy, heart disease (e.g., congestive heart arthrosclerosis and congestive obstructive pulmonary disease), diabetes, and so forth. In addition to those patients with chronic diseases, a subset consists of those who many refer to as medically frail. These are individuals who have medical conditions that often require careful monitoring and the slightest illness, injury, or even disruption in their care routine can lead to significant medical decompensation. Examples of individuals this applies to may include patients with cancer on chemotherapy who cannot fight infection and may have limited nutritional reserves. In a disaster, they are especially vulnerable to infections and to the effects of relocation, including evacuation and altered nutritional sources. Another example might be a diabetic who has difficultly controlling this disease. If, under normal conditions, the diabetes is difficult to control, one can see that when his or her activity and/or diet is altered because of a disaster, that his or her blood glucose levels will certainly get out of control.

- **People with disabilities, including the full age spectrum from pediatric to geriatric:** Disabilities include cognitive, physical, and sensory impairments. (Further definition is discussed later in this chapter.)

- **Age specific:** Children and the elderly (without pre-disaster disability or medical conditions) may have specific and unique needs during a disaster. For example, childhood absorption rates through skin contact differ from that of an adult, they are closer to the ground level, and they may not be able to assist in injury reporting because of their age. Disaster-related trauma and physical injury need to be addressed differently, especially during triage. Many of the standard triage tools are based on verbal response and normal adult vital signs, which would be inappropriate for use with children. There are some modified standards for children, but none have been validated. In addition, children may require systems to be put in place that are not needed for other populations. An example would be the need for systems of identification of children who become separated from their guardians and a reunification process that confirms the identity of their caregivers. A similar system can be used to reunite elderly individuals who have conditions, like Alzheimer's, with their family members.

- **Low income:** Generally, poverty in the United States is determined by the poverty "income line." According to the Institute for Research on Poverty, the 2009 threshold for a family of four is just $22,050.[4] Income issues do not discriminate and include people who have disabilities; the old and the young; people from any religious, racial, or cultural and ethnic background; or people with any sexual orientation; as well as single people or married people with families. All individuals from these groups may be dealing with income problems and poverty issues. Working with low income communities is critical because many people with limited incomes may not have cars; may have limited food and other disaster supplies (if any); and they may have a range of additional challenges, such as the inability to rebuild or find employment after a disaster. Poverty and health are directly related, without question, which results in major impacts from disasters, as well as impacts on a person's ability to prepare for an emergency. If someone is worried about finances for daily living, why would he or she be concerned with preparing for a disaster or obtain the funds for preparedness expenditures? In the economic climate of 2008–2010, this reality only became magnified.

- **Immigrant (both documented and undocumented):** According to *The Free Dictionary*, an online dictionary, a person who is an immigrant "has come into a foreign country to live there permanently, not as a tourist or visitor" (http://www.thefreedictionary.com/immigrant). Immigrants may include political asylums and refugees allowed into the country from conflict regions or individuals and families who have come to work. Immigrants are a significant and important part of the population and have unique needs during disaster. As one example, the Tomas Rivera Policy Institute conducted a study regarding the unique needs of immigrants during a disaster and found that access to information is a key issue.[5] Also, it is clear that status impacts access to health care as well as trust in those who provide the care. Fear may lead to delays in seeking care and obtaining care at different locations, thereby making surveillance difficult and increasing the potential for transmission of certain agents. Further, this may make communicating about critical information more challenging.

- **Non-English speaking/English proficiency:** The non-English speaking population includes people whose first language is not English, but also people who are illiterate or marginally literate and/or have literacy issues. This group may have difficulty receiving and understanding instructions given to the public. Because health literacy may be low, medical information transmitted to the public may be ignored by this group—not because of choice, but because of lack of understanding. The CDC has focused on providing information and resources to healthcare providers in the United States over the last few years on the importance of health literacy and using non-medical language to interact with patients.

- **Homeless:** According to the National Law Center on Homelessness and Poverty, approximately 3.5 million people—including 1.35 million children—are likely to experience homelessness in a given year.[6] Homelessness can be either permanent or temporary. Realistically, the number may in fact be higher; it is difficult, however, to calculate an accurate number, given the level of transience within the population.

DEFINING DISABILITY

All preparedness efforts must be inclusive of the needs of the entire general population, but it is also important to analyze the unique needs of the differing vulnerable groups. Disability, because it comes with specific legal definitions, rules, and guidance materials, should be evaluated as a unique entity. According to the EAD & Associates Special Needs Toolkit,[7] "disability" is its own area, requiring specific attention. The following excerpt from the Toolkit outlines ways in which jurisdictions, healthcare agencies, and hospitals may want to define "vulnerable" and "special needs" populations:

Disability

■ Types of disabilities (includes full age spectrum from pediatric to geriatric)
   ● Physical (i.e., severe arthritis, spinal cord injuries, people who use wheelchairs, people with multiple sclerosis, etc.)
   ● Sensory (people who are blind, deaf, hard of hearing, etc.)
   ● Cognitive (people with mental illness, learning disabilities, mental retardation/developmental disabilities, etc.)

Co-existing disabilities—It is important to keep in mind that some individuals have co-existing disabilities (e.g., physical disability and deafness, blind and deaf, etc.).

Overlap of aging and disability—There is a high correlation between being elderly and having a disability. According to the U.S. Census, there are over 14 million people over the age of 65 who have one or more disabilities.

Medically vulnerable—Some examples include:

■ People who are homebound and not receiving services
■ People receiving home-based care services of any sort
■ People in care facilities (i.e., assisted living, residential care facilities, nursing homes, group homes, etc.)
■ Those dependent on caretakers or life-sustaining equipment (i.e., someone who is bedridden and uses a ventilator)
■ Those with mental illness
■ Homeless populations (since there tends to be an overlap with mental illness and/or health-related illness and homelessness)
■ Alcohol/substance abuse patients

LEGAL STATUS, VULNERABLE POPULATIONS, AND DISASTERS

The law protects vulnerable populations in a number of ways. People with disabilities, for example, are protected under the Americans with Disabilities Act[8] (ADA). The following list identifies legislation and the population segment it protects as well as legislation that related to vulnerable populations during disasters:

- **Americans with Disabilities Act (ADA), 1990 and 2008:** According to the ADA, persons with disabilities are a protected class. An individual is defined as someone with a disability if he or she:
  - has a physical or mental impairment that substantially limits a major life activity; and/or
  - has a record of such an impairment; and/or
  - is regarded as having such an impairment.
- **Post-Katrina Emergency Management Reform Act of 2006:** The Robert T. Stafford Disaster Relief and Emergency Assistance Act (1974) establishes the presidential disaster declaration system and outlines various federal agency functions during a disaster. The Federal Emergency Management Agency (FEMA) is the designated lead and coordinating agency that establishes guidelines and grants for state and local governments in addition to providing assistance during disasters. Prior to Hurricane Katrina, there were no specific provisions in the Stafford Act for people with disabilities. After the horrific events of Hurricane Katrina, however, new legislation was introduced that incorporated the needs of people with disabilities; the Post-Katrina Act specifically makes provisions for the following special needs issues: inclusion of people with disabilities in every phase of emergency management at all levels of government; planning for recovery services to victims and their families; accessibility of temporary and replacement housing; nondiscrimination on the basis of disability; and the establishment of a national disability coordinator position at FEMA.
- **Older Americans Act of 1965 (OAA):** The OAA, similar to the ADA, provides grants to states for community planning and services. In addition, the OAA is an antidiscrimination law that classifies older Americans as a legally protected class.
- **Health Insurance Portability and Accountability Act (HIPAA):** The HIPAA patient-rights-based legislation was passed in 1996 to address the issue of health privacy for patients. The law requires uniform federal privacy protections for individually identifiable health information. The U.S. Department of Health and Human Services recently issued final regulations implementing the privacy provisions of HIPAA, called the "Privacy Rule." This regulation, while protecting patients' health information, does pose challenges during disasters. Examples include barriers to obtaining

medical information in a time of disaster for patients who present outside their normal care facilities and difficulty with sharing patient information for the purpose of identifying victims. Since this time, HIPAA has added certain provisions for emergency preparedness situations, but they do not fully overcome all obstacles.

■ **U.S. Health and Human Services (HHS) and the Pandemic and All-Hazards Preparedness Act, 2006:**[16] "The term 'at-risk individuals' means children, pregnant women, senior citizens, and other individuals who have special needs in the event of a public health emergency, as determined by the Secretary." The Centers for Disease Control (CDC) suggests that many health departments use a similar definition:

> [G]roups whose needs are not fully addressed by traditional service providers or who feel they cannot comfortably or safely access and use the standard resources offered in disaster preparedness, relief, and recovery. They include, but are not limited to, those who are physically or mentally disabled (blind, deaf, hard-of-hearing, cognitive disorders, mobility limitations), limited or non-English speaking, geographically or culturally isolated, medically or chemically dependent, homeless, frail/elderly, and children (CDC, 2004).

It is also important to keep in mind other changes on the federal level that affect emergency planning and special needs populations aside from legislation. This includes the 2004 *Executive Order* and the creation of the *Interagency Coordinating Council*. Known as Executive Order 13347,[10] it is designed to strengthen emergency preparedness with respect to individuals with disabilities; it directs the federal government to address the needs of people with disabilities in disasters and created the Interagency Coordinating Council on Emergency Preparedness and Individuals with Disabilities (ICC).

DISABILITY AND COMPLYING WITH THE ADA

It is expected that all healthcare, emergency management, and government agencies comply with federal law when it comes to accessibility and people with disabilities—especially during disasters. FEMA's report, *Accommodating Individuals with Disabilities in the Provision of Disaster Mass Care, Housing, and Human Services,*[11] outlines key nondiscrimination points for emergency managers and healthcare professionals during disaster, such as the following points:

■ **Inclusion:** People with disabilities must be able to participate in and receive the benefits of emergency programs, services, and activities provided by governments, private businesses, and nonprofit organizations.

- **Integration:** Emergency programs, services, and activities typically must be provided in an integrated setting. The provision of services, such as sheltering, information intake for disaster services, and short-term housing in integrated settings, keeps individuals connected to their support system and caregivers and avoids the need for disparate service facilities.
- **Physical access:** Emergency programs, services, and activities must be provided at locations that are accessible to people with disabilities. People with disabilities should be able to enter and use emergency facilities and access the programs, services, and activities that are provided, including parking lots, entrances, and exits to buildings, shelters, bathrooms and bathing facilities, dining facilities, areas where medical care or human services are provided, and paths of travel to and from these areas.
- **Equal access:** People with disabilities must be able to access and benefit from emergency programs, services, and activities equal to the general population, such as emergency preparedness information, notification of emergencies, evacuation, transportation, communication, shelter, food, first aid, medical care, housing, and long-term recovery assistance programs.
- **Effective communication:** Information must be made available in alternate formats so that people with disabilities can access it.

Brief Sociological Discussion: Medical Model vs Functional Model

The concept of the "medical model" is one that assumes certain characteristics about an individual based on the "condition" or "illness" of the individual. Outside of a well-informed healthcare arena, however, this tells us little about the actual capabilities or limitations of the individual. From this information alone, we are unable to determine if an individual has a disaster-related "special need" that will require some assistance from the community during an actual disaster. The medical model treats the person with a disability as someone with a "problem" or "illness" rather than as an actual person with limitations and capabilities. The focus is often on "diagnosis" and not what the person can do alone or may need assistance to do. According to Simon Brisenden, "The medical model of disability is one rooted in an undue emphasis on clinical diagnosis, the very nature of which is destined to lead to a partial and inhibiting view of the disabled individual."[12]

Therefore, we should approach each population group/individual not as homogenous, but with the expectation that there will be varying levels and types of assistance required during emergencies. This is the basis for the functional model approach that is useful for planning purposes. Planners will work with service providers and individuals with special needs to identify the actual needs that will require addressing in emergency plans. This approach also helps planners to identify appropriate resources and practical solutions that will support individuals in all stages of an emergency. This can only be done well if a partnership is formed among the emergency planning community and participants of varying special needs populations within the community.

The functional model took hold in the United Sates in the 1970s during the Independent Living Movement (ILM), thereby helping to empower people with disabilities (Tierney & Hahn, 1986). The ILM, along with the deinstitutionalization that was occurring simultaneously, meant that people with various types of disabilities were now living in the community rather than in nursing homes or similar types of facilities (Tierney & Hahn, 1986). This enabled and empowered people with disabilities to become a part of society. It also meant dealing with a society that was still holding on to stereotypes and a society in which barriers were not completely removed. Certainly, people with disabilities have seen improvements in the 21st century, mostly resulting from advocacy organizations. However, much still remains to be done in terms of eradicating prejudice, ensuring all communities are fully accessible, and ensuring that appropriate and necessary support systems are strong and accessible. Emergency managers and healthcare professionals must be aware of people with disabilities and other vulnerable populations living within their community. That is why it is critical to plan with and for people with disabilities during disasters.

Some examples, as outlined in the *Special Needs Toolkit* (EAD & Associates, LLC, 2007), demonstrate the functional model approach:

- You may identify the deaf community as a group of people that will likely have special needs that need to be addressed during emergencies. However, just knowing that they are deaf does little to help with planning. Instead, by working with this community, you can begin to identify the actual needs as they relate to emergency situations. For instance, when considering emergency communications, it will be necessary to identify different ways to ensure that emergency notifications and warnings are received and acted upon by individuals who are deaf. In working with the deaf community, you can identify the best modalities that are likely to be used by people who are deaf and incorporate them into your plan.
- For some people who use a wheelchair or scooter, ensuring general population shelters are accessible is a "functional" way to plan. If shelters are not wheelchair accessible, not

only is this a violation of the ADA, shelter managers are potentially placing the individual in harm's way. Further, the person in a wheelchair may unnecessarily be sent away from a general population shelter to a medical needs shelter or perhaps even the hospital. During a crisis or disaster, this further overwhelms an already overburdened system needlessly. If an individual in a wheelchair can self-sustain, it is best to utilize the functional model approach and choose general population shelters that are accessible and ADA compliant.

Healthcare Community

IMPACT OF DISASTER ON VULNERABLE POPULATIONS

- Transfer trauma and other unique issues.
- Disconnection from services/providers.
- Need for medication, medical equipment, and supplies, etc.
- The medically fragile and those with disabilities are often reliant upon specialty services and support. These services and support are often the first to be diverted for disaster surge without any considerations to the impact on special populations. Examples include visiting nurse services:
  - Visiting nurse services are often asked to reassign their nursing personnel to assist with a large disaster response, but in their absence, who is going to care for their patients/client base? While some clients can do without visiting nurse services (VNS) for a short period of time, most cannot self-sustain for the long-term. If you add registered nurses to the hospital from VNS, but in return, cause those patients to seek care in a hospital using hospital resources when they could be cared for at home, you have not added to disaster resources, but in actuality reduced resources available. As such, registered nurse support services like VNS must not be fully removed or these patients will be forced to seek hospital care. At a community level, judgment will need to be made regarding how many nurses to pull from VNS to help with hospital surge but still leave enough to keep home care patients at home.

HEALTHCARE FACILITIES

- **Hospitals:** With regard to hospitals, there are several key issues in addition to the important information regarding special and vulnerable patients presented throughout this chapter. The following issues are included:

- The extent and diversity of those with special needs in our community, who may, in a time of disaster, require emergent care may be understated. This knowledge is vital to ensure appropriate training of staff, stockpiling of medications and medical devices, and sufficient capacity to handle these individuals.

- It is necessary to understand all elements of the population served to allow hospital drills and exercises to reflect the true challenges hospitals will face in times of disaster.

- Plan for the needs of persons who are technologically dependent. One of the large groups of special populations who require assistance in a disaster consists of those who are technologically dependant. The common misconception is their need for medical care when, in fact, they need the items the disaster has often removed. This may be as simple as power, food, water, and, in some cases, medication, equipment, or medial gasses. This misconception often leads to placement of these persons in inpatient units when, in some cases, all they may need is power. For example, a home ventilator-dependent patient who loses power but has no medical issues may be admitted to an intensive care unit when, in actuality, all they need is to be placed in any common room, even an auditorium or cafeteria, that has access to power and space for their normal home caregiver, if one is needed.

- Consideration of persons with disabilities is needed in typical disaster activities, such as decontamination, isolation, and quarantine. For example, do hospitals include in their decontamination plan, a plan for decontamination of a service animal? What about durable medical goods or medical equipment? If they cannot be decontaminated, are replacement procedures in place? These are essential planning considerations for a hospital that the community it serves expects. Other issues exist, such as matters of ADA compliance. While the hospital itself may be ADA compliant, are all surge facilities/sites ADA compliant? If not, this may require a person with a disability to receive care in an acute care area when not medically indicated because the alternate care site is not ADA compliant or does not have the necessary resources to accommodate a blind person or someone who is deaf, for example. This lack of preparedness for persons with disabilities will cause acute and critical care resources to be used for a patient whose medical needs could be met in an alternate care facility or medical needs shelter.

- With regard to quarantine and isolation, one must not only consider the basic needs of patients, but the needs of special populations. With regard to children and the elderly, this is the ability to provide family-based care and keep both children and elderly in quarantine and isolation, if medically appropriate, with their family. This also includes the ability to accommodate service animals in these areas and to involve veterinarians in the process to discuss risk to the service animal and, if needed, prophylaxis or treatment.

Residential healthcare facilities (i.e., nursing homes): The following topics are key issues for these facilities:

- The ability to obtain the necessary resources, such as staff, medicine, and equipment, in times of disaster when they are scarce and may be preferentially provided to acute care facilities is important. This may require preplanning for alternate supply chains and/or stockpiling.
- These facilities may also be used as surge facilities and should be at a minimum prepared to take:
  - patients from other residential facilities who may need to be evacuated;
  - persons from the community who are reliant upon caregivers, VNS, or services that have been disrupted; and
  - patients who would normally be treated in an acute care facility but, because of the numbers of patients seen in a disaster, cannot be accommodated in the acute care facility but still require some level of inpatient medical care.
- Payment and reimbursement issues often arise for patients changing provider services, particularly if the provider is in another state, because many of the public healthcare benefits are administered at the state level and are unprepared to coordinate care provisions in this way. This is true of many of the care system models and complicates the continuum of care efforts.

Other care facilities, such as dialysis centers, methadone clinics, and day treatment centers: Emergency planning must be conducted internally within each of these outpatient facilities, across networks, and with emergency management. The End Stage Renal Disease Network of New York has developed emergency planning guides that, while directed at dialysis centers, can be helpful to other types of care facilities. This information is available at http://www.esrd.ipro.org/index/emergency-planning. According to the American Association of Homes and Services for the Aging,[13] it is estimated that there are more than 1.4 million people living in nursing homes, 900,000 in assisted living residences, 150,000 individuals receiving care and services at adult day centers, and 1.1 million seniors in some type of senior housing communities in the United States. Congregate and residential care facilities include nursing homes, assisted living centers, drug treatment centers, group homes, residential homes, foster homes, adult and childcare facilities, and so forth.

In 2006, the General Accountability Office (GAO) released a report, *Disaster Preparedness: Preliminary Observations on the Evacuation of Vulnerable Populations due to Hurricanes and Other Disasters*, on evacuating vulnerable populations, which states:

> Hospital and nursing home administrators face challenges related to evacuations caused by hurricanes, including deciding whether to evacuate and obtaining transportation. Although state and local governments can order evacuations, health care facilities can be exempt from these orders. Facility administrators are generally responsible for deciding whether to evacuate, and if they decide not to evacuate, they face the challenge of ensuring that their facilities have sufficient resources to provide care until assistance arrives. If they evacuate, contractors providing transportation for hospitals and nursing homes could be unlikely to provide facilities with enough vehicles during a major disaster, such as a hurricane because local demand for transportation would likely exceed supply. Nursing home administrators told us they face unique challenges during evacuations. For example, they must locate receiving facilities that can accommodate residents who may need a place to live for a long period of time.[14]

Preparedness

In your hospital, care facility, or community, one of the ways to assist the special needs populations in getting ready for an emergency is to emphasize the importance of preparedness. The issues that special needs populations might face before, during, and in the aftermath of an incident do not rest on one individual; rather, everyone within the community and vulnerable populations shares the responsibility. Each person and all entities must do their best to be prepared for emergencies with warning (e.g., a hurricane) as well as spontaneous incidents (e.g., an earthquake). Of course, there are those that will not be able to plan for themselves, such as people who are in critical care facilities, people who require close supervision, and others who require a primary caregiver by their side. Individuals living in these facilities or who are living at home will be dependant upon how well prepared and coordinated response and recovery efforts of the facility and/or their caregivers are. It is important for facilities and caregivers to have plans in place with patients and their families. In addition, having a communication system in place with family, friends, and caregivers is essential when dealing with people who are not capable of creating or carrying out plans.

It is vital to collaborate with agencies in local communities that are engaged in emergency preparedness education, such as local American Red Cross chapters, the local emergency management office, the state emergency management office, the United Way, The Salvation Army, and so many others. Also, be sure to include hospitals and care facilities, as well as services such as home-based care, in the planning process. It is vital that hospitals not exclude themselves from the planning process and working with local volunteer organizations and government entities, because this type of planning may very well ensure the survival of patients during disaster. It is important for hospitals to know the patients in their community, including their vulnerabilities and their needs. Without this information, a hospital that is viewed by the community as the safe haven during times of disaster may not have the necessary resources to be prepared for the unique needs of vulnerable populations coming in from their community. In some cases, community organizations can provide additional resources to help hospitals to provide care for segments of their population with less critical needs so that limited medical resources can be directed to the fragile and those in critical need of medical attention. Without these resources, a hospital could be stymied by the worried well and have no capability to care for those truly in need. The worried well may also include those with special healthcare needs that, with preplanning with these organizations, can be cared for in other locations. An example is a ventilator patient typically living at home, who in a disaster may only need a room, available food, and a power strip for their home ventilator, which all could be provided by a community organization. Whereas, in a hospital, they might inappropriately occupy an ICU bed, thus depriving a critical patient of that needed resource. Because the patient maintains good function every day of his or her life at home without a medical environment—just power and basic necessities—all they will need in a disaster may be the same.

Common ways of engaging agencies in the community regarding preparedness are identified in the following list:

- Schedule a meeting with the agencies engaged in emergency preparedness in your community and ensure they understand what messages need to be delivered to the special needs populations living there.
- Do what you can to assist those agencies in getting the word out to the public. This might mean that your agency will need to designate a few people to receive training in delivering the

emergency preparedness presentation and then have them present the material to various audiences, or it might mean your agency will need to make a financial donation to the agency informing the public. However you choose to develop the partnership, simply remember that it is an important one.

- Assist the emergency preparedness agencies in your community in distributing pamphlets, guides, and/or other materials.
- Negotiate a co-branding agreement wherein your agency is permitted to reprint other agencies' materials with your agency's logo.
- **Remember to not always focus on the "needs" of the special needs populations in your community; remember their abilities as well.** Emergency preparedness, response, and recovery begins at the individual level and assisting people in being prepared, where appropriate, will ultimately make your job easier when an incident occurs.

PLANNING GUIDANCE AND CONSIDERATIONS: PLANNING WITH, NOT FOR

The following checklist is for ensuring that special needs issues are integrated into emergency plans and other initiatives. **Please note**: An aggressive public education program must support even the best plans so that the information is disseminated to individuals with special needs as well as the providers and organizations that work with them.

- Identify planning team members using a matrix that recognizes diverse interests, contributions, and resources.
  - Contact key organizations and subject matter experts to review the list and make recommendations.
  - Organize the initial planning team.
  - Establish ongoing meetings and reviews. (Get buy-in from the organizations to continually be a part of the planning and response process; this includes education outreach into the disability and special needs community.)
  - Determine jurisdictional strategies, timelines, and community needs.
- Identify and develop resources to address the needs of special needs populations within your community. This might include examining existing Web sites, hotlines, brochures, flyers, the Emergency Alert System (EAS), 211 systems, media outlets, volunteer groups, and communication technologies (pagers, calling systems, etc.).
- The special needs community is very diverse and not monolithic. As such, there is no "one quick fix" that will meet all

the needs of all members of the special needs populations. Therefore, plans should include a variety of viable options and should be ability-focused (functional approach).

- People from vulnerable populations should be actively recruited and integrated into volunteer emergency management programs, including hospital or nursing home volunteer programs, for example. Consider the following questions:
  - Are seniors and people with disabilities active participants in Community Emergency Response Teams (CERT) or the Medical Reserve Corps (MRC)?
  - Are seniors and people with disabilities a part of emergency management/healthcare planning, awareness education, and preparedness outreach?
  - Are emergency managers and healthcare professionals recruiting from and working with key organizations, such as schools for the deaf or schools for the blind?
- Coordinate with the people from vulnerable populations (such as the disability, aging, and immigrant communities) in establishing cross-training for first responders and the special needs population, as well as with the staff of healthcare services and facilities.
- The medically fragile may be dependent upon their caregivers to plan for, manage, and provide appropriate transportation to various sites, such as shelters or points of distribution. Without a disaster transportation plan for the medically fragile, these individuals could face tremendous risks during major disasters. Local jurisdictions need to take this into consideration when planning. The transportation of the medically fragile may require resources similar to those needed by hospitals for disaster response or evacuation. These critical special and medical needs transport mechanisms and vehicle use must be coordinated by the local Office of Emergency Management (OEM) so the needs of both the hospitals and the medically fragile are met. In addition, the hospitals should advocate for a functional disaster transport system for the medically fragile. If these patients do not have transportation to caregivers and caregivers to them, to medical outpatient appointments and services, or to obtain basic necessities of daily living (including items such as medications and durable medical equipment), their only avenue for help will be getting assistance at a local hospital.
- Consistently reexamine, test, and update systems pertaining to people with disabilities and those with other unique disaster-related needs and emergencies. Each jurisdiction and

their health community should consider including the special needs component during tabletops, exercises, and drills.

SPECIAL NEEDS ADVISORY PANELS AND VULNERABLE POPULATION WORKING GROUPS

Since 2001, several communities throughout the United States, notably New Jersey and Illinois, have started individual groups called a Special Needs Advisory Panel (SNAP). These may have been built on existing planning or may be new initiatives for a community. Others may not call their planning groups or advisory panels "SNAPs" but instead refer to them as special needs planning groups or task forces. No matter what the name, the important aspect is bringing the right people in a community together to plan for special needs populations before, during, and after disasters.

Health professionals should keep in mind that they play an important role in SNAPs and other special needs/vulnerable population working groups and should consider either leading such a group or supporting one. Special needs planning groups bring together an array of stakeholders and emergency management to coordinate and develop plans detailing how the community will address special needs of community members during emergencies. Developing relationships is a key goal for a SNAP or any working group and often is a big step for a community.

Special needs and vulnerable population working groups can help to determine and set priorities for how a community will work before, during, and after a disaster to address special needs. It is important to recognize that the road to a working plan is arduous, but identifying key areas and building the plan step-by-step helps to make it more manageable. In terms of vulnerable population working groups, some communities will break into subgroups, such as one dedicated to disability issues or one dedicated to immigrant issues. These types of working groups can assist agencies with identifying and coordinating resources required for special needs populations before a disaster occurs. Often, the resources needed are limited, even during nondisaster times. Therefore, it is important to pool resources from entities within your community (e.g., government, non-profit, faith-based, and the private sector) and identify gaps so that additionally needed regional, state, or federal resources are identified prior to an incident.

Another important aspect to working groups, and certainly an important aspect to overall emergency management and healthcare planning, is improving the overall ability to communicate preparedness and emergency information to people in the community who have special needs. For example, ensuring that emergency information is in alternate formats, shelters have American Sign Language interpreters, televised press conferences have visible ASL interpreters, and crawl spaces on the television do not block closed captioning, are all critical to people with specific disabilities in receiving emergency information. This also includes making sure information is in other languages, per your community's demographics.

Developing emergency plans for any issue in any community takes time; it takes commitment and you will need to think about new ways to address the issues you will face. Most importantly, you cannot work at this exclusively; you must be inclusive and invite the right people to the planning table. As you will discover, leadership is a shared role in which all stakeholders must actively participate.

PLANNING ASSUMPTIONS AND IMPACT OF DISASTERS ON THE DISABILITY COMMUNITY

There are certain planning assumptions emergency managers and public health professionals alike should consider when planning for emergencies. These may include the following items:

- A need for in-home services (e.g., meals, at-home nursing) will increase, depending on the duration of the event.
- Placements in residential care facilities caused by long-term health effects will increase.
- Mortality rates will increase significantly because of physical and emotional impacts.
- People must access and comprehend information in a variety of different ways and messaging must reflect this approach.
- A comprehensive emergency plan that incorporates the needs of the special needs population not only benefits people with special needs, but the general public as well. Always remain focused on **ability** (functional model). Remaining ability-focused is not just applicable to the disability population, but to all populations.

Community Preparedness and Disaster Education

An integral aspect to planning is education outreach on emergency preparedness for vulnerable populations (e.g., disability, aging, immigrant, homeless). Directly involve experts from the various special needs community groups (such as disability advocacy groups, immigrant advocacy groups, social service organizations, homeless shelters, and soup kitchens) to help educate constituents about plans and individual preparedness roles. It is vital for the general public, as well as people with disabilities, to understand the response plan during an event so they have an appropriate expectation of what the government can and cannot do. Further, early education about an event will allow individuals and their support networks to plan ahead.

Developing Plans Based on the Four Phases: Mitigation, Planning, Response, and Recovery

Discussion of developing hospital emergency preparedness plans is covered in other chapters. The key here is to ensure that the unique needs and considerations elaborated in this chapter are incorporated as an integral part of the preparedness plan and not merely an annex or cursory mention. This planning integration can only be accomplished by inclusion in the planning process of those with expertise in the needs of vulnerable populations and representatives of the vulnerable population community.

Working with the Community

A community assessment, focused on identifying special needs populations, can be accomplished through various methods. Because identifying special needs populations is complex, and some people are affiliated with organizations or agencies while others are not, it is recommended to use several sources of information to get a close-to-accurate picture of your community. The community hospital, viewed by the community as their healthcare safety net and safe haven in times of disaster, in addition to being their backup source for medical care and medical resources (e.g., equipment, pharmaceuticals, and durable medical equipment), needs to understand the variety and numbers of special needs persons in their community. This will also allow the hospital to be prepared to meet these needs and to develop alternatives within their community to address these needs.

It is easier to identify individuals with special needs who are affiliated in some way with a service agency. Working closely with these agencies you can begin to identify:

- the approximate number of people who have special needs
- types of special needs
- resources required to assist those with special needs
- locations that have high concentrations (e.g., a senior residential community and a school for the blind)

Also, in 2004 the CDC developed a workbook, *Public Health Workbook to Define, Locate and Reach Special, Vulnerable, and At-Risk Populations in an Emergency (Draft)*, that provides useful guidance in regard to identifying and defining special needs in your community. The workbook can be found at http://www.bt.cdc.gov/workbook/pdf/ph_workbook_draft.pdf.

COLLABORATE WITH OTHER AGENCIES THAT WORK WITH VULNERABLE POPULATIONS

Various organizations and social service agencies that work with vulnerable populations bring different resources to the table. By pooling resources, you can find creative solutions to gaps or shortages. For example, a working group was finding that it was difficult to handle the administrative work and that no one had time to dedicate to implement strategies they had developed. To resolve this, one group offered a cubicle space with a computer, phone, and printer; another agency offered health benefits; and another agency offered a salary. Together, they were able to bring on board a full-time person dedicated to the working group.

VOLUNTEER SUPPORT

Research and identify volunteer programs that can support your efforts. All over the country, volunteers are involved in disaster mitigation, preparedness, response, and recovery activities, and this includes the healthcare community. They are a tremendous resource for communities. Some examples include national organizations, but do not forget to include the volunteer programs within your own community. With some training and guidance, these volunteers can be great assets to move your vulnerable populations' work forward. The Medical Reserve Corps has successfully integrated volunteers into planning, response, and recovery. Putnam County has a very active and used Medical Reserve Corps that staffs Points of Dispensing (PODs) and provides surge help for community medical shelters and alternate care sites. In addition, by medical providers participating in organized government medical response systems, they are afforded support and protection, such as liability protection, training, and solutions for issues, such as licensure and certification.

- **Citizen Corps:** These are national programs that are implemented in local communities. This includes CERT, Fire Corps, USAonWatch.org, and Medical Reserve Corps.
- **AmeriCorps:** This is a program that assigns volunteers to government, non-profits, and corporate agencies nationwide. AmeriCorps has been involved in emergency management and social services since its inception in 1993. For example: One local emergency management agency that had one individual to work on special needs issues decided to participate in the AmeriCorps program and was able to assign a volunteer to help develop the special needs plan, and another

volunteer to assist with pulling together a Voluntary Organization Active in Disaster (VOAD). Once established, they were able to get new volunteers each year to support these efforts.

Case Study

Hurricane Andrew 1992

Unfortunately, there is no shortage of disasters to look at and specific situations to learn from regarding preparedness, response, recovery, and special needs populations. Although Hurricane Katrina, and to a lesser extent the terrorist attacks of September 11, 2001, brought the needs of special needs populations to the forefront, this issue has been around a long time. Prior to Hurricanes Katrina and Rita, Hurricane Andrew in 1992 was the costliest and most devastating hurricane in the United States. Keep in mind that for this case study, we look back at Hurricane Andrew. However, the issue of nursing home preparedness remains overlooked, underregulated, and not adequate enough, which has yielded devastating results. Consider a report from CNN on nursing home preparedness during Hurricane Katrina:

> Out of 72 nursing homes, only 21 of them complied with the minimum licensing standards for emergency preparedness. Nineteen facilities had one fault in their plans—either they didn't have adequate generators or they didn't have a bus contract to evacuate. Then there are the other 32 nursing homes that had multiple gaps in their emergency preparations—not only did they not have generators, they also didn't have a plan for how or when to evacuate (Towey, 2006).

Hurricane Andrew

On August 24, 1992, Hurricane Andrew hit Homestead, Florida as a Category 5 hurricane, the most powerful and devastating of hurricane categories. The Miami Jewish Home and Hospital for the Aged (MJHHA), a long-term care facility in Miami, survived Hurricane Andrew with some successes and many lessons learned.[15] Staff at MJHHA encountered the following critical challenges after Andrew passed:

- Electric service was disrupted with temperatures in the 90s after the storm and no air conditioning was available. Most residents had to be constantly monitored for dehydration and other complications.
- Water for drinking, bathing, and flushing toilets had to be carried manually to every level within the building.
- Staff members who reported to MJHHA prior to the storm and stayed for the duration were emotionally and physically

drained, especially because most staff members were unable to reach the facility, leaving a small team to manage more than 1,000 elderly patients.
■ According to the Administration on Aging (AOA) report,

> Perhaps the single issue that most traumatized the patients transferred and the staff that received them was the inadequate patient identification. In a number of instances, the caregivers "disappeared" leaving helpless, demented people with no information, as to medication, medical problems and other patient information. Other shelters received large numbers of residents, virtually "dumped" from nursing homes, for their day-to-day care. Many incontinent elderly were brought to shelters with no medications, diapers, or other supplies.

What Worked

MJHHA had seasoned geriatric nurses on staff who helped with both MJHHA patients and those who were ill and were evacuated to the facility from the community. It is critical that trained personnel are available during both an evacuation and a shelter-in-place situation. This asset cannot be taken lightly and should be considered in planning.

Case Study Questions

1. If you were the nursing home administrator, what would you have done differently in the wake of a hurricane?

2. How would you enhance emergency planning?

3. What type of decision tree would you suggest using?

4. How would you work with the loved ones of those in the facility to better ensure disaster preparedness and response?

5. How would you link into the broader healthcare and emergency management community? What would you bring to the table?

Conclusion

This chapter has highlighted the important concepts of addressing the needs of vulnerable populations in both planning and responding to disasters, terrorism, and public health emergencies. It is important that all involved in hospital emergency preparedness understand that one cannot adequately plan for vulnerable populations without an understanding of their unique needs and involvement of both those with expertise in vulnerable populations and members of vulnerable populations. This incorporation of vulnerable populations should not be limited to the emergency plan, but also should include all training, drills, and exercises. Lastly, one must not only consider the vulnerable population preparedness within the hospital, but also consider the preparedness in the community. If the community is not adequately prepared to provide for the needs of vulnerable populations, then many of them may seek care in the hospital. In seeking care in the hospital, these individuals, who with the correct support could be home, will be in the hospital drawing resources away from patients who can only be cared for in a hospital.

Additional Resources

(From EAD/IPHA Toolkit, 2007)

INSTITUTIONAL PLANNING LEVEL

1. National Organization on Disability's Emergency Preparedness Initiative
   Guide on the Special Needs of People with Disabilities for Emergency Managers, Planners & Responders www.nod.org

2. Easter Seals s.a.f.e.t.y. first:
   Working Together for Safer Communities www.easter-seals.org

3. Job Accommodation Network: This is a service of the Office of Disability Employment Policy of the U.S. Department of Labor.
   www.jan.wvu.edu *will provide a document for employee emergency evacuation and also provide free guidance recommendations about workplace evacuation plans customized for a specific employee's special needs.*

4. FEMA/USFA
   www.usfa.fema.gov/usfapubs/index.cfm

5. U.S. Department of Homeland Security *Nationwide Plan Review Phase 2 Report*
   https://www.dhs.gov/xlibrary/assets/Prep_NationwidePlanReview.pdf

6. U.S. Access Board: www.access-board.gov has posted its agency's own planning methodology and plan criteria as an example, as well as providing guidance on the structural requirements under the Americans with Disabilities Act (ADA) pertaining to evacuation.

7. U.S. Center for Disease Control and Prevention (CDC)
   Public Health Workbook to Define, Locate and Reach Special, Vulnerable, and At-Risk Populations in an Emergency (Draft), http://www.bt.cdc.gov/

workbook/. *Also see the CDC's Health Literacy resources at CDC, Health Literacy Resources at* http://www.cdc.gov/healthmarketing/resources.htm#literacy.

8. U.S. Equal Opportunity Office: www.eeoc.gov/facts/evacuation. html will provide guidance about the use of employee medical/disability information for emergency planning by the employer.

9. U.S. Department of Justice: www.usdoj.gov/crt/ada/emergencyprep.html will provide guidance about basic areas of emergency preparedness and response, which must be accessible to people with disabilities as developed and implemented by local authorities.

10. U.S. Health and Human Services and Department of Homeland Security 2006 Conference: http://www.add-em-conf.com Working Conference on Emergency Management and Individuals with Disabilities and the Elderly has many resources, presentations, and information on special needs issues and emergency management.

STATISTICAL RESOURCES

1. U.S. Census: www.census.gov provides demographics on a state, county, and city level. It includes specific information on people older than 65 years of age, people with disabilities, languages spoken, ethnic groups, etc.

2. DisabilityCounts.org: This Web site synthesizes disability statistic information on a state and county level based on the U.S. Census and other sources. It includes some of the following information:
   - county disability demographic data
   - state and county rural/urban disability data
   - urban/rural (Census 2000)
   - metropolitan/nonmetropolitan (OMB)
   - urbanized/nonurbanized (Transit)
   - state and county, disability by age group
   - congressional district disability data
   - Centers for Independent Living data

3. State Data Centers (SDC): The SDCs are official sources of demographic, economic, and social statistics produced by the Census Bureau. The Census Bureau makes these data available to the SDCs at no charge (fees may be charged for customized products). The SDCs make these data accessible to state, regional, local, and tribal governments, as well as nongovernment data

users at no charge or on a cost-recovery or reimbursable basis as appropriate.

4. Use Geographic Information Systems (GIS) to map special needs data. It is likely that your local emergency management has some GIS capabilities or is moving toward this technology. By mapping where people with certain needs are located in your community, you can better plan for evacuations, perhaps consider strategic placement of shelters, and conduct targeted emergency preparedness outreach, among other activities.

INDIVIDUAL PLANNING LEVEL

1. National Organization on Disability's Emergency Preparedness Initiative: www.nod.org/emergency is a repository of continuously updated information for both the disability community and the emergency professional and will provide links to specific preparedness information, checklists, and guidelines for people with disabilities and information about disabilities and disaster planning.

2. The Federal Emergency Management Agency (FEMA), in conjunction with the American Red Cross (ARC), has published many documents for individual disaster preparedness. Those most helpful for people with special needs are listed and may be obtained from your local Red Cross chapter, the FEMA Distribution Center (1-800-480-2520), or www.fema.gov/library; alternate formats are also available.
   - *Disaster Preparedness for People with Disabilities* (ARC—5091)
   - *Preparing for Disaster for People with Disabilities and other Special Needs* (FEMA 476) **Note**: replaces ARC—A4497
   - *Disaster Preparedness for Seniors by Seniors* (ARC—A5059)
   - *Your Family Disaster Plan* (FEMA/ARC—A4466)
   - *Your Family Disaster Supply Kit* (FEMA/ARC—4463)

3. Center for Disability Issues and the Health Professions: http://www.cdihp.org/products.html#eeguide *Emergency Evacuation Preparedness: Taking Responsibility for Your Safety—A Guide for People with Disabilities and Other Activity Limitations*

4. Prepare Now: www.preparenow.org is a California Web site, but links information about disaster preparedness for specific special needs.

5. Three city agencies (NYC Office of Emergency Management, Department for the Aging and the Mayor's Office for People

with Disabilities) sponsored the publication of *New York City's Guide to Emergency Preparedness for Seniors and People with Disabilities* found at http://nyc.gov/html/oem/html/ready/seniors_guide.shtml.

6. www.ready.gov is a comprehensive general emergency planning site maintained by the federal government and the Department of Homeland Security.

7. www.EmergencyEmail.org is one of several free sign-up services that will forward customized geographic emergency information to subscribers via email or alpha pager systems as the information breaks.

References

1. Booz Allen Hamilton. *Technical Memorandum for Federal Highway Administration on Case Studies: Assessment of State of the Practice and State of the Art in Evacuation Transportation Management*. Federal Highway Administration, U.S. Department of Transportation. http://ops.fhwa.dot.gov/publications/fhwahop08014/index.htm. Published February 6, 2006. Accessed August 13, 2009. Publication FHWA-HOP-08-014.

2. Veenema TG. *Disaster Nursing and Emergency Preparedness for Chemical, Biological, and Radiological Terrorism and Other Hazards*. 2nd ed. New York, NY: Springer Publishing Company, LLC; 2007.

3. Phillips BD, Thomas D, Fothergill A, Blinn-Pike L. *Social Vulnerability to Disasters*. Boca Raton, Florida: CRC Press; 2009.

4. Institute for Research on Poverty. Frequently Asked Questions. Institute for Research on Poverty Web site. http://www.irp.wisc.edu/faqs/faq1.htm#hhs. Accessed March 15, 2010.

5. Disaster Preparedness in Urban Immigrant Communities: Lessons Learned from Recent Catastrophic Events and Their Relevance to Latino and Asian Communities in Southern California. Tomas Rivera Policy Institute. http://www.trpi.org/PDFs/DISASTER_REPORT_Final.pdf.

6. National Law Center on Homelessness & Poverty. 2007 Annual Report. National Law Center on Homelessness & Poverty Web site. http://www.nlchp.org/content/pubs/2007_Annual_Report2.pdf. Accessed July 8, 2009.

7. EAD & Associates, LLC. *Special Needs Toolkit*. Brooklyn, NY: EAD & Associates, LLC; 2007.

8. US Department of Justice. ADA Home Page Web site. http://www.ada.gov. Accessed February 4, 2010.

9. Pandemic and All-Hazards Preparedness Act. US Government Printing Office Web site. http://frwebgate.access.gpo.gov/cgi-bin/getdoc.cgi?dbname=109_cong_public_laws&docid=f:publ417.109. Accessed February 4, 2010.

10. 2004 Executive Order and Creation of the Interagency Coordinating Council. Department of Homeland Security Web site. http://www.dhs.gov/xprepresp/committees/editorial_0591.shtm.

11. Federal Emergency Management Agency. Accommodating Individuals with Disabilities in the Provision of Disaster Mass Care, Housing, and Human Services. Federal Emergency Management Agency Web site. http://www.fema.gov/oer/reference/index.shtm. Accessed August 13, 2009.

12. Brisenden S. Independent living and the medical model of disability. In: Shakespeare T, ed. *The Disability Reader: Social Science Perspectives*. London: Continuum International Publishing Group; 2000.

13. American Association of Homes and Services for the Aging. Other Nursing Home Statistics Overview. American Association of Homes and Services for the Aging Web site. http://www.aahsa.org/nursinghomestats/. Accessed June 2009.

14. Bascetta G. *Disaster Preparedness: Preliminary Observations on the Evacuation of Vulnerable Populations due to Hurricanes and Other Disasters*. U.S. Government Accountability Office. http://www.gao.gov/new.items/d06790t.pdf. Published May 18, 2006. Accessed June 2009. Publication GAO-06-790T.

15. Silverman MA, Weston M, Llorente M, Berber C, Tam R. Lessons learned from Hurricane Andrew: recommendations for care of the elderly in long-term care facilities. *South Med J*. 1995;88(6):603–608.

16. Congressional Research Service. The Pandemic and All-Hazards Preparedness Act (P.L. 109-417): Provisions and Changes to Preexisting Law. The National Agricultural Law Center Web site. http://www.nationalaglawcenter.org/assets/crs/RL33589.pdf. Accessed February 4, 2010.

Chapter 20

Altered Standards of Care in Disasters and Public Health Emergencies

John Rinard, BBA, MSCPI

Photo by Ed Edahl/FEMA

Learning Objectives

- Discuss when standards of care may be affected by disasters and public health emergencies.
- Describe the decision-making process of determining when altered standards of care should be considered during or following a disaster or public health emergency.
- Identify the relevant medical and legal considerations with the implementation of altered standards of care.

Case Study

Wednesday evening started as many others had that week in downtown Denver, with community members attending a sold-out event at the Performing Arts Center. However, that is where any similarity with a normal evening ceased for those in attendance. Within 72 hours, that very group of individuals had begun to manifest significant flu and cold-like symptoms, which included cough and fever. As the illness progressed, many decided their best option for medical attention during the weekend was at the local emergency department, and by early afternoon the local health department confirmed the illness not as flu, but pneumonic plague. At day's end, 783 cases of plague were diagnosed and 123 fatalities resulted. More importantly, local hospitals began to report shortages in staff and critical supplies, including antibiotics and ventilators.

The following day, conditions deteriorated further, as presenting cases expanded to 1800 that now included international locations, and fatalities increased to 389. The healthcare system for Denver and the surrounding areas rapidly found itself in a downward spiral caused by the volume of patients and complicated by the rapid depletion of supplies, beds, and staff. By the end of day three, the hospital system, which had recorded 3000 cases and confirmed 795 fatalities, experienced what was, in essence, gridlock and began to shut down. In the initial stages of the event, hospitals within the metroplex documented emergency department visits that were two to three times normal. By the end of the fourth day, the hospitals were inundated with up to 10 times the normal census, as shown in Figure 20-1.

Figure 20-1

Pneumonic Plague Cases and Deaths in TOPFF 2000

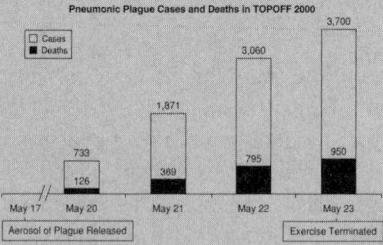

Pneumonic Plague Cases and Deaths in TOPOFF 2000

Association of Schools of Public Health

At completion, Top Officials (TOPOFF) exercise planners estimated 3700 confirmed cases of plague and approximately 2000 fatalities had occurred within the four-day exercise period that began at the time of index patient presentation.[1]

The case you just read represented exercise results and had no actual impact on the citizenry and healthcare system of Denver. While patient numbers paled in comparison to the millions generated by the Spanish Influenza, the results had the same predictable outcome and signaled the reemergence of jurisdiction healthcare issues originally documented in 1919. This exercise is symptomatic of the lethargic

[1] Inglesby TV. Observations from the Top Off exercise. *Public Health Rep.* 2001;116(suppl 2):64–68.

response to known healthcare deficiencies that dog the healthcare system of the United States and will reduce its effectiveness during the next catastrophic event. A report published in 2006, Toner et al., presented data indicating that the 1918 pandemic data modeled to demonstrate an eight-week outbreak and 25% attack rate would generate the following utilization rates:[2]

- 191% census of non-ICU beds
- 461% census of ICU beds
- 198% ventilator usage

As if to add another dimension to concerns raised by this data, the American Hospital Association and the Centers for Disease Control and Injury Prevention released information indicating that hospital emergency department visits had increased by 26% over the period of 1993–2003, while the availability of emergency departments decreased by 14%. Additionally, the United States is facing a shortage of nurses that is estimated to be 116,000 nurses.[3]

This data continues to fuel the debate regarding type and nature of strategy necessary when determining priority of care, access to medication, and staffing options designed to address unexpected increases in demand for service in an overtaxed resource environment. Those issues surround the delivery of mass health care following a catastrophic event.

Altered Standards of Care: What Are They?

"Lifeboat ethics"[4] is a suitable term to describe the concept behind altered standards of care. Some have participated in a management/teamwork exercise that provides a situation where a boat has sunk in shark-infested waters. Several people got off safely and there is only one lifeboat with limited seating capacity that is less than the total number of survivors. All in the water are certain to die if they are not provided a seat in the boat and each survivor has some compelling reason to be granted a seat.

This exercise develops a sense of decision making in a resource-deficient environment, where the key is utilization of an objective system designed around an understood guiding principle.

[2] Toner E, Waldhorn R, Maldin B, et al. Hospital preparedness for pandemic influenza. *Biosecur Bioterror.* 2006;4(2):207–217.

[3] Kaji AH, Koenig KL, Lewis RJ. Current hospital disaster preparedness. *JAMA.* 2007;298(18): 2188–2190.

[4] Krauss CK, Levy F, Kelen GD. Lifeboat ethics: considerations in the discharge of inpatients for the creation of hospital surge capacity. *Disaster Med Public Health Prep.* 2007;1(1):51–56.

In order to fully understand and appreciate altered standards of care, the basic tenant of standard of care must be understood. As one might recall, standard of care consists of standards that dictate the manner in which health care is to be provided by a prudent clinician. The basis for standard of care lies in factors including, but not limited to, local, state, and federal case law; local standards; protocol; and statutory requirements, as well as consideration of how another individual of equal qualifications would act. Standard of care has served as the guiding principle for delivery of health care in emergency situations. However, faced with the changing complexion of health care coupled with an increasing complexity of threats, standard of care has received increased scrutiny from researchers and clinicians regarding its practicality and applicability during mass care events; e.g., the Northridge Earthquake, Hurricanes Rita and Katrina, Madrid train bombings, Beslan school event, etc.

As a result, an understanding has developed that in order for community healthcare delivery systems to remain viable and effective, community resource changes must occur with respect to the manner in which health care is delivered. Hence, the term *altered standard of care* emerged. While there is a lack of a standardized definition for the term, it does suggest a degradation of health care. A concern regarding the term is that it should not be construed to imply a subjective restriction of service or rationing of resources related to clinical care because of the negative connotation coupled with the potential for disparate impact on the population.

GOVERNMENT ACCOUNTABILITY OFFICE RESULTS

In a report dated June 2008, the Government Accountability Office (GAO), reported information following a survey of hospital preparedness efforts implemented as a direct result of federal grant funds during the period of 2002–2007. The sampling methodology utilized to compile assessment results included selecting two hospitals within each of the 10 designated Health and Human Services (HHS) regions for a total of 20 hospitals. One facility within each region had received the greatest level of ASPR funding for that state and the remaining facility represented the one that received the least amount of funding.[5]

The report provides an overview of information regarding the implementation of response and preparedness efforts regarding specific, interrelated functions necessary to meet mass healthcare chal-

[5] US Department of Health & Human Services. The Hospital Preparedness Program (HPP). US Department of Health & Human Services Web site. http://www.hhs.gov/aspr/opeo/hpp/. Accessed April 5, 2010.

lenges following a catastrophic event. The information assessed and presented relative to hospital emergency preparedness included:

- hospital capacity
- alternate care facilities
- electronic volunteer registry
- altered standards of care

HOSPITAL CAPACITY

Federal surveyors indicated that 100% of the 20 reporting facilities had actively implemented expanding physical facilities or coordinating with other state, local, and federal hospital resources to increase availability of surge hospital beds. The ability to effectively implement surge capability is indirectly related to implementation of altered standards of care, which could include implementation of more stringent triage activities, early discharge of patients, and other related functions.

ALTERNATE CARE FACILITIES

The report indicated that 18 surveyed facilities had initiated steps to identify and designate alternate care sites. Alternate care facilities function as an extension to the surge planning process through selection and utilization of locations to serve as a receiving point for overflow patients or those, for instance, who were impacted by exclusion criteria. This type of facility would likely serve as a holding facility for patients with a lower level of acuity, chronic ailments, and/or those who require minimal supervised care. The establishment of alternate care facilities incorporates considerations related to the scope of medical care and staffing necessary to support patients using the prescribed standard of care. Alternate care facilities are also supported by altered standards of care caused by decreased numbers of clinicians and the resulting increased caregiver/patient ratio that exceeds recognized standards.

ELECTRONIC MEDICAL VOLUNTEER REGISTRIES

Among surveyed facilities, 15 had initiated a process of addressing the question of establishing electronic medical volunteer registries. While designed to "pre-certify" potential volunteers, this system also provides a contingency for suspension of the normal credentialing process in times of catastrophic events.

ALTERED STANDARDS OF CARE

Initiation of surge capacity measures following a catastrophic event signals the onset of a situation that, if not addressed through alterations in delivery of clinical care, will rapidly deplete resources. Altered standards of care impact all facets of clinical care and may include staffing/patient ratios, delivery of medications based on a triage-based system, and application of strict clinical guidelines when determining the level of care individual patients receive. This is a relatively new arena and one fraught with pitfalls and unresolved issues for those who proceed through the process in less than an organized systematic fashion. It is no wonder then, that the report indicated only seven facilities had made efforts to address this issue.

Altered Standards of Care: Where Are We and How Did We Establish Them?

Ironically, altered standards of care is not a new concept. It existed for centuries through battlefield-based triage systems. More recently, it was associated with delivery of mass health care during the flu pandemic in 1919–1920. During this event, the situation dictated utilization of extraordinary measures as the healthcare system of the United States struggled to keep pace with wartime demands superimposed with the Spanish Influenza. Efforts to address shortcomings of staff, supplies, and hospital space resulted in a crude implementation of measures we now recognize as altered standards of care. This involved utilization of students to deliver health care, hanging sheets between beds in gymnasiums to create isolation facilities, and utilization of triage guidelines related to hospital admission processes.

Progressing forward, the industry is once again faced with the potential of a pandemic, as well as terrorism and natural disaster-related concerns that, on a relative scale, will result in a mirror image of the concerns, shortfalls, and resource allocation questions faced in 1919. A complicating factor surrounding altered standards of care lies in the fact that it is not a "one size fits all" process. While a general template for implementation, as presented in this chapter, may apply, specific components of clinical care will vary—based on the situation encountered. With that in mind, emergency planners appear to face the impossible task of preparing a response plan, specific to altered standards of care, which will meet a multitude of disaster and infrastructure failure scenarios that might befall their community.

The Hazard Vulnerability Analysis (HVA) provides a practical, reasonably objective evaluation tool to conduct planning and asset prioritization efforts. However, based on the sophistication of the HVA used, it can be a rather complicated, time-consuming process. In 2005, the federal government implemented a capabilities-based planning culture comprised of 15 National Planning Scenarios (NPS); more than 1800 target capabilities on the Target Capabilities List (TCL) that revolve around prevention, protection, response, and recovery; and 36 Universal Task List (UTL)

Table 20-1		
National Planning Scenarios		
Nuclear detonation: A 10-kiloton device	Chemical attack: Toxic industrial chemicals	Radiological attack: Radiological dispersal device
Biological attack: Inhalational anthrax	Chemical attack: Nerve agent	Explosives attack: Improvised explosive device
Biological outbreak: Pandemic influenza	Chemical attack: Chlorine tank explosion	Biological attack: Food contamination
Biological attack: Plague	Natural disaster: Earthquake	Biological attack: Foreign animal disease
Chemical attack: Blister agent	Natural disaster: Major hurricane	Cyber attack

items, which among others, provides a description of capability and desired outcome. Since their initiation, these documents have undergone revision in 2007 and 2009. The NPS (Table 20-1) represent the combined, integrated efforts of federal officials to identify events through inclusion of a wide range of threats, both natural and perpetrated, that have been deemed most likely to occur. Additionally, implementation of planning components for any one of the 15 scenarios can be used to address the remaining scenarios.

Altered Standards of Care: Establishing the Framework

Homeland Security Presidential Directive (HSPD) 21, released in October 2007, provided strategic direction for the development of guidelines designed to govern the delivery of mass care following a catastrophic event. The Directive was designed around the doctrine that the routine healthcare delivery process would fall short in meeting the needs of the public following a catastrophic event, and that disaster medical capability must have the ability to re-orient and coordinate existing resources in an effort to satisfy population needs during a catastrophic health event. In order to achieve this goal, the healthcare system of the United States must "develop a rapid, flexible, sustainable, integrated, and coordinated system which delivers appropriate treatment in the most ethical manner with available capabilities."[6]

Previously documented experiences recorded within the emergency management community, based largely on the culture within the country, required expansion of the general definition of altered standards

[6] Emergency Preparedness: States are Planning for Medical Surge, but Could Benefit from Shared Guidance for Allocating Scarce Medical Resources. US Government Accountability Office.http://www.gao.gov/new.items/d08668.pdf. Published June 2008. Publication GAO-08-668.

of care to ensure that it was as objective as possible. This was obtained through the inclusion of the following additional elements:

- legal considerations
- science or outcomes-based factors
- ethical implications
- policy-based format

LEGAL CONSIDERATIONS

The starting point for formulation of altered standards of care must involve detailed legal research; the desired outcome is development of a legal basis for the adoption, implementation, and utilization of the final product. According to the American Bar Association Checklist for Disaster Preparedness,[7] this would include the following items:

- **Research:** Research, using phrases such as "disaster" or "emergency" *and* specific jurisdiction or level of jurisdiction, such as "state," "municipal," "county," or "town."
- **Use legal indexes of statutes:** Using the bound copies of the index to the general laws in your jurisdiction, look up such topics as *disaster, emergencies, war, civil defense,* and similar terms.
- **Check special acts for the particular jurisdiction:** Many states pass special acts dealing with disaster responses.
- **Check emergency preparedness agencies:** Check with the state and local government emergency preparedness agencies that may have already compiled many of these sources.
- **Check laws:** Check for local laws, ordinances, and regulations on these topics.

A second recommendation is to review the Model State Emergency Health Powers Act (Model Act). This Model Act would grant specific emergency powers to state governors and public health authorities in the course of a large event.

While statutory compliance is directly linked to reduction of personal and corporate liability, a lesser recognized benefit of statutory compliance lies in the ability of healthcare organizations to receive reimbursement for provision of patient care from federal sources, i.e. Medicare and Medicaid. In the absence of statutory support, insurers will likely only reimburse for procedures performed by individuals designated through scope of practice as being qualified to deliver a clinical modality, and may not reimburse for the procedure if done by anyone

---

[7] Agency for Healthcare Research and Quality (AHRQ). *Altered Standards of Care in Mass Casualty Events, Bioterrorism and Other Public Health Emergencies.* Rockville, MD: AHRQ; 2005. AHRQ Publication No. 05-0043.

else. The only exception lies in suspension of regulatory language that addresses scope of practice/credentialing, etc. by the appropriate state or federal agency,[8] such as the state governor. A sample format that meets these recommendations can be found in the state of Illinois, though Public Act 094-0733 has developed just such a process:

> Upon proclamation of a disaster by the Governor, as provided in the Illinois Emergency Management Agency Act, The Secretary of Financial and Professional regulation shall have the following powers, which shall be exercised only in coordination with the Illinois Emergency Management Association and the Department of Public Health:[9]
>
> ■ The power to suspend the requirements for permanent or temporary licensure of persons working under the direction of the Illinois Emergency Management Association and the Department of Public Health pursuant to a declared disaster.
> ■ The power to modify the Scope of Practice restrictions . . . pursuant to a declared disaster.

The example again illustrates the importance of maintaining familiarity with applicable laws, and understanding that successful implementation often hinges on a formal declaration of disaster.

SCIENCE OR OUTCOMES-BASED FACTORS

As previously stated, altered standards of care must be fair, but more importantly, must be based in science. The manner that medicine is delivered on a daily basis is based on clinical evidence, demonstrating that a particular modality is beneficial and clinically sound. In the context of altered standards of care, inclusion and exclusion criteria must be objective and research–based, which demonstrates sound decision making. In order for these standards to be met, it will be necessary to review previous "catastrophic" events—which might, for example, include pandemics and perpetrated and natural catastrophes—in an attempt to understand clinical and epidemiological features that surround and impact the outcome of each event.[10] After conditions and outcomes are understood, a literature review should be undertaken to ascertain the presence of clinical standards that might apply for each parameter in the proposed policy.

[8] Gravely S, Whaley E. The greatest good for the greatest number: implications for altered standards of care. *Hosp Health Syst.* 2006;8(3):10–13.

[9] Illinois General Assembly. Public Act 094-0733. http://www.ilga.gov/legislation/publicacts/fulltext.asp?Name=094-0733. Accessed April 5, 2010.

[10] Houston-Harris County Committee on Pandemic Influenza Medical Standards of Care. *Recommended Priority Groups for Antiviral Medication and Vaccine.* Houston, TX: Houston-Harris County Committee on Pandemic Influenza Medical Standards of Care; September 2008. http://www.hcphes.org/2007forum/resource.pdf. Accessed October 30, 2008.

An example of outcomes-based pandemic flu hospital and ICU triage guidelines can be found in a draft document developed by the Utah Department of Health.[11] Contained within this document are three levels of hospital-based triage that revolve around the stages of a pandemic.

Under this categorization, hospital staff members are provided a series of exclusion criteria designed to provide objective relief associated with delivery of mass care. This includes, as an example, exclusion criteria related to hospital admission for patients with known Do Not Resuscitate (DNR) status, or patients with Glasgow Coma Scale (GCS) score <6, advanced untreatable neuromuscular disease, and chromosomal disease that are uniformly fatal within the first two years of life. Each item discussed in the exclusion criteria represents a triage decision based on documentable outcomes and represents an objective, defensible position for staff and facilities employing this policy. Equally important in the development of altered standards of care is discussion of inclusion criteria that would apply to the hospital in general as well as specialty care units within a facility, such as the ICU. In this instance, the Utah Department of Health identified hypotension refractory to volume resuscitation that requires vasopressor support as criteria for admission into the ICU.

ETHICAL IMPLICATIONS

The initial step in addressing ethical considerations, as discussed in the 2007 CDC document *Ethical Guidelines in Pandemic Influenza*, requires efforts to inform the public of the process, the rationale behind the decision, and what might occur after the policy is implemented. Planners engaged in discussions related to "ethical appropriateness" of altered standards of care guidelines are also reminded to ensure that healthcare concerns for the community are met and that the process retains a large component of fairness. In fact, the procedure should ensure equal application of healthcare standards for all, regardless of race, nationality, or economic factors. If that is not possible, then criteria that are defensible must be utilized. It is for this reason that utilization of "triage-like" criteria, as suggested by Melnychuk and Kenny, be utilized to identify inclusion criteria, exclusion criteria, and minimum qualifications for survival.[12] The

[11] Utah Hospitals and Health Systems Association. Utah Pandemic Influenza Hospital and ICU Triage Guidelines. Salt Lake City, Utah: Utah Department of Health. http://www.uha-utah.org/Disaster%20Prep%20Materials/PANDEMIC%20FLU%20Triage%20Guidelines_081109.pdf. Published March 5, 2008.

[12] Melnychuk RM, Kenny NP. Pandemic triage: the ethical challenge. *CMAJ*. 2006;175(11): 1393–1394.

final aspect necessary when developing an ethically sound procedure is to ensure accountability.[13] Accountability, in this instance, refers to ensuring there is one person who determines when criteria constituting an appropriate environment have been met for initiating the policy, approves activation of the policy, and determines when the policy is deactivated.

An often cited document, produced by the University of Toronto Bioethics Pandemic Influenza Working Group following the severe acute respiratory syndrome (SARS) outbreak, indicates that in order for planners to make ethical decisions, they should ensure that decisions are reasonable, open, transparent, inclusive, responsive, and, as noted previously, carry the trait of accountability.[14] The Santa Clara, California Public Health Department also supports the Toronto recommendations by stating in its policy that "inherently controversial subjects such as determination of social worth, and even triage protocols, should be thoroughly and publically scrutinized *before* a crisis." This is best achieved through utilization of stakeholder planning as well as other public forums where discussions regarding the proposed process may occur.

POLICY-BASED FORMAT

Healthcare administrators and emergency planners must establish a policy designed to govern reconfiguration of resource allocation within a hospital or EMS environment. The plan should address topics that include, but are not limited to the following items:

- When is the plan activated?
- What are the stages or steps for activating the plan?
- How will the public be notified of plan activation?
- What activities are covered by the plan?
- Who is authorized to activate or deactivate the plan?

This rationale for policy development must include a set of assumptions that include the belief that resources will be limited and, further, that new guidelines will be necessary to govern delivery of clinical care in the face of a catastrophic event within the community. Along with these assumptions, it is helpful to also delineate impacts and challenges that might occur as a result of the recognized variables.

[13] Santa Clara Public Health Department. Pandemic Influenza: Ethical Considerations. Santa Clara Public Health Department Web site. http://www.sccgov.org/SCC/docs/Public%20Health%20Department%20(DEP)/attachments/Tool%201-%20Pandemic%20Influenza%20Ethics%20Tool%2012-07.pdf. Published 2007. Accessed December 1, 2008.

[14] Pandemic Influenza Working Group. *Stand on Guard for Thee: Ethical Considerations in Preparedness Planning for Pandemic Influenza.* Toronto, Canada: University of Toronto Joint Centre for Bioethics; 2005. http://www.jointcentreforbioethics.ca/publications/documents/stand_on_guard.pdf. Accessed October 18, 2008.

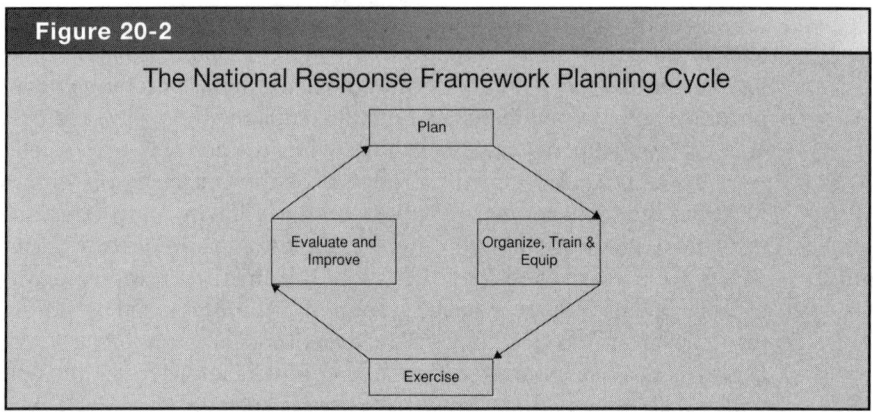

FEMA

The National Response Framework (NRF) presents a planning cycle, illustrated in Figure 20-2, which delineates a process designed to ensure policy development not only meets expectations but is functional.

The initial step associated with initiating an effective policy requires an education component designed to familiarize staff and assess competency regarding the newly developed guideline. While many policies satisfy the initial component, few provide follow-up opportunities, which must be delivered in a continuing education format to ensure maintenance of the desired level of competency. This could occur through an annual refresher, a skills fair, online training, or a traditional didactic offering.

The second component of policy development consists of designing an exercise to "stress" the policy and allow objective assessment of staff competency related to implementation and utilization of the prescribed process. An added benefit to exercising the policy lies in the assurance that the policy, as developed, is not only practical, but also achieves the desired level of functionality.

Altered Standards of Care: Staff, Supplies, Space, and Stuff

Altered standards of care can generally be grouped into one of the following categories: staff; supplies; space; and stuff, a catchall designed to hold all practices not specific to one of the other content areas. This constitutes the "4 S's" necessary to meet demands generated by a catastrophic event.

STAFF

During a catastrophic event, as existed during TOPOFF 1, staffing will become a critical issue because disaster research demonstrates a range of staff

Table 20-2		
Utah Pandemic Plan Level 3 Triage Category		
Triage Level 1: Early	**Triage Level 2: Worsening**	**Triage Level 3: Worst Case**
Increased numbers Recognition of need to surge	Surged to maximum capacity Insufficient beds Increased absenteeism	Altered Standards of Care (ASOC) has been implemented Staff absenteeism of 30–40%

loss of 10–60%, based on the type and duration of the event.[15] These absences will result from a combination of personal illness, concern for individual safety, and concern for their family's safety. This planning assumption has also been expressed in the Utah Pandemic Plan Level 3 Triage Category (Table 20-2).

Regardless of the cause, staff absenteeism will reduce hospital capability and capacity without regard for facility preparedness or resource inventory. As a result, an initial consideration when planning for delivery of mass care must be geared toward staff augmentation/expansion. This may be achieved through several options, including the following actions:

- increased staff-to-patient care ratios
- altered staff shifts
- utilization of "ancillary" credentialed staff
- expanded scope of practice
- utilization of volunteers

Increased Patient Care Ratios

The International Council of Nurses reports the optimum nurse-to-patient ratio as: 1 nurse per 5 patients. This ratio has been adopted in at least one state—the California Department of Health Services enacted legislation recognizing a safe ratio. This established one nurse per six patients as the statutory ratio, starting in 2004, with a reduction to one nurse per five patients in 2005.[16] When assessing the concept of a standardized ratio, it should include the realization that they are wholly dependent on two variables: patient acuity and normal operation conditions.

In the absence of a normal operation environment, it is reasonable to expect a significant increase in the nurse/patient ratio. This altered ratio will be an initial step in stretching available staff resources to meet demands generated in a mass care environment.

[15] Wise RA. The creation of emergency health care standards for catastrophic events. *Acad Emerg Med.* 2006;13(11):1150–1152.

[16] Nurse to Patient Ratios: Research and Reality. NEPPC Conference Report Series No. 05-1; July 2005. http://www.bos.frb.org/economic/neppc/conreports/2005/conreport051.pdf. Accessed April 5, 2010.

Altered Staff Shifts
The presence of an unusually large census, coupled with a decrease of staff up to 40%, and the staffing of alternative care facilities may require an alteration of staffing schedules. This could entail clinic staff working 12-hour shifts and/or a consolidation of staff from a three-shift pattern to a two-shift schedule until the magnitude of the event decreases or staff augmentation options are made available.

Ancillary Credentialed Staff
One form of staff augmentation may involve utilization of appropriately credentialed nonclinic healthcare staff, i.e., nurse educators. Nurse educators, through their positions, are appropriately credentialed healthcare professionals who generally have a background as a clinician.

Expanded Scope of Practice
Utilization of a system that mirrors the fire service "ride up" concept caused by an illness or unexpected absence/assignment may assist in ensuring those with the highest level of skills are used as effectively as possible. It also means that others may be tasked with performing clinic functions traditionally reserved for those of higher licensure or certification levels. In this process, staff would be empowered to function at the next higher level, delivering care that, under normal circumstances, would exceed their scope of practice. An example would be allowing nursing staff to suture, a skill normally reserved for physicians. This effort facilitates increased responsiveness to patients' needs while relieving previously assigned staff to engage in more pressing clinic care assignments. As we have discussed in the past and as was illustrated by the Illinois statute, a formal declaration of disaster at the regulatory level would facilitate implementation of this modified scope of practice. Additionally, the formal declaration would alleviate some, if not all, liability questions related to the described practice.

Volunteers
While other options exist to augment staff, the remaining discussion for this module is the use of previously non-credentialed staff. The federal government has actively taken steps to enhance the credentialing process through implementation of the Emergency System for Advance Registration of Volunteer Health Professionals (ESAR-VHP) system. Designed to ensure compatibility with resource typing utilized by National Incident Management System (NIMS), ESAR-VHP addresses the credentialing of physicians, registered nurses, and five behavioral health occupations. However, from the Spanish Influenza we learn that unlicensed clinical practitioners, as well as other allied healthcare providers, (e.g., medical students, student nurses, dentists, and EMS staff) played a significant role in bolstering the number of clinicians available to support jurisdiction needs. Other existing jurisdiction assets that are available include

Table 20-3		
	Antiviral Administration Recommendations[17]	
Priority	**Group**	
A1	Hospitalized patients with influenza	
A2	Healthcare workers with influenza	
A3	Critical community emergency responders	
A4	Essential infrastructure service workers	
B1	Highest risk outpatients with greater susceptibility to death from influenza	
B2	Increased risk outpatients with more susceptibility to death from influenza	
C	Other outpatients/general population	

retired physicians, veterinarians, etc. There should be a mechanism in place that would allow temporary suspension of normal credentialing processes to allow these individuals to function as clinicians during the mass care event. The effectiveness of this system was demonstrated during Hurricane Katrina when Governor Blanco temporarily suspended credentialing of out-of-state healthcare and law enforcement professionals for a 30-day period to ensure an efficient process for utilizing volunteer emergency responders. Utilized as an emergency process, this system was later submitted for legislative approval and subsequent implementation as a Louisiana statute.

SUPPLIES

With consideration toward supplies, literature focuses on a pandemic event and the subsequent considerations related to distribution of vaccines, antivirals, prophylactic medications, and availability of ventilators. It is safe to say that decisions regarding distribution of medication will result in an ethical dilemma at best. The TOPOFF exercise in 2000 initiated the start of these discussions at the worst possible time—during the event. After much wrangling, the decision was made to offer medications to public safety staff and their families for the promise of remaining at work, a rather lengthy and subjective decision by some standards. Since that time, efforts have been undertaken by some jurisdictions to proactively design and implement a process in advance of the next mass care event. An example can be found in a draft document generated by the Houston-Harris County Committee on Pandemic Influenza Medical Standards of Care. In this example, shown in Table 20-3, priority status regarding receipt of antivirals

[17] Houston-Harris County Committee on Pandemic Influenza Medical Standards of Care. *Recommended Priority Groups for Antiviral Medication and Vaccine.* Houston, TX: Houston-Harris County Committee on Pandemic Influenza Medical Standards of Care; September 2008. http://www .hcphes.org/2007forum/resource.pdf. Accessed October 30, 2008.

and vaccinations has been assigned to groups based on factors that include reduction of disease within the facility as well as maintaining functional components related to maintaining infrastructure.

The principles of controlling the spread of disease within a facility as well as ensuring patency of critical infrastructure espoused by the Houston-Harris County Committee on Pandemic Influenza Medical Standards of Care are not only appropriate but a sound practice.

One of the first authors to address shortages of ventilators and their subsequent "utilization triage criteria" was Dr. John Hick, an ED Physician at Hennepin County Medical Center in Minneapolis. Since publication, many states have followed suit and initiated efforts to develop objective inclusion and exclusion criteria for use of mechanical ventilators. The Texas-based Shore Health System has determined that patients requiring mechanical ventilator support will be categorized into one of three tiers, each containing definition of criteria, as shown in Table 20-4:

Table 20-4
Ventilator Triage Tool
Tier 1 Do not offer **and** withdraw ventilator support for patients with any one of the following: *Multisystem organ failure, failure to respond to mechanical ventilation and antibiotics after 72 hours in context of a biological pathogen, etc.*
Tier 2 Do not offer **and** withdraw ventilator support from patients in respiratory failure requiring intubation with the following conditions, in addition to those in Tier 1:   *Renal failure requiring hemodialysis (related to illness), irreversible neurological impairment that makes patient dependent for personal care, etc.*
Tier 3 Specific protocols to be agreed upon with input from the ethics committee

Additionally, facility administration will be faced with decisions regarding the use and availability of "other" forms of supplies, to include disposable supplies, oxygen, and linen. It may be necessary, because of the volume of patients, to extend usage of these items longer than standard procedures dictate.

SPACE

Patient housing considerations, a continuation of surge capacity, again involves establishment of inclusion and exclusion criteria. In this instance, the very heart of the matter is seated in criteria addressing which patients will be allowed entry into the healthcare facility in general. The state of Colorado has addressed this very issue through release of an Executive Order allowing hospitals to cease admissions and/or transfer patients in order to meet the disaster at hand. This criteria-based triage system should be based on acuity of illness/injury. Those not meeting inclusion criteria will either be directed to return home and self-treat or be redirected to a nearby alternate care facility. In addition to general entry criteria, a further layer of triage will occur with respect to admission to critical care areas of the facility.

Additional actions to enhance available unmonitored bed space consists of evaluation of medical/surgical patients for early discharge, as well as reevaluation of patients housed in critical care beds to determine medical necessity and benefits of continued stays. Additionally, expansion of room capacity and isolation areas, and conversion of common areas to patient care areas serve to illustrate examples of altered standards of care as it relates to space.

STUFF

While sequentially this area is presented last, the ordering is not a reflection of importance. In fact, this category has significant impact on all other discussed areas and includes components related to several areas:

- patient transport
- surgical decisions
- code policies
- decontamination decisions

Patient Transport

The issue of transport includes the ability to transport "credentialed patients" from the scene to a receiving facility, as well as to transfer them from a facility to another one in order to create census capacity. The ability to facilitate early discharge or transfer of patients to step-down facilities is a critical aspect of being able to address surge and its associated components.

In response to facility evacuations caused by hurricanes, the Texas Department of State Health Services (DSHS) developed a process regarding the transportation mode utilized for transfers or transport, which is contained in its Ground and Air Ambulance Utilization Criteria (Table 20-5). Even the underlying key to a successful implementation of this policy is availability of sufficient assets to meet the demands of the assigned task. Designed with the understanding that transport resources will be in short supply, the criteria offers definition and direction for the manner in which patients will travel to or from a healthcare facility.

In addition, as a direct result of Hurricane Rita, DSHS has adopted two additional forms of alternative transport options that include ALS and litter busses. An ALS bus is a commercial bus with a capacity of approximately 35 ambulatory patients. Ambulatory patients are defined as patients who possess the ability to sit up, do not require monitoring, are

Table 20-5	
Ground and Air Ambulance Utilization Criteria	
Ground ambulance transport	patients on oxygen at greater than 4 liters per minute (LPM)
	patients who require hemodynamic and cardiac monitoring
	patients who require continuous IV medication drip that requires monitoring
	orthopedic injuries that require appliances or other acute medical conditions that prevent patients from traveling using alternate forms of transport
Air ambulance transport	transfers from one critical care area to another
	continuous IV vasoconstrictive medications or blood products
	emergency surgical interventions
	acute medical conditions requiring special interventions

not in active labor, and do not have medication-based IV drips or oxygen delivery systems flowing greater than 4 LPM. Additionally, the bus is staffed with at least one paramedic, a jump bag, and a semi automated external defibrillator (SAED). Flexible staffing configurations have been designed to expand the clinic staff to include up to five paramedics and/or registered nurses, based on staff availability. The litter bus resembles what we think of as a mobile army surgical hospital (MASH) style of patient transport, in which nonambulatory patients are attached to stretcher devices mounted on seat tops or slung from the roof of the vehicle.

Surgical Decisions

Additional considerations may include cancellation of not only elective surgeries, but also those that have no immediate determination of survivability, until the event has reached a point where critical care beds are increasingly available to house the patients generated by the surgical event. The *Utah Pandemic Influenza and ICU Triage Guidelines* document provides one example of how surgical procedures are classified (Table 20-6):

Table 20-6	
Classification of Surgical Procedures	
Emergency	Patients whose clinical conditions indicate they require admission to the hospital and/or surgery within 24 hours
Category 1	Urgent patients who require surgery within 30 days
Category 2	Semi-urgent patients who require surgery within 90 days
Category 3	Non-urgent patients who require surgery at some time in the future

Code Policies

In the face of scarce staff and supplies, it will also become necessary to develop altered standards with respect to "code" management. Because code events are both labor- and supply-intensive events, a suspension of established American Heart Association, Advanced Cardiac Life Support (ACLS) protocol may need to happen in the face of a mass care event. Standard resuscitation efforts would then be replaced by limited or modified resuscitation efforts. In this instance, policy may dictate that patients in asystole are excluded from any level of resuscitation efforts and others receive limited efforts to include one round of medications and defibrillation only.

Decontamination Decisions

Another staff-intensive category that may require alterations are facility-based decontamination efforts. Facility policy, under normal operation parameters, may initially dictate that decontamination efforts occur for everybody following a hazardous materials release. However, in context of staff shortages and a mass care event, this policy may be modified such that decontamination efforts might be limited to only symptomatic patients who have been documented to have been within the impact area. A further alteration to the policy may be that anyone who had previously undergone decontamination would be considered clean and no longer possess a contamination threat.

Summary

As noted in a New York State Department of Health Task Force on Life and the Law document, planning is not optional; rather, it is an obligation. In this case, it carries with it the very survival of the community healthcare system as well as protection from legal proceedings and financial ruin.

The ability of a jurisdiction healthcare system to remain functional is based largely on the ability of community and professional leaders to effectively integrate their efforts with stakeholders representing the state and federal governments in an effort to develop and exercise a cohesive plan in advance of a catastrophic event. This integrated effort is best illustrated by The Joint Commission, in its document *Health Care at the Crossroads: Strategies for Creating and Sustaining Community-wide Emergency Preparedness Systems.* Within this document, a list of consensus tactics (Table 20-7) that must be addressed in order to meet mass care demands is provided and further illustrates that the policy implementation regarding altered standards of care does not rest solely with a single entity, regardless of the level of government it represents. It is only through a coordinated, cooperative effort that healthcare facilities will be able to sustain operations in the face of an austere environment.

Table 20-7	
Health Care at the Crossroads: Strategies for Creating and Sustaining Community-wide Emergency Preparedness Systems	
Tactic	**Accountability**
Maintain the ability to provide routine care	Healthcare professionals Healthcare organizations Community organizations
Make provisions for the graceful degradation of care in all emergency preparedness plans	Healthcare organizations Community organizations
Provide for the waiver of regulatory requirements and other standards expectations under conditions of extreme emergency	Federal and state government agencies Accrediting bodies

It is hoped that this overview has provided readers with a sense of the work that must be undertaken to think through and implement a policy regarding altered standards of care. Further, that procrastination in engaging in these discussions will only hasten potential liability and financial exposure if a mass care event occurs prior to acceptance and implementation of an appropriate policy.

References

Agency for Healthcare Research and Quality (AHRQ). *Altered Standards of Care in Mass Casualty Events, Bioterrorism and Other Public Health Emergencies.* Rockville, MD: AHRQ; 2005. AHRQ Publication No. 05-0043.

Altered standards of care workgroup. Region 8 Public Health Preparedness Update. http://www.bfhd.wa.gov/bio/pdf/May%2008.pdf. Published May 2008. Accessed October 21, 2008.

Center for Health Policy, Columbia University School of Nursing. *Adapting Standards of Care Under Extreme Conditions: Guidance for Professionals During Disasters, Pandemics, and Other Extreme Emergencies.* Silver Spring, MD: American Nurses Association; 2008. http://www.nursingworld.org/MainMenuCategories/HealthcareandPolicyIssues/DPR/TheLawEthicsofDisasterResponse/AdaptingStandardsofCare.aspx. Accessed October 2008.

Emergency Preparedness: States are Planning for Medical Surge, but Could Benefit from Shared Guidance for Allocating Scarce Medical Resources. US Government Accountability Office. http://www.gao.gov/new.items/d08668.pdf. Published June 2008. Publication GAO-08-668.

Gravely SD. *Altered Standards of Care: An Overview* [slide show]. Troutman Sanders, LLP. http://www.vdh.state.va.us/EPR/pdf/Health_and_Medical_Subpanel.pdf. Accessed November 12, 2008.

Gravely S, Whaley E. The greatest good for the greatest number: implications for altered standards of care. *Hosp Health Syst.* 2006;8(3):10–13.

Houston-Harris County Committee on Pandemic Influenza Medical Standards of Care. *Recommended Priority Groups for Antiviral Medication and Vaccine.* Houston, TX: Houston-Harris County Committee on Pandemic Influenza Medical Standards of Care;

September 2008. http://www.hcphes.org/2007forum/resource.pdf. Accessed October 30, 2008.

Illinois General Assembly. Public Act 094-0733. http://www.ilga.gov/legislation/publicacts/fulltext.asp?Name=094-0733. Accessed April 5, 2010.

Inglesby TV. Observations from the Top Off exercise. *Public Health Rep.* 2001;116(suppl 2): 64–68.

The Joint Commission on Accreditation of Healthcare Organizations. *Health Care at the Crossroads: Strategies for Creating and Sustaining Community-wide Emergency Preparedness Systems.* Oakbrook Terrace, IL: JCAHO; 2003.

Kaji AH, Koenig KL, Lewis RJ. Current hospital disaster preparedness. *JAMA.* 2007; 298(18):2188–2190.

Kelen GD, McCarthy ML. The science of surge. *J Acad Emerg Med.* 2006;13(11): 1089–1094.

Kinlaw K, Levine R. *Ethical Guidelines in Pandemic Influenza—Recommendations of the Ethics Subcommittee of the Advisory Committee to the Director.* Centers for Disease Control and Prevention. http://www.cdc.gov/od/science/phec/panFlu_Ethic_Guidelines.pdf. Published February 15, 2007.

Koenig KL, Cone DC, Burstein JL, Camargo CA Jr. Surging to the right standard of care. *Acad Emerg Med.* 2006;13(2):195–198.

Krauss CK, Levy F, Kelen GD. Lifeboat ethics: considerations in the discharge of inpatients for the creation of hospital surge capacity. *Disaster Med Public Health Prep.* 2007;1(1):51–56.

Melnychuk RM, Kenny NP. Pandemic triage: the ethical challenge. *CMAJ.* 2006; 175(11):1393–1394.

Moriber MR. On the Survivability of the Citizens of the State of Texas [Handout for GETAC Medical Directors Committee]. http://www.dshs.state.tx.us/emstraumasystems/SurvivabilityofCitizensDocument.pdf. Published May 8, 2008. Accessed October 12, 2008.

Nurse to Patient Ratios: Research and Reality. NEPPC Conference Report Series No. 05-1; July 2005. http://www.bos.frb.org/economic/neppc/conreports/2005/conreport051.pdf. Accessed April 5, 2010.

OHA Insurance Solutions. Liability coverage questions during disaster planning. OHA Insurance Solutions Web site. http://www.ohainsurance.com/riskmgmt/newsdisliabcovFeb2007.pdf. Published February 2007.

Pandemic Influenza Working Group. *Stand on Guard for Thee: Ethical Considerations in Preparedness Planning for Pandemic Influenza.* Toronto, Canada: University of Toronto Joint Centre for Bioethics; 2005. http://www.jointcentreforbioethics.ca/publications/documents/stand_on_guard.pdf. Accessed October 18, 2008.

Salinsky E. Strong as the weakest link: medical response to a catastrophic event [background paper]. Washington, DC: The George Washington University; August 8, 2008. http://cdm266901.cdmhost.com/cgi-bin/showfile.exe?CISOROOT=/p266901coll4&CISOPTR=1628&filename=1518.pdf. Accessed March 11, 2010.

Santa Clara Public Health Department. Pandemic Influenza: Ethical Considerations. Santa Clara Public Health Department Web site. http://www.sccgov.org/SCC/docs/Public%20Health%20Department%20(DEP)/attachments/Tool%201-%20Pandemic%20Influenza%20Ethics%20Tool%2012-07.pdf. Published 2007. Accessed December 1, 2008.

Shore Health System. Critical Care and Ventilator Triage Guidelines During a Disaster Event. Shore Health System Administrative Policy. http://doctors.shorehealth

.org/policies/TX/TX-57-CRITICAL%20CARE%20VENTILATOR%20TRIAGE-08-08.pdf. Published August, 2008. Accessed October, 2008.

Thompson A. Stand on guard for thee: ethical considerations in preparedness planning for pandemic influenza [slide presentation]. Toronto, Canada: University of Toronto Joint Centre for Bioethics; 2005. http://www.aohc.org/aohc/index.aspx?CategoryID=16&lang=en-CA. Accessed March 11, 2010.

Toner E, Waldhorn R, Maldin B, et al. Hospital preparedness for pandemic influenza. *Biosecur Bioterror.* 2006;4(2):207–217.

US Department of Health & Human Services. The Hospital Preparedness Program (HPP). US Department of Health & Human Services Web site. http://www.hhs.gov/aspr/opeo/hpp/. Accessed April 5, 2010.

Utah Hospitals and Health Systems Association. Utah Pandemic Influenza Hospital and ICU Triage Guidelines. Salt Lake City, Utah: Utah Department of Health. http://www.uha-utah.org/Disaster%20Prep%20Materials/PANDEMIC%20FLU%20Triage%20Guidelines_081109.pdf. Published March 5, 2008.

Wise RA. The creation of emergency health care standards for catastrophic events. *Acad Emerg Med.* 2006;13(11):1150–1152.

Chapter 21

Mass Fatality Management

Barbara A. Butcher, MPH and Frank DePaolo, RPA-C

Learning Objectives

- Discuss ways to manage mass fatalities during or following a disaster or public health emergency.
- Identify potential methods of altered operating procedures to accommodate mass fatalities following a disaster or public health emergency.
- Discuss planning considerations for a mass fatality event.
- Describe the process of handling and processing contaminated remains.
- Describe the issues concerning disposition of remains and family support services following a mass fatality event.

Overview

The importance of fatality management is frequently overlooked, and yet recent events since 2001 have shown that disasters frequently overwhelm the traditional systems designed to care for the deceased, exceeding the ability of local authorities to manage mortuary affairs. Although life safety issues always take precedence over the recovery of the dead, advance planning for fatality management will prevent errors that may prolong the effects on a grieving populace. The governing authorities' ability to identify and return human remains will better enable the community's recovery following a disaster. After Hurricane Katrina, the sight of dead bodies floating in the streets of New Orleans, some for months, shocked the world and helped precipitate a crisis in the national government.

A failure to recover and identify decedents in a timely fashion will produce legal ramifications that are additionally burdensome to grieving families. For example, families may be unable to obtain insurance and inheritance benefits. Following the World Trade Center attack of September 11, 2001, it was soon acknowledged that the extensive fragmentation of human remains could delay the identification of victims by years, and in turn delay the issuance of death certificates. Many widows and widowers with children were unable to pay mortgages and bills without the ability to make insurance claims based on death certification. The New York City legal and judicial community intervened and instituted "death certification by judicial decree" based on sworn affidavits and evidence in the absence of a body. Such steps were required to ease the burden on grieving families and provide some degree of assistance.

Proper planning and preparedness capacity can begin to anticipate such challenges, and develop systems to respond as effectively and efficiently as possible. The following text is designed to alert the mass fatality manager to the range of issues to consider in developing appropriate response plans.

The objectives of this chapter are to provide an overview of mass fatality management (MFM), identify issues in mass fatality events, and give the disaster manager a basic framework for developing strategies to cope with such events in a healthcare or community setting.

Case Study

Case Study and Discussion

In 2005, the United States government began new efforts for the development of plans to prevent, mitigate, and manage the effects of pandemic influenza (PI). This nationwide effort was sparked by the discovery of a deadly Avian Influenza in the Far East, an H5N1 viral strain that has a high mortality rate among birds and fowl, and a greater than 60% death rate among the humans infected by direct or indirect contact with the species.

In 1918, the Spanish Flu, an H1N1 virus, caused a world-wide pandemic resulting in more than 50 million deaths; 675,000 of them in the United States. These and other such pandemics, by their sheer numbers, overwhelmed the healthcare system and paralyzed mortuary operations all over the world, further demoralizing the stricken population.

To understand the magnitude of such a PI event, using an infection rate of 25% and a fatality rate of 5-7% of those infected, the Army's United States Northern Command Joint Task Force-Civil Support (JTF-CS) estimates 3,612,500 deaths in addition to the 2.4 million deaths that occur annually in the United States. New York City, using a lower fatality rate of 2.1%, estimates having to manage an additional 50,000 deaths over an 8-week period—in addition to the usual 6000 deaths occurring from other causes during that same time. This may be repeated in two or three waves throughout the pandemic life cycle of 12–18 months.

Discussion

It is estimated that 67% of PI deaths in New York City (NYC) would occur in the city's 68 hospitals; 12% in the 200 assisted living centers; 19% in private residences; and 2% in other locations, such as prisons. Most hospitals have very limited morgue capacity. Those hospital personnel who are not ill will be stretched to the limit in caring for the living; funeral directors and cemetery workers will be similarly taxed and unable to remove decedents from hospitals, nursing homes, and residences. In fact, every service, such as food distribution, electrical power, law enforcement, and the burying of the dead may be so impacted as to bring ordinary life to a standstill. Nevertheless, we can create strategies and operations plans to manage what we can.

Using your own city or region as an example, what strategies could you employ to manage the fatalities from such an event? Are there plans in place for hospitals, medical examiners, and funeral homes? From whom could you expect help, and what resources would you need? Who will be in charge, and who will do the work? These and other questions will be addressed throughout the text.

> "The people of America will not settle to see fellow Americans going to waste on the street. (Thus,) we must take the mission of mortuary affairs right behind saving lives, (and) its execution must be implemented concurrently."
> —Lieutenant General Russell L. Honore, Commanding General of the U.S. First Army, Former Commander of the Joint Task Force-Katrina

Introduction

Fatality management is as old as death itself, and ranges from the mummification processes used by ancient Egyptians to preserve their pharaohs, to the elaborate rituals and beautiful cemeteries of old Europe, to today's technologically sophisticated DNA identification of fragmented remains from terrorist bomb attacks. All nations, cultures, societies, and religions have developed their methods of caring for the dead; most often designed with a single death in mind. On those occasions when societies were overwhelmed by mass fatalities, as in earthquakes, fires, or storms, traditions and rites were often abandoned out of the necessity of using limited resources to care for the living. As we shall describe, modern technology and political imperatives no longer permit such dispensation. Even the most resource-challenged must struggle to care for the dead in as dignified a manner as the citizenry demands.

Mass fatality events are not a rare occurrence; in the first half of 2008 alone, 101 natural disasters were reported, killing 229,043 people in seven countries. Storms and floods were responsible for 72% of these deaths; the remaining 38% were the result of the May earthquake in China. While Asia was hardest hit by these disasters, the West is not immune; in 2003, a heat wave swept Western Europe, killing more than 35,000. Despite sophisticated warning systems, more than 1800 people died in Hurricane Katrina in the United States in 2005.

Terrorist attacks present a particular challenge to recovery workers because the use of improvised explosive devices (IED) causes fragmentation and commingling of remains, making identification (and separation of victim's remains from terrorist's remains) very difficult. The 1993 and 2001 attacks on the World Trade Center, the train bombings in London and Madrid, and the insurgent attacks in Iraq and Afghanistan have pushed fatality managers to develop an unwanted expertise in re-association of decedents' bodies.

CHALLENGES IN MASS FATALITY MANAGEMENT— A FEW EXAMPLES

In a mass fatality context, even the simplest forms of identification become suspect when put to the test of overwhelming numbers and circumstances. Following the 2001 attack on the World Trade Center (WTC), for example, firefighters seeking survivors, their colleagues, and friends desperately tore through a seven-story pile of burning rubble. At times, they would find the body of a fellow firefighter, unidentifiable except for his heat-resistant turn-out gear, labeled with his name and fire company. They would announce the identification to each other, which spread to the families and the media. Unfortunately, these often proved incorrect as it became apparent that many responders ran into fire stations and grabbed whatever gear was available, regardless of what name was on the helmet or coat.

In at least two instances during 9/11, medical personnel, finding themselves without survivors to treat, attempted to help by setting up temporary body collection points (BCP) without notifying the Office of Chief Medical Examiner (OCME). They documented external findings on remains and removed jewelry and ID cards for safekeeping. Though well-intentioned, they inadvertently destroyed the ability to confirm or establish identification by personal effects.

THE TSUNAMI OF 2004—LESSONS LEARNED

In the Tsunami of 2004, at least 250,000 people were killed by waves surging inland for miles, reaching more than 30 feet high, and sweeping out again with everything from homes, to trees, animals, and even the soil. The greatest impact was in some of the poorest countries in the world. More than 2 million people were left homeless, without food or water. In Indonesia alone, 130,000 died, 40,000 were missing, and 500,000 people were displaced. The world response was swift, and aid came rapidly for the living. The dead, however, came to rest among the trees and wreckage where villages once stood, and floated in and out with the tides on fouled beaches.

In Thailand, more than 5400 people were killed, approximately half of them foreign tourists. Thailand's major industry is tourism, and numerous beach resorts and local craft industries had been ruined. Still reeling from the devastation and grief, Thai authorities quickly became aware that the European and Scandinavian nations, from which most of the tourists came, wanted the bodies of their citizens identified and repatriated swiftly. In recognition of both economic and political imperatives, the Thai government initiated the concurrent recovery and identification of the dead, even as the region struggled to bring care to injured survivors and restore basic services.

Although Thailand has a robust capacity for public health disaster response, there were few resources or plans to care for deceased victims. Volunteers, military personnel, law enforcement, and others began locating bodies and removing them to makeshift morgues, where the intense heat caused rapid decomposition. Lacking a fatality management plan, no one documented where they found the bodies; they were not labeled or numbered correctly, and often no photos were taken. Fortunately for some areas, the police took over quickly and began directing location documentation, numbering, and photos where possible. Police began taking fingerprint impressions and developing files on each body recovered. Because most Thai citizens are fingerprinted after the age of 16 years, the authorities at least had some possible reference data from which to work.

In the absence of clearly defined roles and responsibilities, confusion among agencies and authorities soon ensued. Overall authority shifted from the Ministry of the Interior, to the Royal Thai Police, to the Ministry of Public Health, and then back to the Ministry of the Interior. As an example of the aftermath created by conflicting policies and directions, a well-known and well-intentioned medical examiner arrived on the scene and directed that all identification efforts cease, save for the taking of DNA swabs, because "DNA was the most accurate method" for identifying bodies. This had the unfortunate result of delaying the crucial work of recording physical characteristics before the bodies decomposed.

Indeed, the utility of DNA-based identification methods under these circumstances was questionable. Most direct reference samples to the victims had been swept away by the flood waters and, absent recovery location records, searching for such samples was next-to-impossible. Not surprisingly, DNA played almost no role at all in post-tsunami victim identification (0.4%). In fact, dental comparisons proved most useful, resulting in 85.5% of all identifications, as numerous Thai dentists volunteered to compare decedent x-rays to records provided by international authorities and some local clinics. Fingerprints were most useful for the local Thai victims, given that most dental records had been lost or destroyed in the wreckage.

By mid-January of 2005, Interpol Disaster Victim Identification (DVI) teams from 29 countries had arrived in Thailand and began working with the Thai authorities under the direction of the Ministry of the Interior, forming the Thai Tsunami Victim Identification (TTVI) team. Disaster portable mortuary units (DPMU) and family assistance centers (FAC) were set up, protocols established, and data management systems uploaded to accession, antemortem, and postmortem data. Working together, the Thais and the international responders made remarkable progress in the face of an overwhelming task.

Storage of the decedents, both temporary and long-term, was a critical issue because the heat and humidity of the region caused the bodies to decompose within days, leaking fecal matter into the water supply and sending noxious odors into the surrounding areas where survivors hunted for their family members. At first, bodies were brought to area temples and laid outside on the ground. This served the dual purpose of having centrally located known sites, as well as the ability to perform Buddhist rites over the dead, giving relatives the comfort of knowing that even if they never received their loved ones back for burial, the souls of the dead would be at rest. (See Figure 21-1.)

After a week, morgue workers tried using dry ice banked around the bodies, but this was impractical. Dry ice is difficult to obtain and handle, causing "cold burns" to workers, and as it evaporates, toxic carbon dioxide is emitted in dangerous quantities, especially in enclosed

Figure 21-1

Temporary morgue at a temple in Thailand

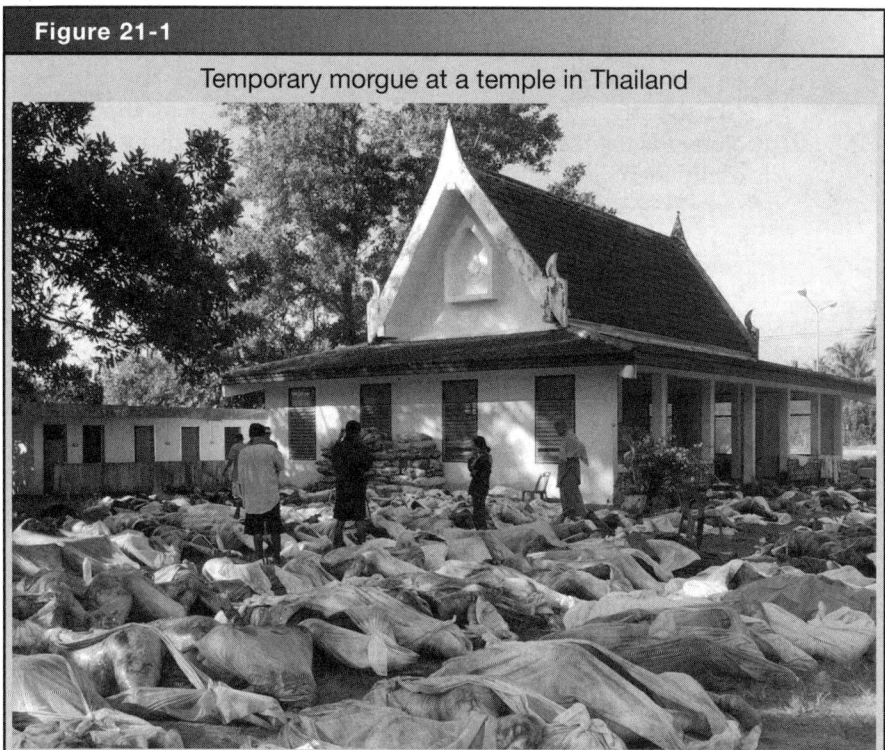

© Aprichart Weerawong/AP Photos

spaces. Soon, trenches were dug and labeled decedents in marked body bags were temporarily interred in fields near the temples.

As the DVI teams arrived, refrigerated shipping containers were obtained and off-loaded at the DPMU sites. After being fitted with racks for body storage, they proved to be most effective at retarding the already advanced decomposition of decedents. These containers are not without their own problems, however, because the logistics of placement, powering or fueling, and sanitation may prove too difficult for heavily impacted or resource-poor areas.

Final disposition of unidentified and unclaimed bodies proved equally daunting. Cremation was attempted, but a lack of dry wood and old tires precluded any significant efforts. In many cases, memorialized temporary internment sites would be the long-term solution for many victims. Other affected nations, such as Indonesia, were not able to spare their limited resources for fatality management, and had to resort to mass burials.

The preceding case provides a window to a myriad of logistical, technical, material, and political issues to be considered in preparing for mass fatality scenarios. It is, of course, impossible to anticipate all contingencies, but studying past response operations and gleaning lessons learned should certainly be a component of planning and preparedness activities.

In the pages that follow, we present an all-hazards approach to planning for and managing a mass fatality event, while maintaining the flexibility necessary to adapt to varying resources and imperatives.

Definition of a Mass Fatality Incident

A mass fatality incident can be defined as follows:

- any event having the potential to produce 10 or more fatalities
- any situation in which there are more human bodies or human remains to be recovered and examined than can be routinely handled by available resources
- any situation in which remains are contaminated by biological, chemical, or radiological agents
- an incident or other special circumstances requiring a multi-agency response in support of mortuary operations
- an incident involving a protracted or complex remains recovery operation

Hazard Analysis

Based on this definition, the impact of almost any hazard can result in a mass fatality event. Hazards such as a terrorism incident, heat emergency, fire, aircraft disaster, hurricane, or disease outbreak all have the potential to yield mass fatalities. For mass fatality management operations, the scale and nature of the incident will determine the extent of the response. Mass fatality incidents or events will be either localized or regional and may include special conditions resulting from chemical, biological, or radiological contamination, and/or fragmentation from large explosions.

Examples of incidents that cause localized mass fatalities include a terrorism incident, a major building collapse, a severe multivehicle accident, a vehicle-borne improvised explosive device, and a chemical agent release. Responses to localized events should be guided by the protocols laid out under the National Incident Management System (NIMS), the federal government's framework for coordinated disaster response. Response efforts will typically include the establishment of an Incident Command Post, an Operations Section, and, in some cases, area-wide coordination through an Emergency Operations Center (EOC). The Incident Action Plan (IAP) must include fatality management objectives.

Particular conditions that require specialized response techniques may occur in either a localized or a citywide mass fatality incident. In the case of decedent contamination in a radiological event, for example, a safety concern for those who handle contaminated remains and for the public must be considered. Public health concerns begin at the time of contamination/disease and continue through the human remains processing and final disposition phases. Individuals who handle contaminated remains must have the capability to prevent exposure to the contamination or disease and have the capability to decontaminate or isolate the remains.

The authority responsible for fatality management (often the medical examiner or coroner), in coordination with other agencies (such as the health department, law enforcement, and others), must incorporate the necessary steps to mitigate any further public health threat that could result from the handling and disposition of contaminated remains, or those infected with a highly contagious disease. The wishes and religious beliefs of the decedent's family will be weighed against the continued risk to the public health, and special restrictions may apply to the funeral services and final disposition of human remains.

Jurisdiction Authority and Roles

Fatality management falls within the jurisdiction of the local authority in all cases. Most often, the medical examiner or coroner and department of health will direct and manage operations with assistance from supporting agencies. These may be local agencies, such as police and fire departments, or state and federal agencies, depending on the magnitude of the incident.

Among federal supporting agencies are the Department of Homeland Security (DHS) and the Federal Emergency Management Agency (FEMA). Together, they oversee the National Response Plan (NRP), which unifies national resources necessary to mitigate the effects of an incident that has been designated a Presidential Declared Disaster. Assets must be requested through the state governor.

The Department of Health and Human Services (DHHS) is the lead federal agency for mortuary services and medical care under Emergency Support Function #8 (ESF #8). Within DHHS are the National Disaster Medical Service (NDMS) and the Disaster Mortuary Operational Response Team (DMORT), consisting of regional volunteers who are federalized as they are deployed. As the lead agency, DHHS has the authority to ask the DHS and the Department of Defense (DOD) for assistance. DOD has expertise in mortuary affairs, but available resources can be limited; for instance, availability of personnel and assets at any given time is subject to current deployment.

The 2006 White House report, *The Federal Response to Hurricane Katrina: Lessons Learned*, states: "Federal and state officials struggled to locate, recover, and identify the hundreds of deceased victims. While mortuary affairs are generally a state and local responsibility, the NRP is unclear about the appropriate federal role, leading to substantial confusion." Mortuary affairs still does not have its own ESF.

Key Planning Issues

Health and safety plans will cover a host of items, including personal protective equipment (PPE), exposure/work time, worker certification for different tasks, monitoring equipment for hazardous conditions, emergency evacuation procedures, and decontamination requirements. It is important that these plans are in place prior to the start of operations; prevention is the only way to avoid worker injury and negative long-term health effects. Each health and safety plan must meet the standards established by regulatory agencies, such as the Occupational Safety and Health Administration (OSHA) and Environmental Protection Agency (EPA).

Training and continuing recertification of workers will ensure that operations go smoothly in the event of a disaster. Numerous training programs have evolved since 9/11, and are generally available through the Department of Homeland Security at no cost to government agencies.

All plans, whether all-hazards or incident-specific, will include a *concept of operations* (ConOps) that will provide a high-level overview of the operation. Flexibility must be built into the plan to account for unanticipated disasters (airplane guided missile) and changing conditions (hurricane-broken levees flood). A modular approach will enable the incident commander to broaden or shrink the operation, saving resources.

Although *command and control* will be consistent with the Incident Command System (ICS), the National Incident Management System (NIMS) does not *specifically* address fatality management. Local response efforts must, therefore, conform to local protocols if available. In the author's jurisdiction, for example, a fatality management branch is established and placed under the Operations Section; forensic investigative functions of MFM fall within the Human Remains Group under the Intelligence and Investigative section.

A *personnel notification system* is necessary not only to bring in workers, but to prevent "free-lancing" or self-dispatching. These actions will result in worker injury and preclude the commander from holding reserves for a phased response or extended operations. Job Action Sheets for each task or position are held by the section chiefs to give to workers. Although team members should know their roles prior to an incident, we cannot assume that those workers will be available, and should be prepared for just-in-time (JIT) training. In mass fatality management, job aids can be crafted for positions such as the agency's incident command positions and specific job functions, such as the forensic section chief, fingerprint technician, recovery transport operator, pathologist, photographer, scribe, DNA sampler, and others.

Schematics should lay out more than workstations or equipment placement; they should also demonstrate a work flow. In addition to pull-out sheets in plan binders, poster-sized printouts attached to workspace walls will enable the staff to set up workstations quickly, and assist new workers in understanding their part in the operation.

Fatality management will often require extended operations because initial resource supplies will be directed toward response and rescue of the living. It is important that planners take resource allocation issues into consideration when assessing operation needs and sources of equipment and personnel. In larger urban areas, emergency management (EM) may coordinate resources—if planning has taken place to pre-identify necessary assets. Indeed, it may be advantageous for jurisdictions to identify specific vendors and suppliers for items such as body bags or wooden coffins. During a crisis, logistics teams can then more easily acquire and deploy resources, pulling from pre-established lists with contact numbers. It should be noted that this type of inventory, known as "just-in-time" will likely be insufficient if the event involves a large geographic area crossing multiple jurisdictions. For example, body bag suppliers are limited in the United States. It is likely that federal, state, and local governments will attempt to make purchases from the same vendors, resulting in higher pricing and limited or first-come availability. A more effective method of emergency procurement that can occur in advance of an incident is called "contingency contracting." Contingency contracting is in widespread use in places such as the United Kingdom where the central government has contracts in place that provide a turnkey solution for a "resilience mortuary." It is likely that this type of contracting will replace procurement methods currently in place in the United States.

Phased responses are critical to conserving human resources. Staging and redundancy minimize the possibility for exhaustion to undermine the first wave of response. In large-scale events, however, it is not likely that there will be sufficient numbers of trained mortuary workers. Planners are advised to meet with other supporting agencies in advance to enhance their surge capacity. By identifying a potential worker pool that can function under the direction of MFM experts, managers can build in human resource potential. For example, medical students are excellent scribes and autopsy assistants, sanitation workers will be able to move coffins and bodies readily, and corrections officers may provide security for sensitive areas.

Functional Areas of Mass Fatality Management

CENTRALIZED MISSING PERSONS REPORTING

In the first hours after a major incident, emergency operations will be focused on life safety issues, with one notable exception for MFM. As the incident evolves, thousands of people will attempt to call government agencies and healthcare facilities to locate family members and friends. The 911 emergency lines, community assistance offices, and hospital emergency rooms will have their telephone lines swamped with calls. The absence of a centralized mechanism for a local government to communicate with its citizenry in the hours and days following an incident will further complicate the problem. In the aftermath of the London Underground bombing of 2005, the United Kingdom's Casualty Call Center received more than 4000 calls in the first hour the system became operational. Eventually, the call center handled more that 121,000 calls for the 56 people killed and 850 injured. London and NYC are two of only a few cities in the world with the ability to set up a centralized casualty call center. Following the 2001 attack on the World Trade Center, more than 25,000 people were reported missing; 2752 actually died.

Communications chaos can be expected for "open manifest" incidents, in which the event occurs in areas accessible to the public—such as a train station or open-air venue; it is impossible to know up front who was in the area at the time. A "closed manifest" incident, by contrast, is one in which there is an available list of names for those present, such as the passenger list in an airplane crash.

Two major factors will influence a jurisdiction's success in managing missing persons reporting: (1) avoiding use of emergency lines needed to report ongoing events, and (2) formation of an accurate missing persons list. The first issue is reporting by the public. It is relatively easy to establish a dedicated line for use in disasters, but trained operators must be available. In some jurisdictions, an information number already in daily use can be converted to an emergency call center with a predesigned missing person's protocol, complete with trained personnel and preloaded software for data collection. Another option would be to contract with a commercial call center. In New York City, for example, the City's 311 citizen's help line is fully staffed 24/7; 311 personnel have been trained to use NYC's emergency casualty call system.

Developing and managing a missing persons (MP) list is the other primary concern. Specialized missing persons reporting software must be in place prior to the incident and may be used to catalogue the data as it comes in. Typically, this software will generate known missing persons lists that can then be used by the medical examiner or coroner for identification purposes. Reports may be assigned a relative priority based on proximity to the incident and likelihood of being present; however all reports must be fully investigated.

Access to group lists are provided to police detectives and medical examiner/coroner (ME/C) personnel who gather additional information from the scene, hospital emergency departments, the morgue, the family assistance center, and the callers themselves. These personnel will refine the list as additional information becomes available; callers are also asked to call back if the missing person returns home, further clearing the list. The continually refined list of missing persons and the identifying information gathered will form the basis of antemortem data for each victim.

SCENE OPERATIONS

If the community has a well-developed mass fatality response plan, command and control issues will have been previously addressed, and fatality management operations will be coordinated within the ICS. The staging of fatality management personnel and equipment should occur in such a way that guarantees full access for life safety operations. Too often, emergency response is not staged appropriately, leaving roads blocked, equipment inaccessible, and operations personnel caught in hazardous situations.

MFM resources at the scene will generally include body collection points (BCPs) set up at the periphery and tents for personnel and equipment. Each event will dictate the setup, but safety will always be the overriding concern. This requires the full characterization of potential hazards at the site prior to beginning MFM operations. This characterization is generally performed at the direction of the incident safety officer. After a hazard assessment is complete, a health and safety plan is developed. A complete safety briefing is required, along with the issuance of appropriate personal protective equipment (PPE).

Contaminated Remains

If the remains are contaminated by chemical or radiological materials, as in a terror attack or industrial accident, they must be decontaminated by trained hazmat-certified forensic personnel. In the event that decontamination is not possible, a containment strategy may be employed. Decontamination may be achieved through a variety of mechanisms that involved either the removal (displacement) or the neutralization of the contaminant. Runoff or effluent resulting from the decontamination process may prove hazardous to those in the area. Any such operation must be carried out by well-qualified teams, in conjunction with safety officers, Environmental Protection, and Emergency Services Units.

It is possible to carry out all mortuary functions in a hazardous environment, including autopsy, but special equipment and training is required. It is unlikely that many ME/C offices will have this capability, but several urban centers do, and regional planning may enable them to share resources. In a local or regional event, the Disaster Mortuary Operational Response, Weapons of Mass Destruction Team (DMORT-WMD) can provide a limited number of trained personnel and resources. In addition to the remains, all personnel operating at the scene must undergo decontamination as well.

Although dead bodies do not spread disease, biological agents may also complicate operations. Smallpox, anthrax, viral hemorrhagic fevers, and other organisms require special handling and must be isolated and contained. Any processing of fatalities under these circumstances must be guided by the Centers for Disease Control and Prevention (CDC) and health subject matter experts.

A plan for remains recovery will be developed in conjunction with the command element, and may be enacted after the immediate hazards have been cleared, provided that this is a natural disaster and no forensic investigation is needed. If criminality is suspected, as in a terrorist incident, then the ME/C must work with law enforcement to conduct an appropriate investigation prior to body removal. It is seldom urgent to remove decedents from a disaster scene, especially if doing so will destroy forensic evidence or endanger workers.

Fragmentation

It is useful to grid the area and flag remains for overall documentation of their location. Each remain must be securely tagged with a unique identifier in waterproof material, noting the location, date, time, and involved personnel. Each remain should be photographed in situ with the label visible. Jewelry and wallets or other personal effects should not be removed. The exterior of the body bag must be labeled in waterproof ink with the same number as the remains tag. Any body part found must be treated as an individual, tagged and bagged separately, and not re-associated in the field. Following an explosion or building collapse, there may be extensive commingling of remains, which will be separated later by anthropologists, pathologists, and others at the morgue.

Remains Transport

Remains may be brought to a BCP for collection and transport to an established fixed mortuary site, or they may be brought to an off-site mortuary for preprocessing and examination. Regardless, every step should be fully documented and all remains transported should be accompanied by a manifest. Each photograph or document should be labeled with the same unique identifier as the remains. These will form the basis of the postmortem charts, just as the missing person's reports and information collected at the family assistance center form the basis of the antemortem charts. As information is added to each, the antemortem and postmortem charts will be compared, eventually resulting in a match for the identification of each victim.

If the disaster is widespread, as in pandemic influenza (PI), there may be a need for numerous BCPs and body recovery teams, as well as facilities for temporary storage. In an urban setting with numerous healthcare facilities, refrigerated trailers (reefers) could be placed at each hospital, and picked up when full. The bodies can be transported to remains storage facilities and held in refrigerated shipping containers, tents, or prefabricated units. In Hurricane Katrina, the large high-ceiling tents and chillers did not work because of the extreme heat and humidity of the region; in the even greater heat of Thailand following the tsunami, shipping containers worked very well.

DISASTER MORTUARY OPERATIONS

Prior to commencing mortuary operations, a primary objective, and the strategies for achieving it, must be determined. In any death investigation, practitioners look to answer the following questions regarding the decedent: Who are you, where were you, what happened to you, who was involved, when did it happen, how did it happen, and why? Answering these questions can guide decisions about how to proceed in a mass fatality scenario.

For instance, in the 9/11 attack on the WTC, we knew where it happened, what happened, when, how, who did it, and even why. The only outstanding question was "who are you?" Consequently, identifying the victims was the primary mission. It then became clear that autopsies were less necessary than careful external examinations were. Histology studies were of no help, but DNA testing, fingerprinting, and forensic odontology were.

In Hurricane Katrina, autopsies *were* performed because many different causes of death were possible, from drowning to overdose by injection. Identifications were further complicated because the flood waters breached the above-ground cemeteries common in New Orleans' high water table areas. Caskets opened and old remains floated away, mixing with the decomposed bodies of the storm's victims.

In the case of pandemic influenza, the deaths are natural and not within the typical jurisdiction of the ME/C; death certification will be the responsibility of the treating physician or hospital. However, because of the high number of decedents, it will likely fall to the ME/C to manage the mortuary functions of storage and disposition of decedents as the system rapidly becomes overwhelmed.

In the preceding three cases, answering the preliminary questions helps to determine the primary objective of disaster mortuary operations, which, in turn, guides resource allocation and critical logistical decision making.

After the primary objective has been established, the mortuary area can be set up so that work processes flow most efficiently to achieve this primary objective. At intake, the remains should receive the postmortem chart with labeled forms and any information gathered at the recovery site. At triage, a checklist of stations for appropriate examinations can be filled in. These may include x-ray, external exam by a pathologist, photography, DNA sampling, evidence/personal effects collection, anthropology exam, fingerprinting, forensic odontology, cataloging and separation of personal effects, and others. Each and every exam is documented, and all samples taken are labeled with the same unique identifier as the victim. A decedent escort will transport bodes from station to station and ensure that the chart and forms stay with the remains. As each test result and exam is entered into a data collection system, a complete postmortem chart will be constructed.

After all processes are completed, and the corresponding checklist initialed at each station, the remains will either go to temporary storage or be released to the funeral home if possible. A mortuary supervisor must keep an accurate tracking system for all remains stored or released.

FAMILY ASSISTANCE CENTER OPERATIONS

The family assistance center (FAC) is the place at which all antemortem information and exemplars for comparison will be collected. This location is not to be confused with the Disaster Assistance Service Center (DASC), which may help families and victims with a myriad of services. Although they may be located in the same area, the FAC should be kept separate for the relatives and friends of deceased or missing persons. Here relatives and friends will be asked to provide extensive information about the decedent, and items which may be useful in identification. Among these items are dental records, toothbrushes, and other personal items for direct DNA comparison, photographs, fingerprint cards, medical records, or swabs from family members for DNA kinship analysis. FAC personnel must be trained to obtain, handle, and package exemplars appropriately. It is also advisable to have a scientist present to select the best possible combination of family members for the collection of DNA reference samples.

Information gathered will be extensive and will require a software system to manage the accessioning of all data. Systems such as DMORT VIP, NYC UVIS, and PLAAS are just a few of the options available, and are currently in use by DMORT, New York City, and Interpol, respectively. Although the systems vary, all require accurate physical descriptions that include documentation height and weight, clothing size, and body type. Tattoos, scars, surgical procedures, broken bones, hair length and color, eye shape and color, jewelry worn, watch brand, clothing brands, even fingernail type are recorded.

Each program attempts to use standard descriptive language to facilitate comparisons. A uniform checklist of choices is thus often used. The information obtained will form the antemortem chart, to be compared with postmortem data in the hopes of a match. DNA comparison software operates in much the same fashion, but is far more complex in that it must select from billions of pieces of information contained within the profiles entered.

Although data management systems may produce potential matches from the antemortem and postmortem comparisons, trained Disaster Victim Identification (DVI) teams must make the final identifications. DVI teams generally consist of one member from each forensic discipline, e.g. pathology, forensic dentistry, radiology, fingerprints, DNA, and investigations. As each potential match is made, the antemortem and postmortem information is presented to the team for review and verification of an ID. In order of ease, speed, and resource requirements, visual identification of the body is possible if the decedent's appearance is unchanged, followed by photo, fingerprints, and comparison of teeth to dental records. Characteristics such as tattoos or surgical implants are helpful, but are not always definitive. Of all identification methods, only DNA comparison is definitive, but it is costly, time-consuming, and sometimes difficult in the case of decomposed remains.

LONG-TERM STORAGE

It is inevitable that some remains will not be identified in a large-scale incident, or will undergo repeated attempts at identification as technology and science advances. This is presently the case with the WTC 9/11 remains, which were fragmented and degraded to the point that just over half the victims have been identified at the time of this writing, 8 years later. Despite these difficulties, efforts to make new IDs continue; this requires that the remains are stored properly and kept accessible. In order to prevent further decomposition, the WTC 9/11 remains were preserved through a drying process that does not degrade DNA. They are housed in a memorial facility adjacent to the laboratories where scientists continue their work.

There are other methods of long-term storage, such as embalming, refrigeration, freezing, and chemical preservation. Each must be evaluated for the effect it will have on the ability to continue identification efforts as well as any potential hazards. Long-term storage decisions will, of course, also be constrained by resource availability.

FINAL DISPOSITION

Issuing an accurate death certificate is the primary objective of the disaster mortuary process. In the absence of an identified body, how is it possible to certify a death and allow the family to collect necessary benefits? Following the 2001 WTC attack, it became apparent that some victims would never be found, and so death certification by judicial decree was established. Assisted by volunteer attorneys, families would gather evidence such as WTC employee ID cards, payroll stubs, and sworn statements from colleagues who survived. The attorneys compiled the evidence and drafted affidavits to the courts, petitioning for a declaration of death. After the courts investigated and accepted the petitions, an order was given to the medical examiner to produce a death certificate.

There are other issues in certifying death that may become apparent in a natural outbreak such as PI. Will physicians be able to issue death certificates, and will there be enough clerks working to register them at burial desks? Will there be funeral home and cemetery personnel available to inter the deceased, or will they be interred temporarily? What of the unidentified dead, or those found at home? In a contagious illness such as PI, the professionals we count on will usually become as sick as the patients and be unable to work. Indeed, many may choose not to go to work, staying instead with their families in an effort to avoid the infection. In any planning effort involving infectious disease, we must factor in for a greatly reduced workforce.

Following death certification, the final disposition of remains will be determined based on their characteristics and the status of external factors in the disaster. If the remains are unidentified, they must be kept either in storage for continued processing or temporarily interred. When cold storage resources are exceeded, it is best to inter remains in the ground to retard the decomposition process, at a depth sufficient to remain cool—generally 4 to 6 feet. Bodies should be placed in a single layer in body bags; if coffins are available they may be stacked no more than three deep. Of course the internment trenches should be located at least 800 feet from the water supply, and well-marked.

Identified remains should be released to families as quickly as the staff is able; this may not be possible if external factors prevent them from being claimed. The family members may be too ill to make funeral arrangements, or funeral homes may be unable to keep up with a large number of deaths. There are instances where families do not want to claim the body for personal reasons, and the governing authority must provide internment.

In discussions and planning sessions on mass fatality management, it is often stated that cremation will be the choice when labor resources have been exceeded. This is seldom realistic, because even large urban areas do not have a sufficient number of crematoria to process more than 100 bodies per day.

However, certain categories of contaminated remains will require restricted, controlled burial or mandatory cremation. Currently, the CDC recommends that remains contaminated with smallpox or viral hemorrhagic fevers be double-bagged, washed down with a 0.5% hypochlorite solution, and cremated. Given the dearth of crematorium capacity, some planners have explored air curtain or plasma incinerators. These are used to cremate cattle following death from hoof-and-mouth disease or other equally contagious agents. The incinerators rapidly and efficiently reduce remains to a small amount of a glass-like substance, and can handle large numbers daily. One such plasma torch on a mobile platform resides at Georgia Tech, and there are others in veterinary use, each costing upwards of $3 million. Obviously, this method is distasteful to most people, given the association with cattle and the seeming impersonality of the process; it would require planning and extensive outreach with the religious community in order to make this a palatable solution.

Another alternative for disposition of Category A contaminated remains is burial within a sealed, welded casket, such as a Ziegler case. These containers are expensive, heavy, cumbersome, and prone to leakage if mishandled.

Remains infected with anthrax can be interred in the ground, but there is concern among biologists that the cadaver can become an efficient bioweapon incubator, in that the spores will remain viable for as long as 100 years. It is conceivable that secure cemetery facilities could be established, but at great cost financially and great emotional distress to families.

It is generally acknowledged that other contaminants, such as radioactive dust, can be washed away with soap and water, and will not harm workers if appropriate PPE is used and decontamination is thorough. It may not be possible to decontaminate chemical weapons like sarin or VX. Off-gassing may occur from the cadaver, and supplied air will be necessary for all workers. Extreme hazmat situations like these require highly trained certified personnel with extensive operations support teams.

It is likely that bodies contaminated with chemical, radiological, and some biological agents will undergo a form of restricted disposition that will prevent families from conducting the customary funeral rites and services. To preclude the emotional damage this may engender, it is helpful for the manager to engage the religious community in the planning process prior to any MFM event. With foreknowledge, religious leaders may find appropriate dispensations in canon law that may be applied during a disaster, affording some degree of comfort to observant or devout relatives. For instance, the tenets of the Jewish faith require burial before sundown and prohibit cremation, yet in a PI event, it may not be possible to observe these religious laws. Communications through area rabbis would help their constituents to cope with these distasteful necessities.

Psychological Factors

The entire population of a region will be psychologically and emotionally affected by a MF incident, but none more than the workers handling the remains, and the families of the victims. The care of these two groups should be approached very differently.

Following the WTC 9/11 attack, our nation and much of the world mourned the victims and grieved for their families. The firefighters, police officers, construction workers, and volunteers who worked on the rubble pile were hailed as heroes.

At the New York City Office of Chief Medical Examiner (OCME), where the remains were taken for identification and processing, weekly meetings were held with families to keep them apprised of progress. A family hotline was established and manned 24 hours a day so that relatives could call for information, ask questions, add data, or just talk with the people who were working on finding their loved ones. The Members of Service (MOS) from police and fire departments had their own representatives at the OCME to ensure that their families were appropriately cared for. After 7 years, the OCME still meets with victim's relatives, holds ceremonies, and answers the hotline.

The common theme in any service provided to families is communication—open, constant, and honest. If the next-of-kin wanted to know the exact condition of the remains, or what happened to them, they were told straightforwardly that it might be painful to hear, and to be absolutely sure they wanted the details. Surprisingly, most did, and many even saw photos. Many said that it was better to know the facts than to imagine untold horrors.

Communication to the general public is also important to ensure cooperation, maintain order, and avoid the rumors that can unnecessarily frighten people. Following any MF event, the public needs to be reminded that dead bodies do not spread disease. After the Asian Tsunami, the bodies and the ground at the mortuary were sprayed with disinfectants by workers clothed in Level C PPE; it was a waste of time and manpower, but also an inducement of fear in those who had neither PPE nor disinfectant. Public communication of the government's plans for MFM will reassure the community that their deceased loved ones will be treated with dignity and respect.

Involvement of the religious community while writing MFM plans will aid in cooperation for difficult decisions ahead. It may be necessary at some point to inform religious groups that their funeral rites are prohibited because of a ban on mass gatherings, or recommend cremation to those whose beliefs prohibit it. Nongovernment organizations (NGOs) will make a major contribution toward the psychological care of the victims' families, and provide support in multiple areas of family assistance.

Support for those working in mortuary affairs is different, and more difficult. First, we are asking personnel to remain in the midst of the disaster for a prolonged period, long after the fires are put out and the first responders have left. MFM requires a large influx of nonmortuary workers, e.g., truck drivers, identification specialists, photographers, scribes, body movers, and others not used to the constant sight and smells of the dead. Some psychologists studying the military write that soldiers working as medics or in mortuary affairs may have a comparatively high incidence of post-traumatic stress disorder (PTSD) after seeing mutilated or grossly wounded bodies. Those who work with the families of victims may become numb or even depressed from the constant outpouring of emotion and the empathy they feel. Some families lash out in anger at those trying to help them, especially when bureaucratic hurdles cannot be surmounted easily or expectations cannot be met.

If we accept that those working in mortuary affairs will be adversely affected by what they experience, yet must continue working in that setting for a prolonged time, what measures can we take to mitigate the psychological effects of MFM? If staff cannot be removed from duty, at the least they must be rotated out to other work assignments at regular intervals. Rest breaks have to be enforced because staff working on adrenalin may make mistakes and injure themselves. NGOs are excellent support systems in many aspects; often providing hot food, shelter, cots, dry clothes, and a place for workers to gather on breaks.

A gathering place for workers is especially important because it provides an arena for peer support. Disaster experts have noted reluctance among first responders and emergency workers to obtain outside counseling or therapy following a disaster, attributable perhaps to the culture of their individual units or a desire to "remain strong." Many police departments have instituted mandatory debriefing following a stressful incident, as have other uniformed services. Peer support has always been a mainstay of disaster workers because those working side by side have seen the same horrors and felt the same emotions. Encouraging colleagues to talk about the work will help relieve mental and emotional stress; of course, outside support services should be made available as well. It may even be possible to "embed" a mental health worker or counselor into fatality management operations, much as armed forces units utilize chaplains.

The location of a food and break area for workers must be out of sight and hearing of the public and victims' families. Mortuary affairs personnel and all disaster workers must be able to laugh among themselves, often at things that those outside would consider highly inappropriate. It is the responsibility of team leaders to maintain worker morale during what may be the most stressful times of their own lives; they will do well in setting the example by talking, resting, seeking help, and laughing even more than the others. As stated in the first paragraph of this chapter, life safety issues will always take precedence over fatality management, and that begins here, with us and our coworkers.

References

Blakeney RL. Providing Relief to Families After a Mass Fatality: Roles of the Medical Examiner's Office and the Family Assistance Center. *OVC Bulletin*, Department of Justice. http://www.ojp.usdoj.gov/ovc/publications/bulletins/prfmf_11_2001/welcome.html. Published November, 2002. Accessed November, 2008.

Centre for Research on the Epidemiology of Disasters. Disaster data: a balanced perspective. *Cred Crunch*. 2008;14:1–2. http://www.cred.be/sites/default/files/CredCrunch14.pdf. Accessed November, 2008.

Devlin S, Gavin C, Lyle B, et al; for US Northern Command's Joint Task Force-Civil Support. *White Paper—Morgue Operations, Identification, and Command and Control of Mass Fatalities resulting from a Pandemic Influenza Event in the United States*. http://www.ofdamrt.org/panflu/whitepapers/MorgueOperationsWhitePaper.pdf. Accessed October, 2008.

Guidance on Dealing with Fatalities in Emergencies. Home Office Communication Directorate. http://www.cabinetoffice.gov.uk/media/132748/fatalities.pdf. Published 2004. Accessed October, 2008.

Hirsch C, Brondolo T, Butcher B. Assessment of Victim Identification Operations, Thailand Tsunami Disaster. Report to the Minister of Public Health, Thailand, and the World Health Organization. WHO 2005.

Interpol Disaster Victim Identification Guide. Interpol Web site. http://www.interpol.int/Public/DisasterVictim/guide/default.asp. Accessed November, 2008.

Larsen J. Record heat wave in Europe takes 35,000 lives: far greater losses may lie ahead. Earth Policy Institute Web site. http://www.earth-policy.org/Updates/Update29.htm. Published October 9, 2003. Accessed November, 2008.

McArdle D, Dubouloz M, Arafat R, et al. *Mass Casualty Management Systems; Strategies and Guidelines for Building Health Sector Capacity*. World Health Organization; 2007.

Morgan OW, Sribanditmongkol P, Perera C, et al. Mass fatality management following the South Asian tsunami disaster: case studies in Thailand, Indonesia, and Sri Lanka. *PLoS Med*. 2006;3(6):e195. http://www.plosmedicine.org/article/info:doi%2F10.1371%2Fjournal.pmed.0030195. Accessed January, 2009.

Pan American Health Organization. *Management of Dead Bodies in Disaster Situations*. Washington, DC: Pan American Health Organization; 2004. http://www.crid.or.cr/digitalizacion/pdf/eng/doc15631/doc15631.pdf. Accessed October, 2008.

Tun K, Butcher B, Sribanditmongkol P, et al. Forensic aspects of disaster fatality management. *Prehosp Disast Med.* 2005;20(6):455–458.

United States Congress. Select Bipartisan Committee to Investigate the Preparedness for and Response to Katrina. A Failure of Initiative—Final Report of the Select Bipartisan Committee to Investigate the Preparedness for and Response to Katrina, Washington, DC: U.S. Government Printing Office; 2006. Report 109-377.

Ursano RJ, McCarroll JE. Exposure to traumatic death: the nature of the stressor. In: Ursano RJ, McCaughey BG, Fullerton CS, eds. *Individual and Community Responses to Trauma and Disaster:The Structure of Human Chaos.* New York, NY: Cambridge University Press; 1994:46–71.

USAMRID, Department of Justice, and Office for Domestic Preparedness. *Capstone Document: Mass Fatality Management for Incidents Involving Weapons of Mass Destruction.* http://www.ecbc.army.mil/hld/dl/MFM_Capstone_August_2005.pdf. Published August, 2005. Accessed October, 2008–January, 2009.

US Army PPE and WMD guide. http://www.dtic.mil/cgi-bin/GetTRDoc?AD=ADA451952&Location=U2&doc=GetTRDoc.pdf. Chapters 2,3,7,8. Accessed November, 2008–December, 2008.

US Department of Health and Human Services. *HHS Pandemic Influenza Plan.* http://www.hhs.gov/pandemicflu/plan/pdf/HHSPandemicInfluenzaPlan.pdf. Published November, 2005. Accessed November, 2008–January, 2009.

US Department of Health and Human Services. Centers for Disease Control and Prevention. Official CDC Health Updates. Centers for Disease Control and Prevention Web site. http://www.bt.cdc.gov. Accessed November, 2008–January, 2009.

US Department of Health and Human Services. Centers for Disease Control and Prevention. Decon and PPE. Centers for Disease Control and Prevention Web site. http://www.bt.cdc.gov/planning/personalcleaningfacts.asp. Accessed November, 2008–January, 2009.

US Department of Health and Human Services. Disasters. Department of Health and Human Services Web site. http://www.hhs.gov/disasters/index.shtml. Accessed November, 2008–January, 2009.

US Department of Homeland Security. Federal Emergency Management Agency. Emergency response plans. Federal Emergency Management Agency Web site. http://www.fema.gov/rrr/frp. Accessed November, 2008–January, 2009.

US Department of Homeland Security. National Response Framework. Homeland Security Web site. http://www.dhs.gov/nrp. Accessed November, 2008–January, 2009.

US Department of Justice. *Mass Fatality Incidents: A Guide for Human Forensic Identification.* Washington, DC: Office of Justice Programs NIJ; 2005.http://www.ojp.usdoj.gov/nij. Accessed November, 2008–January, 2009.

US Department of Justice. *Lessons Learned from 9/11: DNA Identifications In Mass Fatality Incidents.* Washington, DC: Office of Justice Programs; 2006.

Wright KM, Ursano RJ, Bartone PT, et al. The shared experience of catastrophe: an expanded classification of the disaster community. *Am J Orthopsychiatry.* 1990:60(1):35-42.

World Health Organization. *Avian Influenza: Assessing the Pandemic Threat.* World Health Organization Web site. http://www.who.int/csr/disease/influenza/WHO_CDS_2005_29/en/index.html. Published January, 2005. Accessed November 2008.

Chapter 22

Research in Emergency and Disaster Medicine

Kobi Peleg, PhD, MPH and Michael Rozenfeld, MA

Photo by Ed Edahl/FEMA

Learning Objectives

- Discuss the challenges that disasters pose to the healthcare system.
- Explain the importance of proper disaster research to hospital preparedness.
- Outline the process of conducting disaster research.

Case Study

On December 7, 1988, a series of successive earthquakes with maximum magnitude of 6.9 on the Richter scale hit Armenia, resulting in 25,000 deaths and 18,000 injured. A major international relief effort was directed to Armenia in order to help the local authorities deal with the situation. Because of the lack of proper planning and preparation for the mass convergence of unsolicited international humanitarian assistance, this relief effort became known as Armenia's "second disaster." Out of 5000 tons of drugs and consumable medical supplies, 20% had to be destroyed and an unknown percentage was stolen by local authorities. Traffic jams on land and in the air resulted in major delays and, finally, in two planes crashing, killing 85 members of a relief expedition. Local medical personnel were sometimes undertrained and unwilling to participate on emergency teams. Before the event, low seismic resilience of prevalent building patterns, already known after Tangshan earthquake in China, together with major tremor predictions by Soviet seismologists, were totally ignored by the authorities.

About one year later, on October 17, 1989, a 7.1 magnitude earthquake struck California, resulting, amazingly, in a much smaller volume of casualties (65 deaths, 3000 injured). The obvious difference in outcomes between the two events could be safely explained by the better preparedness of California communities in terms of mitigation efforts and response capabilities.[1] A crucial part of this successful preparedness effort was the careful studying of previous events, including the Armenia earthquake of 1988, in connection to local context.[2]

Q: What are the benefits of epidemiologic research to hospital preparedness for disasters and other emergencies?

A: It is the only tool that can provide the involved authorities with reliable evidence-based information so existing resources can be utilized to maximum effect.

Health Care: Impact of Disasters and Importance of Disaster Research

Disasters pose a major challenge to a healthcare system. In addition to causing mortality and overcrowding the hospitals with injured, they disrupt communication and transportation, cause power and water shortages, and sometimes endanger the medical personnel directly, diverting the focus from treatment attempts. In the chaos created by a disaster, the limited medical and human resources could be wasted in uncoordinated relief efforts, further aggravating the situation.

A general myth exists about emergencies in general and about disasters specifically: they happen suddenly and their most characterizing feature is chaos; therefore, no systematic knowledge could be obtained in order to ease their impact. Actually, most disasters, or at least the casualties they bring, are preventable.[3] In order for that to happen, credible data considering the disasters should be acquired before, after, and as they happen, so logical conclusions and feasible recommendations can be derived. The probability of a disaster and its possible impact should be assessed. Vulnerable populations must be discovered and regarded within the general effort to strengthen community preparedness. Agencies entrusted with the responsibility of responding to a disaster, including the healthcare system, are to be provided with clear guidelines for action, together with an understanding of required resources. This information helps to acquire specific resources according to calculated future needs in order to channel them efficiently during times of emergency. The list of possible tasks for a researcher can continue much further, but total indispensability of data collection and analysis in preparation for disaster response is made clear by these examples.

The best known instrument for this sake is *epidemiological research*, the interest of which is the measuring of occurrence, distribution, and determinants of health and decease cases in a given population.[4] But, like any instrument, it should be used according to specific needs, posed by the task at hand: preparing for disasters as an extreme case of medical emergency.

Epidemiological Profile of Disasters

The first important issue of disaster research is that there are major differences in epidemiological profile (levels and types of mortality and morbidity) of different disasters. The immediate meaning of this fact is that hospital preparedness for disasters would differ among geographic regions, because most disasters, even those that are man-made, are peculiar to specific regions.[3] The prospects of a volcano eruption would have lower priorities in large river deltas, especially compared to floods, the same as tsunamis are less of a threat in mountain regions, compared to earthquakes and volcano eruptions. Settlements situated near nuclear reactors or chemical plants should be better prepared for technological disasters than rural areas. Some definite areas of the globe provide the majority of conflict-related emergencies.

If patterns of morbidity and mortality specific to the different types of disasters could be understood, the healthcare system of any region could be provided with specific recommendations about its preparedness to handle disaster outcomes. Injuries are the most immediate outcome of disasters, but some long-term outcomes, such as contagious disease and post-traumatic stress disorder (PTSD) could be present. Disasters could also aggravate existing chronic conditions, such as cardiovascular problems, or cause miscarriages and premature births in pregnant women.[3]

Reliable estimation of expected casualties in different scenarios is crucial for preparedness efforts, but it is complicated to achieve because disasters vary, not only by type, but also by magnitude, which is hardly predictable. Despite that, the rule of thumb is that water-related disasters usually result in high mortality and low morbidity, wind-related disasters result in low mortality and moderate morbidity, while earth-related emergencies are the most severe in both outcomes.[3] Terror-related events also usually have a high injury profile, but differences could exist between different mechanisms, such as a car explosion, suicide bombing, or mass shooting. It is important to understand that the ratio of mortality and morbidity is an important piece of data, because those injured who are still alive are the ones who receive medical treatment, and, therefore, the resource planning should be concentrated on this population. Another epidemiological issue of disasters is that their impact could vary by orders of magnitude between developed and developing countries (caused by vast disparity in resources for prevention and response). In addition to already mentioned differences in the outcomes of the Armenia earthquake of 1988 and the California earthquake of 1989, there are less obvious issues. For one, during disasters in developed countries the nutrition of the population is rarely an issue, while, in developing regions, it could become one of the most prominent issues of the response effort. Transportation capabilities are a major factor: a developed country enjoys greater flexibility in vehicle types and transport facilities. Heavy-duty army trucks can bring supplies even if there are no roads left, and a fleet of helicopters can reach almost any destination.

Secondly, because epidemics could become the major threat of the century, the differences in immune system adaptability between developed and developing countries are to be considered because history knows many examples of entire populations being wiped out by a disease previously unknown in the region.[5]

Disasters are also varied in their direct and indirect influence on the healthcare system (in addition to crowding them with multiple patients of different severity). Earthquakes are the greatest challenge, physically destroying the hospitals, hindering evacuation attempts by disrupting transportation arteries, and aggravating the situation by power shortages. But the same problems, even if on a smaller scale, could be caused by other emergencies. Strong winds may cut the power supply and jam approach routes with debris. Hospital buildings could be struck by bombardment or even occupied by militant forces in conflict scenarios.

Issues of Interest in Disaster Research

Despite the mentioned variations among different kinds of disasters, there exist a number of issues, generally common to disaster research, differentiating this field of research from other fields where epidemiology is applied. The main reason for this differentiation is the low level of control the researcher of disasters has over the studied context, leading to compromises in accepted method of data collection and statistical analysis.

RESEARCH METHODS

The immediate result of the low level of control over the studied context is that disaster research is usually based on *surveys* and not on *experiments*.[6] The main difference between these two primary methods of research is that in surveys, information is systematically collected without deliberate intervention on study subjects used in experiments. A survey can be used to provide a snapshot picture of the situation (a *cross-sectional* study) or to link the outcome and cause in a longitudinal study (*prospective* follow-up from exposure or *retrospective* investigation from outcome to cause). When surveys are used to monitor the health situation in a population in the long term, they are referred to as *surveillance*.

The establishment of a successful surveillance system is largely dependant on relevant *case definitions* and trained personnel. A case definition should be both *sensitive* (able to include all relevant cases) and *specific* (able to exclude all irrelevant cases). The issue of personnel becomes evident as sheer volumes of information proceeding through surveillance systems are understood. This information should be collected by competent interviewers and, after processing, is to be aggregated and stored by proficient database specialists. This is not always the case.[7]

It should be also noted that, as disaster epidemiology is distinctive in the fact that it connects data collection and analysis to immediate decision-making process, it uses management research methodology in addition to clinical and epidemiological research.[8] The most prominent application of management research to disaster medicine is *risk analysis*.

Risk analysis is performed in situations with a low level of certainty about "what to expect" derived from the need to prepare the response and prevention efforts. The use of analytical tools is dedicated to identification of possible risks in a number of areas connected to medical aspects of disaster management. A distinctive example of risk analysis application is measuring clinical risks, such as possible mistakes in diagnosis and treatment. Those mistakes could be generated by different aspects of the treatment process, some of which are listed in Table 22-1.

Risk analysis could be both prospective, looking for possible hazards that have not yet presented themselves, and retrospective, basing its recommendations on past events. Regrettably, retrospective risk analysis seems to be more prevalent in the field, because virtual hazards considered in prospective analysis tend to be regarded as unreal and irrelevant. But, because environments are dynamic, sometimes changing

Table 22-1	
Target Areas for Risk Analysis	
Area for applying risk analysis	**Main aspects**
Personnel	Availability, training, functioning
Environmental hazards	Type, probability, volume, timing
Resources/Needs	Availability, relevance, spending, gaps
Equipment/Needs	Availability, relevance, spending, training
Mission profile	Level of emergency, timing
Command, control, organization	Chains of command and responsibility, communication
Agencies involved	Cooperation, responsibility
Interfaces of above-mentioned areas	Probability, impact

very rapidly, a previously unknown threat appears in areas that were not exposed to it before. For example, floods are now striking regions previously protected by "natural sponges" such as marshes and mangroves, which were able to accept large volumes of water, but are now being removed for agricultural and industrial purposes.[9,10] If no risk analysis is applied in areas where "natural sponges" are being cleared, a sudden flood comes as an unpleasant surprise to those that regarded it as irrelevant because it never happened before.

Of course, the role of retrospective risk analysis is not to be underestimated. It has the advantage of being context-rooted—measuring the efficiency of response by certain agencies to certain events. Lessons learned in this way are easier to present to decision makers and are better apprehended by personnel because personal experience is integrated into the "story that the numbers tell." Clear measurement of outcomes, which could be judged as satisfactory or not, also adds to the value of retrospective risk analysis.

TIME FRAME

Another prominent issue is the time frame for research. Different data becomes available as the disaster unfolds, adding to data that was available before it began. Multiple new questions arise to be answered. Therefore, the research priorities will differ between disaster stages, which could be described as pre-event, immediate response, and recovery. Many other gradations of disaster stages are known to specialists in the field, but because our focus is on the disaster research more than on other issues, this view of the timeline seems to be the most helpful.

The research in the pre-event stage could focus on both the future and the present situation. It could serve in assessing the current level of population and organizational preparedness, as well as the level of information-gathering systems. In addition, it could be pointed into the future, in order to assess risks and hazards, and to plan mitigation efforts according to this assessment. Hospitals benefit directly from this kind of research because they are provided with estimations of patient flow volumes in different scenarios and the volume of resources needed to treat those patients. Mitigation efforts could become very specific and goal-oriented. For example, a very troubling finding became known in Israel during the first Gulf War: the medical personnel in major cities were unwilling to report for duty under rocket barrage. The prevalent reason for this was found to be the war-related disruption of daycare services for children.[11] Because daycare services were established in main hospitals during the next decade, no problems of staff participation were encountered during the Second Lebanon War of 2006. Despite claims that war may not exactly be a disaster, we would like to underline the fact that, in terms of hospital preparedness, this question is irrelevant, because the strain war puts on the healthcare system could be a hard one, even when fighting overseas.[12]

The research in the response phase is concentrated on measuring the immediate impact outcomes and supervising the ongoing management of the event. In some cases (9/11 attacks are the most prominent example), this is the only way of getting a clear picture of what actually happened. Exact knowledge of inflicted injuries enables the direction of the wounded to hospitals that are more ready to receive them (closer, more available, better prepared to deal with specific threats) and better management of evacuation resources (ambulances and helicopters).

In the recovery phase the research could be focused on all time frames—past, present, and future. As more data becomes available and the atmosphere of chaos subsides, a clear understanding of the event can be obtained and lessons can be learned from preparedness/response assessment. In many cases, a dedicated surveillance system should be established to indicate unanswered population needs and possible long-term health-related effects of the event. Resources and timetables for restoration efforts are planned at this stage.

AVAILABILITY OF DATA

As was mentioned, *availability of data* is an issue closely connected to the time frame. The ability to answer the research questions largely depends on the existence of the source, which becomes questionable in the atmosphere of fear and chaos created by a disaster. Some data must be gathered as soon as it is available because it becomes distorted or irrelevant with time (e.g., information about immediate population needs), while other data, such as a complete injury profile of the event, which would be used in *mitigation* planning, should wait until its completion.

Surveillance provides a constant stream of data, helping to monitor population needs and health *indicators*, such as doctor visits and occupational/academic absence. It is also important to obtain *baseline* data about the studied population before the event, so comparison with later measurements could be made in order to evaluate the volume of impact and the change in population needs. Baseline data is also crucial for proper *sampling*. Large-scale population movement during some disasters adds to the problem of obtaining *denominator* data, because, in this case, the existing records do not cover the actual population present in the area.

Caution should be exercised when using existing data from medical or public records because the researcher may be unaware of deficiencies in their management. Some of the known problems include: *insufficient case definitions*, leading to over- or underreporting of mortality and morbidity cases; exaggeration and other distortions of money-spending reports (also relevant to volumes of requested relief resources); and unknown levels of *missing data*.

Aggregation of data (combining data from different sources), as well as separate analysis of different sources with further comparison, could be used to overcome these problems. In order to acquire valid aggregated databases on disasters, initiatives for international registry systems with uniform coding are promoted.[13] Other innovative data collection systems, such as surveillance by means of Internet search engines, were proposed recently.[14] Table 22-2 depicts the main research priorities and the availability of data sources according to disaster stages.

Table 22-2

Research Priorities and the Availability of Data According to Disaster Stages

	Pre-event	Immediate response	Recovery
Research priorities	Preparedness evaluation	Volume and profile of casualties	Long-term effects
	Hazard assessment	Volume of damage	Resource management
	Surveillance evaluation	Evaluation of management	Rebuilding effort
	Populations at risk	Population needs	Population needs
	Population preparedness		Lessons learned
	Possibilities for mitigation		Total mortality and morbidity
	Estimation of resources		Epidemics
			PTSD
Availability of data	Emergency drills	"Quick and dirty" surveys	Reports
	Medical registries	Video	Surveys
	Surveys	Personnel debriefing	Personnel debriefing
	Public registries	Event log	Medical registries

REGIONAL PECULIARITIES

Another issue that distinguishes disaster research is *regional peculiarity*. Disasters can strike communities in countries all over the globe, which could have many differences among them in their culture, resources, and *modus operandi* of institutions. This diversity could impair the applicability of *research methods* and of *previous knowledge* gained in different contexts or even antagonize the locals towards the researchers. The latter issue is especially important because researchers are dependent on the willingness of the population to participate in the study, as well as on the cooperation of local authorities. Problems could arise, even within the borders of the same country, in cases when local officials are interested in suppressing the event-related information flow to the federal government.[15] Researchers may find themselves "unwanted," being seen as federal representatives.

Another region-rooted issue that could haunt researchers, even in their native country, is language. The need for successful written and verbal communication in a local language is obvious when working in a foreign context because data is usually collected through interviews and questionnaires. But the problem of translation could arise even in the native country, because some areas could be crowded with work immigrants or other ethnic communities not speaking the researcher's tongue. Finding interpreters fluent in both languages is an obvious solution, but caution should be applied when translating questionnaires because some important issues could be actually "lost in translation."

The consideration of regional peculiarities becomes especially important in response evaluation. Because the effectiveness of a response should be measured according to the resources available to responders at the time of event, the effort could be misjudged by rating its effectiveness according to irrelevant standards.

Important Choices in Different Stages of Research

During the research process, the researcher is frequently faced with choices that sometimes could be difficult to decide upon. Figure 22-1 summarizes the most prominent choices according to stage of research.

DEFINE ISSUE OF INTEREST: FOCUSED VS. GENERAL

This choice has a general influence on the research process because it defines most of the consequent choices, including that of data collection. If the problem was defined in broad terms, the researcher would strive to collect as much data as possible, while with a focused definition, a limited set of wanted variables is acquired, bringing a risk of missing a variable that was not seen as crucial in the beginning.

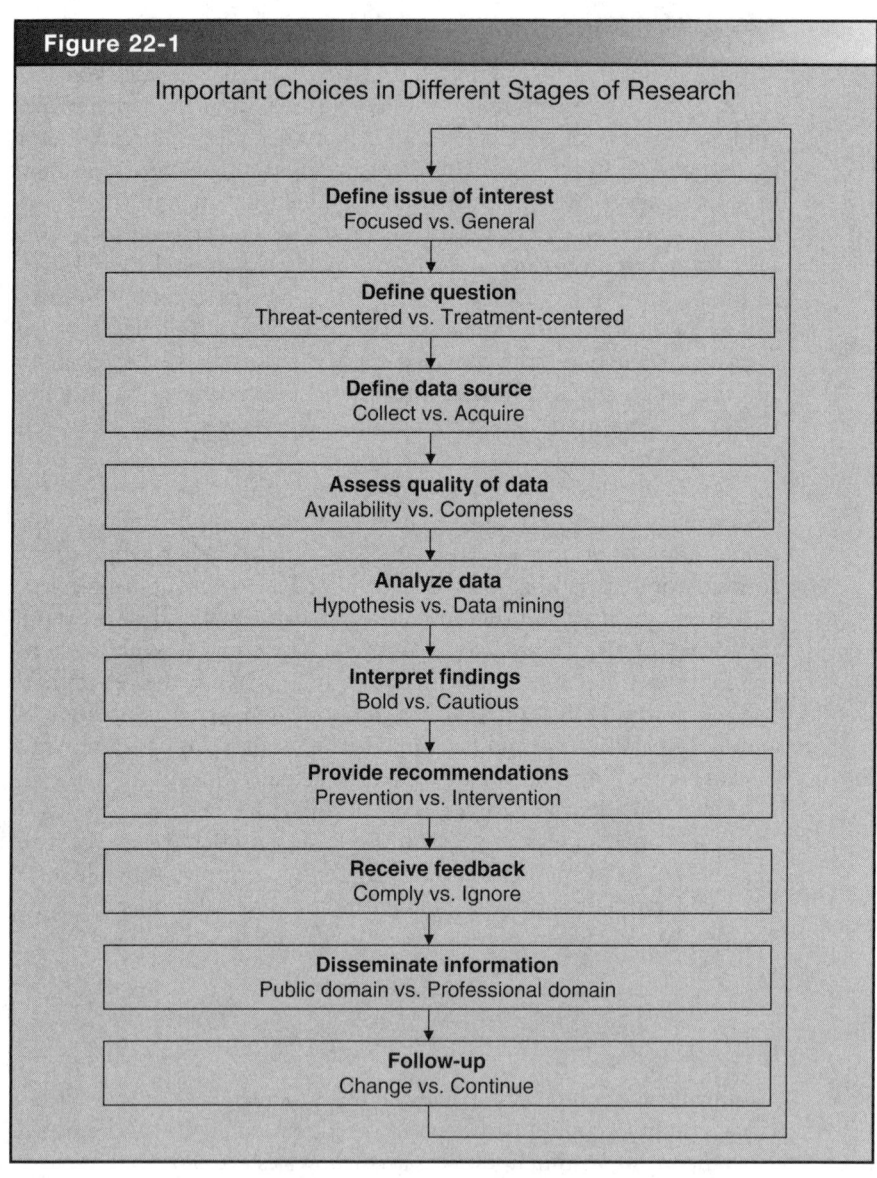

Figure 22-1

Important Choices in Different Stages of Research

Define issue of interest
Focused vs. General

Define question
Threat-centered vs. Treatment-centered

Define data source
Collect vs. Acquire

Assess quality of data
Availability vs. Completeness

Analyze data
Hypothesis vs. Data mining

Interpret findings
Bold vs. Cautious

Provide recommendations
Prevention vs. Intervention

Receive feedback
Comply vs. Ignore

Disseminate information
Public domain vs. Professional domain

Follow-up
Change vs. Continue

Let us take, for example, the emergency treatment of mass casualty events (MCE). In the first stage, the problem could be defined in such broad terms as "the challenge of MCE to emergency healthcare," providing the researcher with vast varieties of possible research questions, or it could be defined in a much more focused way, like "the sudden influx of severely injured patients after an MCE," "head injuries in an MCE," "multiple penetration wounds in an MCE," and so on. This kind of definition, though narrowing the general view of the problem, is much more helpful in actually deciding *what to research*.

DEFINE QUESTION: THREAT-CENTERED VS. TREATMENT-CENTERED

Clear understanding of the problem under scrutiny brings the researcher to formulating the research questions. It is possible to be interested in describing the "threat," that is, the impact of the problem from the view of emergency medicine by describing injury volume patterns; rating the severity of injuries caused by a primary/secondary/tertiary blast; estimating need for surgical capacity; and looking for similarities, or the lack of them, in the time/space context of specific events. On the other hand, questions could be asked about the treatment of the problem: the effectiveness of different kinds of treatment, the priorities for triage, the organization of emergency departments, and so on. Of course, some questions will try to connect between threat and treatment factors, but even in those cases, the focus on one of them will stand out.

DEFINE DATA SOURCE: COLLECT VS. ACQUIRE

The next step is data collection, but it does not always have the genuine right to be called so. The reason for this is that a researcher does not always collect his or her own data by means of survey or experiment, but instead relies on existing databases, available from hospital registries, surveillance studies, government agencies, and nongovernment organizations (NGOs). Both methods have their advantages, because *acquired* data tends to include more cases, while *collected* data could be (but not always is) tailored specifically for the study's needs. When using different data sources for the same study, problems of nonuniversal coding could arise during the aggregation process. Creation of international databases under one roof is proposed as a remedy to this problem.[13]

A known way to facilitate collection of data during the response phase is to prepare a research protocol and to train survey teams before the event, saving precious time. The responsibility for collection of different types of data could be prospectively divided between relevant agencies for the same goal of saving time.

ASSESS QUALITY OF DATA: AVAILABILITY VS. COMPLETENESS

The validity of collected or acquired data is always an issue in research. The collection process could be inherently biased, the coding as well as aggregation processes are subject to machine or human error, and even well-collected data could become outdated if the situation is dynamic. All of these and other deficiencies of data sets are influenced by the choice between completeness, which is the acquirement of all desired data despite costs in time and resources, and availability—using only data already available, even if not full. The impact of this choice on quality of data is context-sensitive. If all injured in an MCE were brought to the same hospital that has a well-developed registry system, it is natural to use this data exclusively, but if the injured were divided between a number of hospitals, and we still use only the first registry, based on its quality—the picture could be distorted by misrepresentation. On the other hand, if the quality of data from other hospitals is so low that it could distort the picture even further, an easily available dataset would be preferred. Sometimes the race for completeness leads only to filling the dataset with more missing cases.

ANALYZE DATA: HYPOTHESIS VS. DATA MINING

When the dataset is found to be acceptably valid, the researcher proceeds to analyzing the data with the variety of known research methods, guided by one of two very different approaches. The researcher can make a hypothesis about relationships between variables in a dataset, such as: "a sudden influx of severely injured patients in an MCE will lead to higher mortality caused by the inability of the emergency system to provide quality treatment for everyone," using statistical methods to verify or to refute the hypothesis. It is also possible not to make any assumptions before approaching the data. In this case the researcher looks for relationships between all or most variables in the dataset, then tries to explain the relationships that were found, after choosing the most prominent ones. The last method is claimed to be unscientific by some, but it must be stated that relationships unsuspected by the researcher and not mentioned in literature could be revealed this way, helping to formulate better hypotheses in the future.[16] The hypothesis approach holds the advantage of being better protected from biases, because the formulation of a hypothesis is naturally a more conscious process than data mining.

INTERPRET FINDINGS: BOLD VS. CAUTIOUS

It is important to remember that the findings of the study, no matter how significant, are of little value to emergency medicine if they are not translated into clear recommendations that can be presented to and understood by decision makers. The most prominent choice in interpretation of the findings into conclusions and recommendations is between being bold or cautious. The choice is further complicated by known uncertainty of generalization from sample to population. A large sample and validated methods can help the researcher to be more confident about the contribution of the study to the field, but it is necessary to decide how far to go with the findings. If it was found that MCE patients have higher in-hospital mortality than other patients, it is possible to explain the finding by the influence of a crowded emergency department on quality of treatment, providing recommendations for better ED protocols and expansion of emergency services. The cautious way of interpretation would be to guide the focus of further research onto prehospital activity: the field triage and treatment and the evacuation process, because in-hospital mortality is not necessarily explained by in-hospital factors.

PROVIDE RECOMMENDATIONS: PREVENTION VS. INTERVENTION

The real recommendations are those presented to decision makers, who control the flow of limited medical and human resources. The researcher must have a clear understanding about the relevance of his or her findings to either the prevention of emergency casualties or the intervention—the actual response to challenges of a specific emergency. Of course, recommendations for both prevention and intervention could be based on the same findings, but the researcher must have a clear understanding of the distinction between the two if the recommendations given are to be understood and accepted by the decision makers. The recommendation to prepare the emergency services to an MCE by adding manpower or making other organizational changes in order to reduce mortality by prevention of overcrowding of emergency departments by injured. Developing better triage and treatment protocols based on distinctive features of MCE injuries is done for the sake of reducing mortality by means of better medical intervention.

RECEIVE FEEDBACK: COMPLY VS. IGNORE

The feedback given by decision makers to a researcher's findings, conclusions, and recommendations could span the entire range, from positive through ambivalent to negative. The results could be found to be too bold and revisionist, irrelevant or unwanted, too long and/or costly to apply in the field. In any case, the researcher must choose between complying with received feedback by checking the findings once again and modifying the conclusions, or ignoring the feedback by defending the study or even presenting it to a different authority. It should be stated that in the business of saving lives, which is emergency medicine, both options are relevant as long as the researcher sees his or her study as crucial to the field.

The most constructive way to deal with feedback is to integrate as much feedback as possible from specialists in relevant fields, so the results of the study can be seen in a broader context. Instead of a mere assessment of a study's relevance, different specialists would be able to state their needs for information on the subject, judging the study by its ability to provide those needs. This would be especially helpful when planning further research.

DISSEMINATE INFORMATION: PUBLIC DOMAIN VS. PROFESSIONAL DOMAIN

The new knowledge gained in the study process should be disseminated to a wider audience through media, special issue reports, and academic journals, either to professionals or to the general public. The principles guiding the choice are *relevance* (should they know?), *interest* (do they want to know?), and *usefulness* (would it do any good if they knew?). For example, the information about the need to develop new treatment protocols could be interesting to the general public, but is not very relevant and even less useful to them, while it is both relevant and useful to medical personnel. The information about survivability-increasing conduct on an impact site is relevant, interesting, and useful to both professionals and general public. Because it seems that, in any case, the professional should be informed anyway, and knowing that some scientific findings are reported in the media after being academically published, the need for choice between the two domains could be questioned. Another principle, called *urgency*, reveals another aspect of the problem: during some emergency situations, especially natural and technological disasters, the public should be the first to know because it could be the best way to reduce mortality and morbidity.[17,18] The Chernobyl nuclear disaster is a known example of failure to disseminate crucial information in time.[19]

FOLLOW-UP: CHANGE VS. CONTINUE

The last important choice the researcher is to make in order to continue the cycle of acquiring new knowledge is whether to keep the existing study format or to change something in the process, maybe even changing the focus to a totally new subject. Undoubtedly, this decision is heavily influenced by the feedback the study received.

There is a possibility that the flow of events has already made the study irrelevant, because the emergency-related field is rarely static by definition. Accordingly, the case could be the opposite—the study discovered an important issue, which must be further explored. The researcher should also look for new research methods, including data collection instruments and analytic tools.

Conclusion

Neglect of proper disaster research endangers the whole preparedness and response effort by creating redundancies in some areas and deficiencies in others. On the other hand, shrewdly planned and executed research based on valid data could provide decision makers with epidemiological profiles for disasters in different regions, analysis of risks of different hazards and their treatment, recommendations for prevention and intervention, and other indispensable information for enhancing the preparedness of the healthcare system for emergencies.

A number of peculiarities separate disaster research from other areas of epidemiological studies. A different set of research tools is used by researchers, because they exercise very little control over the studied context. Therefore, surveys without the involvement of deliberate intervention are preferred to experiments, where such intervention is practiced. Data is sometimes received from less reliable sources than the norms of epidemiology would approve, but reliability and completeness of data become secondary to the issue's existence. When the need to know is dire and immediate, selective personnel debriefing or a hastily executed survey are the best tools a researcher may have. The accent on urgency underlines the specific time frame issues of disaster research, because the questions asked and tools used vary greatly between pre-event, response and recovery phases. They also generate diverse results, which are selectively relevant to hospital preparedness.

The relevance of research is further stressed by regional peculiarities, such as culture, operational patterns, available resources, and center-periphery relations. All those peculiarities are to be considered if the researcher is interested in the cooperation of local factors and in stating the relevance of the study's conclusions to a broader context.

The research process involves making many important choices that arise consecutively during different stages. Compromises are sometimes made based on priorities set by the researcher and the task on hand. Regardless of the priorities involved, the goal of the research stays the same: to provide decision makers with a better understanding of the situation in order to better prepare for emergencies.

References

1. Palafox J, Pointer JE, Martchenke J, et al. The 1989 Loma Prieta earthquake: issues in medical control. *Prehospit Disaster Med.* 1993;8(4):291–297.
2. Noji EK. The 1988 earthquake in Soviet Armenia: implications for earthquake preparedness. *Disasters.* 1989;13(3):255–262.
3. Noji EK. The nature of disaster: general characteristics and public health effects. In: Noji EK, ed. *The Public Health Consequences of Disasters.* New York: Oxford University Press; 1997:3–20.
4. Abramson JH. *Survey Methods in Community Medicine.* 4th ed. Edinburgh: Churchill Livingston; 1990.
5. Wisner B, Blaikie P, Cannon T, Davis I. At risk: Natural Hazards, People's Vulnerability and Disasters. 2nd ed. New York: Routledge; 2003.
6. Peleg K, Aharonson-Daniel L. Research in Disaster Medicine. In: Hogan DE, Burstein JL, eds. *Disaster Medicine.* 2nd ed. Philadelphia, PA: Wolters Kluwer/Lippincott Williams & Wilkins; 2007:464–474.

7. Spaite D, Benoit R, Brown D, et al. Uniform prehospital data elements and definitions: a report from the uniform prehospital emergency medical services data conference. *Ann Emerg Med.* 1995;25(4):525–534.

8. Binder S, Sanderson LM. The role of the epidemiologist in natural disasters. *Ann Emerg Med.* 1987;16(9):1081–1084.

9. Abramovitz JN. Averting unnatural disasters. In: *State of the World 2001: A Worldwatch Institute Report on Progress Toward a Sustainable Society.* New York: W.W. Norton and Company; 2000:123–142.

10. Dahdou-Guebas F, Jayatissa LP, Di Nitto D, Bosire JO, Lo Seen D, Koedam N. How effective were mangroves as a defense against the recent tsunami? *Curr Biol.* 2005;15(12):R443–R447.

11. Shapira Y, Marganitt B, Roziner I, Shochet T, Bar Y, Shemer J. Willingness of staff to report to their hospital duties following an unconventional missile attack: a state-wide survey. *Isr J Med Sci.* 1991;27:704–711.

12. Engel CC, Hyams KC, Scott K. Managing future Gulf War Syndromes: international lessons and new models of care. *Philos Trans R Soc.* 2006;361(1468): 707–720.

13. International Council for Science. *A Science Plan for Integrated Research on Disaster Risk.* International Council for Science Web site. http://www.icsu.org/Gestion/ img/ICSU_DOC_DOWNLOAD/2121_DD_FILE_Hazard_report.pdf. Published 2008. Accessed January 12, 2009.

14. Ginsberg J, Mohebbi MH, Patel RS, et al. Detecting influenza epidemics using search engine query data [published online ahead of print November 19, 2008]. *Nature.* 2009;457(7232):1012–1014. doi:10.1038/nature07634.

15. Waugh WL Jr. The political costs of failure in the Katrina and Rita disasters. *Ann Am Acad Political Soc Sci.* 2006;604(1):10–25.

16. Mayer T. Data mining: a reconsideration. *J Econ Methodology.* 2000;7(2):183–194.

17. Pearce L. Disaster management and community planning, and public participation: how to achieve sustainable hazard mitigation. *Nat Hazards.* 2003;28: 211–228.

18. Rattien S. The role of the media in hazard mitigation and disaster management. *Disasters.* 2007;14(1):36–45.

19. Rahu M. Health effects of the Chernobyl accident: fears, rumours and the truth. *Eur J Cancer.* 2003;39(3):295–299.

Appendix: Universal Checklist

I. Emergency Declarations

A. PUBLIC HEALTH EMERGENCIES

1. Has the state or local government adopted a statutory or regulatory definition of a "public health emergency" or other similar terms (e.g., public health crisis or catastrophe)?
2. Does the state or local government have procedures that must be followed for the governor or other primary political authority to declare a public health emergency?
3. Do the procedures to declare a public health emergency require specificity as to the type, nature, location, and duration of the emergency?
4. After a public health emergency has been declared, is there statutory or regulatory authority to grant specific emergency powers to state or local public health agencies and other relevant entities to facilitate emergency response efforts?

5. Do the granted public health emergency powers include immunity or indemnification for volunteer health professionals who are assisting in emergency response efforts?
6. Does the state statutorily define the term "volunteer" (or other similar terms) to include health professionals within an emergency management context?
7. Is there statutory or regulatory authority that permits the governor or other political authority to terminate the public health emergency or that provides for automatic termination after certain conditions are met?

B. GENERAL EMERGENCIES

8. Has the state or local government adopted a statutory or regulatory definition of an "emergency" and/or "disaster" (or other similar terms)?
9. Does the state or local government have an emergency management system in place?
10. Does the state or local government's general emergency provision also cover emergencies that affect public health?

C. DUAL DECLARATIONS

11. Has the state or local government adopted conflicting statutory or regulatory definitions of a "public health emergency," "general emergency," and/or "disaster?"
12. Do state or local laws and regulations grant authority to different agencies based upon a declaration of "public health emergency" or "general emergency?"
13. Does the statutory or regulatory scheme require or provide for coordination of emergency response efforts among the various state and local agencies involved in the emergency response efforts?

II. Licensing, Credentialing, and Privileging

A. LICENSURE REQUIREMENTS

14. What type of professional is required to have state licensure or certification to practice in the state?
15. Does state law provide civil and/or criminal penalties for healthcare professionals who practice without a license?
16. Has the state adopted provisions for reciprocity of state licensure and/or certification requirements for health profession-

als acting in response to an emergency, including physicians, nurses, and behavioral health professionals, who are licensed in another state?

17. Has the state entered into reciprocity agreements or compacts providing for the recognition of out-of-state licenses and/or certifications for health professionals?

B. CREDENTIALING AND PRIVILEGING REQUIREMENTS

18. Does state law require hospitals to establish medical staff by-laws including provisions for credentialing and privileging in response to emergencies or disasters?

19. Are hospitals required to adopt disaster privileging policies that comply with JCAHO requirements?

20. Does state law require hospitals to have an emergency management plan that governs the hospital's response to a declared emergency?

III. Civil Liability, Immunity, and Indemnification

21. Are civil liability protections explicit in the state or local public health emergency statutes and regulations or other relevant laws?

22. Has the state entered into any intrastate or interstate mutual aid agreements that address civil liability?

23. Does the state tort claims act abrogate sovereign immunity for state actors related to emergency response activities?

24. Does the state tort claims act provide civil liability protection for "discretionary acts" by state actors (e.g., government public health agencies, responders and volunteers working on behalf of the state, private sector entities working under contract with the state) during emergencies?

25. Do conflicts of laws and rules address which state's law will apply when an out-of-state healthcare volunteer commits an act giving rise to liability in another state?

A. VOLUNTEER HEALTH PROFESSIONALS

26. Does state law explicitly provide volunteer health professionals with immunity from civil liability (e.g., volunteer protection acts, Good Samaritan laws, state emergency statutes and compacts) when responding to an emergency?

27. Does the state volunteer protection act provide volunteers with liability protections that exceed protections provided by the federal Volunteer Protection Act?
28. Do state sovereign immunity protections apply to the actions of volunteer health professionals who are employees of the state?
29. Does the state Good Samaritan law apply to the actions of volunteer health professionals and, if so, under what circumstances?
30. Do state emergency statutes or compacts (e.g., MSEHPA, MIMAL, EMAC) provide civil liability protection for volunteer health professionals?
31. Do state laws that provide volunteer health professionals with immunity from civil liability apply to compensated and uncompensated volunteers?
32. Are there exceptions to civil liability protections for volunteer health professionals for acts that rise to the level of gross negligence, recklessness, or willful or wanton misconduct?
33. Are entities employing volunteer health professionals, including government agencies, required to defend and indemnify volunteers for tortious acts committed within the scope of their duties?

B. HEALTHCARE ENTITIES

34. Do healthcare entities face potential civil liability for their own tortious acts committed in association with the use and application of a registration system?
35. Do healthcare entities face potential civil liability for the tortious acts of their employees, agents, and volunteers?
36. Does state law immunize healthcare entities utilizing volunteers who engage in negligent acts (e.g., volunteer protection acts, Good Samaritan laws, state emergency statutes and compacts)?
37. Does state law immunize healthcare entities for negligent acts associated with the use and/or administration of the registration system?

C. ADMINISTRATORS OF A VHP REGISTRATION SYSTEM

38. Do state sovereign immunity protections apply to government agencies administering a registration system?
39. Do state sovereign immunity protections apply to private contractors associated with the administration of a registration system?

IV. Workers' Compensation

40. Is a volunteer health professional recognized by state law as an employee of the state or healthcare entity for whom he/she is providing emergency healthcare services?
41. Are volunteer health professionals required to register with the state or other political subdivision in order to qualify for workers' compensation benefits for injuries sustained in the performance of their duties?
42. Are existing "home" employers of volunteer health professionals required to provide workers' compensation coverage for injuries sustained in the course of performing their duties as a volunteer?
43. Do conflicts of laws rules provide guidance as to whether the workers' compensation laws of the home or host state apply to an out-of-state volunteer health professional's claims for injuries sustained in the course of his/her duties?
44. Do the applicable workers' compensation laws provide for the coverage of occupational diseases contracted in the course of the performance of volunteer activities (e.g., outbreaks of infectious diseases, bioterrorist attacks)?

V. Criminal Liability

45. Does state law provide criminal penalties for health professionals practicing their trade without a license?
46. Are criminal actions exempted from the immunity protections granted to healthcare volunteers under volunteer protection acts, Good Samaritan laws, and state emergency statutes and compacts?
47. Do sovereign immunity protections apply to criminal actions engaged in by employees or agents of the state?

Source: The Centers for Law & the Public's Health: A Collaborative at Johns Hopkins and Georgetown Universities. Legal and Regulatory Issues Concerning Volunteer Health Professionals in Emergencies. Universal Checklist. http:// www.publichealthlaw.net/Research/PDF/ESAR%20VHP%20Universal%20Checklist .pdf.

Index